Bioethical
Decision Making
for Nurses

Bioethical Decision Making for Nurses

Joyce E. Thompson, R.N., C.N.M., D.P.H., F.A.A.N.
Director, Graduate Program in Nurse–Midwifery,
School of Nursing, University of Pennsylvania,
Philadelphia, Pennsylvania

Henry O. Thompson, M.Div., Ph.D.
Senior Fellow in Ethics, School of Nursing,
University of Pennsylvania, Philadelphia, Pennsylvania

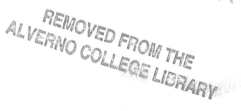

APPLETON-CENTURY-CROFTS/Norwalk, Connecticut

0-8385-0650-X

Notice: The author(s) and publisher of this volume have taken care that the information and recommendations contained herein are accurate and compatible with the standards generally accepted at the time of publication.

Copyright © 1985 by Appleton-Century-Crofts
A Publishing Division of Prentice-Hall, Inc.

85 86 87 88 89 / 10 9 8 7 6 5 4 3 2 1

Prentice-Hall of Australia, Pty. Ltd., Sydney
Prentice-Hall Canada, Inc.
Prentice-Hall Hispanoamericana, S.A., Mexico
Prentice-Hall of India Private Limited, New Delhi
Prentice-Hall International, Inc., London
Prentice-Hall of Japan, Inc., Tokyo
Prentice-Hall of Southeast Asia (Pte.) Ltd., Singapore
Whitehall Books Ltd., Wellington, New Zealand
Editora Prentice-Hall do Brasil Ltda., Rio de Janeiro

Library of Congress Cataloging in Publication Data
Thompson, Joyce Beebe.
  Bioethical decision making for nurses.

  Bibliography: p.
  Includes index.
  1. Nursing ethics. 2. Nursing ethics—Case studies.
  3. Nursing—Decision making. I. Thompson, Henry O.,
  1931-   . II. Title. [DNLM: 1. Bioethics—nurses'
  instruction. 2. Decision Making—nurses' instruction.
  3. Ethics, Nursing. WY 85 T473b]
  RT85.T478 1985   174'.2   84-28355
  ISBN 0-8385-0650-X

Design: M. Chandler Martylewski

PRINTED IN THE UNITED STATES OF AMERICA

This text is dedicated to the following:

In Memoriam

Edward V. Sparer
Orrin S. Thompson

In Honorium

Mary Lenzi
Elizabeth Nester Thompson

Contents

Acknowledgements xi

Introduction xiii

PART I. THEORETICAL BASES FOR BIOETHICS 1
1. Ethics, Morals, Bioethics, and Professionals 3
   Introduction / 3; Ethics, Morals, and Metaethics / 4;
   Bioethics: Ethics and Life / 8; Professionals in Health and
   Illness / 11; Conclusions / 17; Notes / 18

2. Ethical Systems: Right and Wrong 27
   Utilitarianism or Teleology: The Bottom Line / 28;
   Deontology: The Principled Way / 31; Natural Law: Does
   Is Mean Ought? / 37; Moral Theology: Religion as Source
   and Reason / 40; Conclusion / 43; Notes / 43

3. Moral Development: How People Grow 49
   Jean Piaget's Intellectual and Moral Stages / 49; Lawrence
   Kohlberg's Six Stages / 51; James Rest's Defining of the
   Issues / 61; Pro and Con / 64; Notes / 68

4. We are Moral Beings 75
   Personal Value Set: Who Am I? / 77; Professional Value
   Set: What is a Good Nurse? / 80; Summary / 84;
   Notes / 84

PART II. A BIOETHICAL DECISION MODEL 87
5. The Decision Model 89
   Critical Inquiry and Reasoned Analysis / 89; Decision
   Theories for Health Professionals / 92; Recognizing
   Ethical Issues and Dilemmas / 93; Evaluation of Process
   and Outcome / 97; A Bioethical Decision Model / 97;
   Notes / 99

6. **Step One: Review the Situation** 103
   What are the Health Problems in the Situation? / 105; What
   Decision(s) Needs to be Made? / 106; What are the Ethical and
   Scientific Components of the Decision(s)? / 107; What
   Individuals are Involved/Affected by the Decision(s) / 108;
   Summary / 109; The Case / 110; Notes / 111

7. **Step Two: Gather Additional Information** 113
   What Further Information is Needed? / 114; What Further
   Information can be Obtained? / 117; Summary / 118; The
   Case / 119; Notes / 120

8. **Step Three: Identify the Ethical Issues** 121
   What is the Historical Basis of the Ethical Issue? / 123;
   What is the Philosophical Basis of the Ethical Issue? / 123;
   What is the Theological Basis of the Ethical Issue? / 124;
   Summary / 124; The Case / 125; Notes / 127

9. **Step Four: Identify Personal and Professional Values** 129
   What are Your Personal Values on the Issues? / 130; What
   are Your Professional Values on the Issues? / 131; What
   Guidance Does the ANA *Code for Nurses* Offer? / 132;
   Summary / 133; The Case / 133; Notes / 134;

10. **Step Five: Identify the Values of Key Individuals** 135
    Why Bother With the Moral Positions of Others? / 136;
    How Does One Identify Value Positions of Others? / 137;
    Summary / 140; The Case / 140; Notes / 142

11. **Step Six: Identify the Value Conflicts, If Any** 143
    What are the Value Conflicts? / 144; What is the Value
    Hierarchy? / 148; Summary / 149; The Case / 149;
    Notes / 150

12. **Step Seven: Determine Who Should Decide** 153
    Who Owns the Problem? / 154; Who Decides Who
    Decides? / 157; What is the Role of the Nurse? / 160;
    Summary / 161; The Case / 162; Notes / 163

13. **Step Eight: Identify the Range of Actions and
    Anticipated Outcomes** 165
    What is the Range of Actions? / 166; What are the
    Anticipated Outcomes of Each Alternative? / 166;
    Summary / 167; The Case / 167; Notes / 168

14. **Step Nine: Decide on a Course of Action and Carry It Out** 171
    Application of Ethical Theory to Each Action / 173;
    Weighing the Goods and Harms / 176; Choose One
    Action / 178; Summary / 179; The Case / 179; Notes / 182

15. **Step Ten: Evaluate the Results** 185
Did the Decision or Action Produce the Intended
Results? / **185**; Is Another Action Needed? / **186**; What
Information is Transferable to Other Situations? / **187**;
Summary / **187**; The Case / **189**

Appendix A. Case Studies in Nursing 191
Pregnancy Decisions / **191**; Neonates and
Advocates / **197**;   Children, Consent, and Research / **199**;
Adolescent Care / **200**; Health Care for Adults / **202**;
Illness and Old Age / **204**; Health Care Professional
Relationships / **206**

Appendix B. Codes of Ethics..209
International Council of Nurses Code for Nurses (1973):
Ethical Concepts Applied to Nursing / **209**; American
Medical Association Principles of Medical Ethics / **210**

Appendix C. Models of Ethical Decision Making..213
Brody Act-Utilitarian Ethical Method / **214**; Brody
Deontological Ethical Method / **214**; Payton Pluralistic
Ethical Decision-Making Model / **215**

Glossary..217

Annotated Bibliography 233

Index 249

Acknowledgments

It is a joy to take this opportunity to say thank you to Diane Adler, Dale Drucker, Phil Greiner, Edna Rainone Knowsley, Warren Knowsley, Arlene Konicki, Mary Lenzi, Anne M. O'Malley, Ann O'Sullivan, Gloria Sarto, Edward Sparer (d. 1983), Eileen Sullivan, Judith Smith, Warren G. Thompson, and to all our colleagues and students for their help with this text. They not only shared their knowledge but also gave of their moral support along the way. Several have used the decision model and shown that it works. In their minds and hands it has moved from theory to pragmatics and changed from an idea into a useful, functional tool in the vital process of ethics in nursing. At the same time, we hasten to take responsibility for the final product. Any errors or omissions are our responsibility.

Books can stimulate thinking and offer suggestions; only people can make decisions.

Joseph Fletcher[1]

Introduction

Nurses and other health care providers are vitally concerned with promoting health, curing disease, and supporting the health and illness needs of their clients or patients. Nurses want to do the "best" or "right" thing for society and for the individuals within society whom they serve and care for. Usually nurses do this very well. Sometimes, however, the best or right thing is not clear or easily discernable. One of the most common, yet most difficult, areas for knowing what is the right or best thing to do involves the ethical dimensions of health and illness care.

STATEMENT OF PURPOSE

This book was written to provide nurses and other health care professionals with a practical model for making ethical decisions. The focus is on the *process* of ethical decision making.

REASONS FOR THE TEXT

It has become increasingly difficult for health care professionals to know what is best or what should be done for a given patient. One of the major reasons for this is the availability of treatment options never imagined relatively few years ago. New technologies, new methods of diagnosis, and new forms of treatment of health and illness conditions have created new choices for patients and professionals alike. To put it another way, the success of modern health care has brought up the ethical question "Just because we can do something, should we?" Educational efforts for ethical decision making have not kept pace with the need for making these increasingly complex decisions in health care.

Wanting to do good, or the "best" thing, for clients is not synonymous with actually doing good. Just as being a competent nurse or physician required study and practice, making ethical decisions requires study and practice. Health professionals have had limited exposure to this type of ethical study in years past. This book was written to help narrow the gap between what we say and what we do.

In 1976 the American Nurses' Association published the fifth revision of the *Code for Nurses*, now with interpretive statements.[2] The first ANA code was written and adopted in 1950.[3] The concern for ethical practice, however, has been a part of organized nursing from the beginning. A 1926 statement is one illustration of the profession's commitment to ethical nursing practice. It included a desire to "create a sensitiveness to ethical situations and to formulate general principles which . . . create the individual habit of forming conscious and critical judgment resulting in action in specific situations."[4] This commitment continues today.

Commentators throughout the seventy-five years of the development, creation, and revision of the code have recognized that the code does not tell a nurse exactly what to do in every specific nursing situation. Indeed, no code could. Rather, a profession's code of ethics is concerned with broad principles or rules of conduct for the professional's responsibilities, duties, and obligations to clients and society. A code provides guidance for carrying out one's professional role, rather than direct instruction or a set of packaged answers to current ethical concerns.

Our second reason for writing this text is based on our understanding of and commitment to nurses and nursing. We have worked with this particular group of health professionals for over ten years, discussing, exploring, and facing head-on the challenges of what it means to be a good nurse and to practice in an ethical manner in today's society. We are aware of the long history of nursing's commitment to ethical practice and wish to further the educational commitment to both learning and the application of sound principles of moral reasoning in making ethical decisions. The ten-step decision model described in this text in intended to expand the guidelines for ethical decision making in health care explicated in the ANA *Code* while also recognizing that the final answers remain with the individuals involved in the situation.

OVERVIEW OF THE BOOK

Part I includes four chapters on the theoretical bases for bioethics. Part II has an introductory chapter on the decision model, followed by chapters describing each of the ten steps of the decision process. Appendix A presents a series of actual cases involving nurses and other health care professionals for application by the reader of the decision model.

One characteristic of a professional is understanding. The professional not only knows how to do something, but also why he or she is doing it. Part I reflects this concern for understanding. Professionals must understand the terminology of ethics, ethical theories, moral development, and the moral nature of human beings. Part I offers a summary of ethical theory. Additional study can be found in the authors' *Ethics in Nursing* (New York: Macmillan, 1981) and in other works listed in the Annotated Bibliography. Those already familiar with such theory may find the review helpful, or they may choose to move directly to Part II and the decision model.

Part II of the book presents the decision model. This model has been successfully used with a variety of health professionals. It is pluralistic, recognizing the variety of moral views of professionals and clients in our society. It allows for differences in personal and professional values. It allows for change over time in our views of what constitutes ethical practice in health care. The guiding principle is reasoned analysis or critical ethical inquiry that can be shared whether people agree or disagree. How a decision is made may be more important than who finally makes that decision. The "how" assumes the use of moral reasoning. That reasoning, in turn, includes the recognition that one person (the patient, for example) may be a more appropriate decision maker than another.

Chapter 5 provides the theoretical framework for the model and criteria for recognizing the ethical dimensions of nursing practice. The ten-step decision model is a process for bioethical decision making rather than a failsafe formula for choosing one action to follow in all situations. A separate chapter is devoted to each of the ten steps of the decision model. Each chapter includes the reasons for the step, how each step relates to the others, and suggestions on how to carry out the steps. As an aide to the reader, each decision step is applied to a paradigm case called "Birth of a Family," presented in Chapter 6.

The case studies in Appendix A offer the reader an opportunity to apply the decision model to some representative nursing care situations. The cases are organized according to the life cycle. They have been contributed by experts in each area. They are actual situations, with names and locations changed to protect the confidentiality of all persons involved. The first case is analyzed by the authors as an additional demonstration of the decision model. The rest of the cases are for self-study.

Appendices B and C include professional codes of ethics and three examples of other models for ethical decision making, respectively. A Glossary of Terms is included for ready reference; the annotated Bibliography is a guide to further study.

SUMMARY

The decision model is based on the use of reason as an aide to making ethical decisions. However, the ethical dimensions of health care also require a delicate balance of emotion, art, and science. A balance is needed between "anything goes" or "doing whatever feels right" and being frozen into inaction by what may appear to be a vast network of ethical theory. Decisions are made in health care. They need to be made with the awareness of the balances needed. They need to be made, also, with the awareness that each situation is unique because of the unique individuals involved. Yet the final step in decision making requires a reasoned analysis of the ethical commonalities. It is our pleasure to share this text with others. We invite your critical evaluation and encourage your interest and efforts in ethical decision making.

J.E.T.
H.O.T.

NOTES

1. Fletcher, Joseph. "Foreword," In Brody, H. *Ethical Decisions in Medicine*. Boston: Little, Brown, 1976, p. v.
2. *Code for Nurses With Interpretive Statements*. Kansas City, MO: American Nurses' Association, 1976.
3. Sward, K. "An historical perspective." In American Nurses' Association, *Perspectives on the Code for Nurses*. Kansas City, MO: American Nurses' Association, 1978, pp. 1–9.
4. "A suggested code: A code of ethics presented for the consideration of the American Nurses' Association." *AJN* 26(8): 599–601, 1926.

Bioethical Decision Making for Nurses

Theoretical Bases for Bioethics

The first section of this text is devoted to discussion of some of the theoretical foundations of bioethics. In order for individuals new to the study of philosophy and bioethics to understand this theory base, we begin with our definitions of ethics, morals, metaethics, and the systems of ethical theory. We also refer the reader to the Glossary of terms at the end of this text. The chapters on moral development and moral personhood provide the rest of the foundation for study of bioethical decision making. We are moral beings and value laden. As professionals we need to understand how our personal and professional values and level of moral development may potentially influence our decisions in practice. We wish to do the best for each of our clients or patients, and this understanding of the moral nature of self and others facilitates ethical practice.

There is a wonderful word—"Why?"—that children, all children, use. When they stop using it, the reason too often is that no one bothered to answer them. No one fostered and cultivated the child's innate sense of the adventure of life.

—*Eleanor Roosevelt*[1]

We cannot give the final answers to our human problems, because it is we human beings who are the problem.

—*Eugene B. Borowitz*[2]

CHAPTER 1

Ethics, Morals, Bioethics, and Professionals

INTRODUCTION

Definitions are necessary as we begin the theoretical background for the 10-step decision model. Definition of a relatively simple sounding word, such as ethics, may prove to be very confusing and somewhat frustrating, however. This is especially true for health care professionals steeped in the scientific method who have limited or no exposure to philosophy or philosophical inquiry. We urge you to bear with us as we attempt to clarify the key concepts and definitions relative to bioethical decision making.

Whether one reads moral theology or moral philosophy, there are times when one wonders if there are as many definitions of ethics as there are ethicists![3] At first, this may be discouraging to the novice in ethics. But is this not so in most if not all fields of human endeavor? One nurse educator deliberately withholds alternative viewpoints or procedures during the early phases of learning, "lest the student be confused." In a pluralistic age, that kind of matriarchal paternalism is intriguing and may be destructive. We note, however, that after the initial training, the educator just mentioned brings in alternate procedures.

We shared this anecdote only to have another nurse educator respond with, "What alternatives?" Just as there are those philosophers who know only one ethic—theirs—so there are nurse educators who know only one procedure—theirs. Others, however, are aware of alternatives. Some see only a few, but those with a knowledge of history are aware of numerous alternatives, not merely in procedures but in opinions about the very essence of nursing. What is a nurse? The physicians' maid? Is the nurse a professional? What is a profession? One question often leads to another, like the child's "Why?" which, when answered, leads to another "Why?" Sometimes the exasperated parent or adult ignores the child, or snaps "Because I said so, that's why." The nurse educator who snaps in similar fashion to the nursing student is following a long precedent in authorities—in health care, in philosophy, science, religion, politics, and so on.

There are times when most of us have submitted or will submit to authority.[4] In an emergency, we need to respond to the matter at hand. Debates over authority can be left aside until the emergency is over. Some prefer to rely on authority for all ordinary things and even at all times. The writers pretend to no expertise in nuclear physics and have no plans to become experts in this area. We are content to accept the authority of the experts, with some limitations. At other times, on other subjects, and in other circumstances, one might be permitted or even obligated to ask "Why?" There seems to be some type of curiosity in the human animal, perhaps not totally dissimilar to the curiosity that killed the cat. Some would reverse that metaphor and suggest that we had better be curious or we will indeed be killed, whether by nuclear holocaust or by a prejudicial one.

The "Why?" of the child becomes the philosophical reasoning of the adult. In our teaching, workshops, and seminars, we comfort and encourage parents who are "climbing the walls" with their children's infinity of whys to stop and rejoice because they have a budding philosopher on their hands![5] The philosopher's "Why?" is a step beyond the childlike wonder, however, for it is a reasoning process. The process can become quite complex and obtuse at times and lose sight of its clarifying intent. At that point, it becomes part of the problem rather than the solution that philosophy on occasion claims it offers.[6] One strain of philosophical thought, however, does not claim to offer answers to life's problems. It is up to us to find the answers, whether from the authorities or from ourselves. What philosophy offers, according to this other tradition, is not better answers, but better questions. It may even help us choose the appropriate questions in the first place.[7] Among these questions are the foundational ones: What are ethics, morality, and metaethics in the first place? We stand in this tradition as we propose a model for bioethical decision making.

ETHICS, MORALS, AND METAETHICS

Ethics consists of the why, *morals* consists of ought, and *metaethics* is that which is beyond the why.[8] For some, the three are interchangeable. The word "ethics" comes from the Greek *ethos*, and the English "morals" comes from the Latin *moralis*. In their origins, the two terms are the same word in different Indo-European languages. Linguistically, it is appropriate to use the two English words interchangeably. The reader will note that this common usage appears in this text. However, on occasion it is helpful to consider an alternative. Morals are the "shoulds" and "oughts" or "should nots" of life, culture, society, religion.[9] This is what we "should" or "should not" do. The Ten Commandments of Judaism and Christianity are obvious examples. Ethics in this view are the moral philosopher's or the moral theologian's "Why?" What are the reasons for the moral "should" or "should not?" A concern with reasons goes back at least to Socrates (c. 469-399 BC).[10]

There are many alternatives to these definitions. John Ladd says that there is no standard distinction of meaning between ethics and morals. Ethics may mean professional ethics or Jewish ethics or Plato's ethics.[11] Another definition is *descriptive ethics*, which describes what is, for example, the anthropologist who describes a primitive tribe. There is a *normative ethics*, or applied ethics, which prescribes what "ought" to be or to be done, somewhat like our use of the term "morals." Some say bioethics or health care ethics is applied ethics.[12]

Metaethics

It is not unusual for philosophers, like parents, to reach the end of their explanations, and so they end with their version of "Because . . . ." Such submission may carry us "beyond ethics," the meaning of the Greek *metaethics*. However, Aiken says "It is always legitimate, if often fatiguing, to ask 'Why?' when a particular moral judgment is proposed."[13]

In religion, such a "beyond" may be God or the will of God, or it may be the "One," or the "All," or "nature." Philosophers may use such metaphysical ultimates also. Some philosophers prefer a nontheistic Nature, or an "Ideal" or a "prima facie" reason. The "first face" or "on the face of it" means an end to reasoning. Why should we care for people in their illness? Because it is good (whatever that is) or because nurses are committed to do good or to do no harm (whatever that is) or because of a commitment to the greatest good for the greatest number (whatever that is) or out of self-interest ("Do unto others as you would have others do unto you"). We will come back to these reasons in the Chapter Two as we talk about systems of ethics. Here we note that some reasons are intermediate, while others are ultimate, that is, final or unquestioned. Kohlberg sees justice as the ultimate principle. All other moral principles are intermediate.[14] Margaret Cotroneo suggests that trust is the focus for nursing ethics—the ultimate.[15] Others propose ultimates, such as love, care, and so on.[16]

We might say an action is for the good of society, and the budding philosopher may ask why should we be concerned for the good of society. One of the Ten Commandments says, "Thou shalt not murder." If we ask "Why?" we might move immediately to the ultimate—it is the will of God. For those who believe in God, this is usually beyond ethics, beyond question. Others might say that we should not murder because we cannot live in society without such a moral or law. The budding philosopher may then ask why preserve society only to be told that God created us to live in society. On a nontheistic level, one might answer that it is human nature to be gregarious and leave it at that ultimate metaethic.

Metaethics is sometimes seen as linguistic analysis, attempts to define the "good" or to set up the rules for discussion. "Is this an ethical question?" "Why be moral at all?" These are metaethical questions.[17] It has been suggested that if ethics discusses the reasons for morals, metaethics discusses the reasons for ethics.

Some see metaethics as the position that asks if a given situation is really a matter of ethics.[18] In health care, it is not unusual to see an issue or a decision as a matter of clinical judgment rather than as an ethical or moral issue. This concept begs several questions. Is there an ethical issue here? There is at least some evidence to suggest that clinical judgments masquerade as objective, scientific decisions of health care, when in fact they are expressions of values that the practitioner will not admit.[19] This may be viewed as deception, and deception is often seen as unethical in contrast to the ethical principle of truthfulness.

Moral is the Nature of Human Beings

But suppose there is no masquerade? Is it simply ignorance that does not see the moral dimension of our humanity? Jacques Barzun has noted that "moral" is the nature of human relationships, i.e., (all) human relationships have a moral dimension.[20] One could go further and say that human beings are moral creatures. Robinson Crusoe was a moral being before Friday. This definition of morality is different from moral rules. This is the morality of the person as *moral agent* rather than the morality of the thing—action, event, decision.[21] The moral agent is part of situation ethics, an "act utilitarianism" described in Chapter Two. The psychology of moral development will be explored in Chapter Three. It can be said that moral equals human.

The nonmoral or amoral person is seen as a psychopath or sociopath, one lacking in an essential ingredient of humanness. Moral as a matter of nature, including human nature, is explored further in the discussion of natural law in Chapter Two. Another dimension of this is human rights.

There is, however, an old saying that "Everyone's business is no one's business." If everything is a matter of ethics, we may end up with nothing. We note here for later discussion (Chapter Four) that ethics becomes an issue when we are faced with a dilemma, such as a choice among ethical principles. The principles of ethics will be described in Chapter Two under deontology (the study of rules or principles). Here we observe that while all human relationships have a moral dimension, a given clinical judgment or situation may not have a significant moral or ethical dimension. We say this, however, aware that one person's significance may be someone else's trivia, and someone's trivia may be someone else's significant issue.[22]

One of the subsets in the discussion of ethics is the legitimacy of various kinds of ethics. Eric Fromm has observed that there are only human ethics.[23] Others claim that animals have rights too.[24] Still others think that life has rights, and we must practice what Indian thought calls "ahimsa"—nonviolence, or reverence for life.[25] Still others claim that rocks and rills and templed hills have rights, and ethics must extend to the entire world, nonanimate as well as animate.[26] We speak of universal rights, and perhaps our discussion should extend to the stars and the right of space not to be littered with our junk until it looks like planet earth. Environmental ethics is a crucial concern for humanity, but for the moment we will try to keep our feet on the ground.[27]

Moving in the opposite direction, there are those who object to the proliferation of ethics. We have business ethics, political ethics, legal ethics, medical ethics. Is it appropriate to have a baker's ethics or a butcher's ethics? The Automobile Dealers of America have a Code of Ethics.[28] Is this appropriate? Some say yes, and others say no. One variation on the theme is to look at a given type of ethics, such as medical ethics, and claim that it is appropriate to speak of medical ethics but only as a variation of ordinary ethics. It is ethics as applied to the field of medicine.[29]

If such a distinction is valid, it would appear valid to speak of nursing ethics as a distinct type or genre of ethics. Is there a nursing ethics that is something other, or more than, ordinary ethics as applied in the nursing situation? That is a much more debatable subject to which we do not yet have an answer. However, one could compare an analogy. In religious history, Christianity was originally a Jewish sect or cult. Two forms of Judaism survived the Second Jewish Revolt of 132–135 AD (or CE, Common Era). One was Pharasaic Judaism, which eventually produced the Talmud and the religion known as Judaism today. The second consisted of the followers of Rabbi Joshua of Nazareth, commonly called by his Greek name, Jesus. At some point in history, many commentators believe Christianity became a separate religion. It is commonly so treated today. At what point in the application of ethics to the field of nursing does nursing ethics become a distinct ethics and not just ordinary ethics applied in the nursing situation? It is a question that does not need to be answered here, but it is one that we continue to ponder. We do not pretend to have all the answers in ethics in general nor in nursing ethics in particular.

It may be helpful to add one more thought. It has been said, "To know the good is to do it." Aristotle said we become just by doing just acts. An Iowa farmer was asked if he wanted help to be a better farmer. He said, "No." The surprised county agent asked, "Why not?" The farmer answered, "I already know how to farm better than I'm doing." Personal experience suggests that many people, if not most of us, already know how to do better than what we do. Leah Curtin and many others have cited the disparity between what nurses say and what they do,[30] and one suspects the same could be said about other health care professions. Davis and Aroskar have pointed out that theory is concerned with knowing, and practical interest is concerned with doing.[31]

Some see normative or applied ethics as deciding or helping people to decide what to do. This may not be a matter of dictum so much as a matter of helping to clarify what is involved with the final decision made by the practitioner. At the same time, we are under no illusions that all nurses or health care providers are agreed on even the importance or value of ethics. The study of ethics is seldom required in educational programs, for example. Hence there is often an element of consciousness raising in health care ethics.[32] Before making ethical decisions, one needs to recognize the significance of the ethical. Both aspects appear in the text that follows.

BIOETHICS: ETHICS AND LIFE

The prefix *bio* means "life." In this sense, bioethics means ethics concerning life. That includes all animate matter, and one could say it includes all that affects life. As noted earlier, this is the broad view of ethics, as in the Indian concern of "ahimsa"—nonviolence or reverence for life. It includes a concern for the environment. The first use of the term "bioethics" is credited to Van Rensselaer Potter who used it with reference to the environment and to population control.[33] Warren T. Reich said bioethics "can be defined as the systematic study of human conduct in the area of the life sciences and health care, insofar as this conduct is examined in the light of moral values and principles."[34] In practice, the word has come to be practically interchangeable with medical ethics or biomedical ethics, that is, the ethics of health care. While for Potter, bioethics was the use of the biological sciences to improve the quality of life, current practice focuses more on the medical sciences. We would add that this latter concept can include all 268 health care professions, though we here focus primarily on nursing.

In his overview, Clouser[35] notes a vast conglomeration of subject matter loosely tied together to form the discipline of bioethics. The *Encyclopedia of Bioethics* consists of four volumes with a total of 1933 pages. It is only one example of a vast and burgeoning literature in the field.[36] Clouser suggests, however, that one should not get lost in the vast network of issues. The basic aim is to decide how humanity "ought to act in the biomedical realm affecting birth, death, human nature, and the quality of life." Earlier, he claims that medical ethics is only an application of ordinary ethics. So is bioethics, but it is a more general case. It has a wider concern than those of a particular guild, and it connotes both the ethics and the science–technology out of which the issues grew.[37]

The growth metaphor is certainly appropriate. There is a long history of ethical concerns with life, a history that stretches back to biblical times and probably to the prehistoric period of human existence. The roots of our ethical concerns certainly go back to the beginnings of human culture, and not infrequently those beginnings are lost in the mists of time. Others can be pinpointed to particular people and times, like Moses and Jesus, Buddha and Muhammad, Socrates, Plato, Aristotle, and Confucius. But bioethics is perhaps the more immediate product of the population explosion, the knowledge explosion, and the technology explosion of the twentieth century.[38] At the turn of the century, 95 percent of the babies born were born at home. Now that percentage is born in hospitals. At the turn of the century, 95 percent of the people who died died at home. Now, over 80 percent die in a hospital or some other institution. "The concentration of specialized medical care in hospitals encouraged an impersonal organizational approach to medical care."[39]

The specialized knowledge is part of the knowledge explosion, which itself is part of the development of scientific medicine. Scientific medicine developed out of the nineteenth century discoveries in bacteriology, pathology, and physiology, but such a scientific approach did not take hold in medical schools until after the famous Flexner report of 1910.[40] The real impact, however, did not come until the post-World War II development of antibiotics. Along with these new treatments came increasingly sophisticated and complicated machinery and techniques. "The fascination of scientific knowledge and techniques drew many physicians into narrower fields of concentration."[41] Patients lost their status as people and became "that interesting liver in Room 501." Ironically, the nursing profession has turned more and more to the scientific, the technological, the specialization of care, in its educational programs, even as some reassessment is taking place in the education of physicians.[42] Historically, as Patricia Munhall has pointed out, nursing has cherished the individual patient.[43] It is oriented to a humanistic philosophy rather than statistics.

Public reaction to the dehumanization of health care has had its effect on health care ethics. A century ago, this was a matter of etiquette and professional courtesy. Early nursing ethics were concerned with conduct becoming to a lady and obedience to the physician and hospital authorities. In 1927, Chauncy D. Leake took note of this classic health care ethic and called for a real ethics that would apply the traditions of moral philosophy to health care.[44] Roman Catholics had been doing this for centuries. A series of writings in the 1940s and 1950s gave this approach a louder voice. In 1949, the US Catholic Hospital Association issued its "Ethical and Religious Directives for Catholic Health Facilities" (revised 1954 and 1971).[44] The US Protestant Hospital Association published standards for religious work in hospitals, but it was Joseph Fletcher's *Morals and Medicine*[45] that sparked serious attention to bioethics by Protestants. Jewish ethics go back to Moses and earlier but came to prominence in the United States with such works as those of Immanuel Jakobovits and Fred Rosner.[46] The change Leake called for finally began to appear in the professional codes of ethics. The revisions in the codes and the development of codes of ethics were a part of the background to the rise of bioethics in the 1970s.[47]

However, the emphasis here needs to be on the success of modern health care. This is the most forceful impetus to the growth of bioethics. Renal dialysis developed to help those with kidney failure. One of the first centers was established in Seattle, Washington, but the number of machines were limited. How were the limited number of patients to be chosen? A committee was set up in 1962 to make the selection. Older people were eliminated. Children were eliminated (dialysis may stunt their development; the kidney failure merely kills them!). Two thirds of those chosen were males—they can be helped to maintain their jobs and support their families. Not everyone approved such criteria. The matter was presumably solved when the federal government began financing dialysis and kidney transplants in 1972. Today, 60,000 people are on dialysis at a cost of $2 billion a year. The technology continues to raise questions, such as the justification for spending this kind of money when there are other health needs. There are enormous profits in the dialysis business, and people in permanent coma and the totally senile are being transported to the centers for dialysis. The cost-benefit ratio is part of this question, but so is a much older issue called the "Is–Ought" problem. Because we can do dialysis, must we do it to everyone with kidney problems? Britain does not offer dialysis to those over 65. That would not be acceptable in the United States, but are there some limits?[48]

The issues have continued to increase astronomically. Experiments, such as giving retarded children hepatitis, the aged live cancer cells, and black males with syphilis a placebo instead of real treatment, have raised issues about experimenting with human beings. The recent history of the Nazi doctors and their so-called experiments add an urgency to this concern, as they do to the issue of informed consent. While death remains more sure than taxes, the grim reaper has been held at bay to a greater extent than before thanks to new knowledge, new machinery, new techniques ranging from antibiotics to heart transplants. When the quality of life (QOL) is enhanced, this has generally been seen as good. When a person ends up with the heart kept pumping by a machine, some have suggested that this is less than good. Reproductive technology has changed enormously. Contraception is still officially murder in some circles. It "wastes the seed," the "precious fluid" of medieval attitudes. Now it is widely practiced, and there are those who think it should be more widely practiced yet. Abortion has become safer (at least in the first trimester) than giving birth, but the health care changes have brought only a partial change in attitudes. For many, contraception and abortion are murder. The development of the Neonatal Intensive Care Unit (NICU) has saved many infants, but some of the saved have a less than optimal QOL, leading to the charge that the NICU is the new horror chamber of the modern era.[49] From the beginning to the end of life, "things they are a-changing!"

Nurses are a part of that change. For one thing, nurses take care of the patients who are the objects [sic!] of the experiments, the machinery, the new technologies, the impersonal care, the prolonged dying. For another thing, there are changing perspectives on what is a nurse. We will come back to this later. Here we want to consider several developments.

PROFESSIONALS IN HEALTH AND ILLNESS CARE

Codes of Ethical Behavior

Codes of health care ethics are fairly ancient. One of the oldest is the well-known Hippocratic Oath. It dates officially from the Greek Hippocrates (460–377 BC), though more recent research credits much of it to the Cult of the Pythagoreans in the fourth century BC. It has a stricter morality than that of Greek law or Platonic and Aristotelian ethics. It was not widely honored in the West until the Middle Ages. It may have influenced Indian traditions, known from a later time in the student's oath, "Charaka Samhita," c. 1 AD. Both traditions put an emphasis on loyalty to the teacher and profession. Both put the patient's well-being above that of the practitioner.[50]

A very influential code was that of Percival's *Medical Ethics*, published in 1803 and republished by Chauncy Leake in 1927.[51] Thomas Percival's gentlemen's ethic was the basis of the Code adopted by the newly formed American Medical Association in 1847. (See current AMA Code in Appendix B) Percival stands in the Hippocratic tradition. He urged physicians to keep their heads clear and their hands steady by observing the strictest temperance. His emphasis on professional etiquette was in marked contrast to the "quarrelsome conduct" of practitioners in that day. The AMA used it to exclude those not of their school, the so-called irregulars who had a new lease on life when Jacksonian democracy eliminated professional licensing laws. Increasingly from 1870 on, the Code was also used to eliminate blacks and women from the physician role, an exclusion that the Flexner Report helped to near completion.[52]

Modern nursing stems from the work of Florence Nightingale (1820–1910), who focused on responsible obedience to the physicians. The test came in the Crimean War (1854–1857), when the physicians would not allow the nurses on the battlefield, and she withheld her "troops" until the physicians were assured of that obedience. More recent research has stressed that she did not call for blind obedience. The Florence Nightingale Pledge long used in nursing says, "With loyalty will I endeavor to aid the physician in his work, and devote myself to the welfare of those committed to my care." Current emphasis is on intelligent obedience, as in the 1965 Code for Nurses of the International Council of Nurses (ICN). (See Appendix B for ICN Code.)

The concern for a code of ethics was present from the beginnings of the American Nurses' Association, but no formal code was promulgated until 1950. It was revised in 1976 (Table 1-1) and dropped the concept of obedience, as did the 1973 revision of the 1965 ICN Code. The ANA Code for Nurses speaks to collaborative relationships with members of the health professions and other citizens in order to meet the health needs of the public. The new emphasis is on professional responsibility and accountability. The ICN code has a fourfold responsibility to promote health, to prevent illness, to restore

TABLE 1-1. AMERICAN NURSES' ASSOCIATION CODE FOR NURSES, 1976

1. The nurse provides services with respect for human dignity and the uniqueness of the client unrestricted by considerations of social or economic status, personal attributes, or the nature of the health problem.
2. The nurse safeguards the client's right to privacy by judiciously protecting information of a confidential nature.
3. The nurse acts to safeguard the client and the public when health care and safety are affected by the incompetent, unethical, or illegal practice of any person.
4. The nurse assumes responsibility and accountability for individual nursing judgments and actions.
5. The nurse maintains competence in nursing.
6. The nurse exercises informed judgment and uses individual competence and qualifications as criteria in seeking consultation, accepting responsibilities, and delegating nursing activities to others.
7. The nurse participates in activities that contribute to the ongoing development of the profession's body of knowledge.
8. The nurse participates in the profession's efforts to implement and improve standards of nursing.
9. The nurse participates in the profession's efforts to establish and maintain conditions of employment conducive to high-quality nursing care.
10. The nurse participates in the profession's effort to protect the public from misinformation and misrepresentation and to maintain the integrity of nursing.
11. The nurse collaborates with members of the health professions and other citizens in promoting community and national efforts to meet the health needs of the public.

Reprinted with permission of the American Nurses' Association.

health, and to alleviate suffering. The ANA code has an expansion in its Interpretive Statements. Ronald S. Gass notes the code's "distinctiveness among codes of ethics." Though its form is hortatory, "The nurse provides . . . ," "The nurse safeguards . . . ," "The nurse acts . . . ," it goes beyond prescriptive statements to advocate accountability to the client. The statements reflect an awareness of shifting roles and the complexity of modern health care. They identify the values and beliefs behind the ethical standards. There is a remarkable breadth of social and professional concern within the ANA Code for Nurses.[53]

One might compare the code itself to the concept of morals described earlier, the normative or applied ethics of other interpreters. The Interpretive Statements might then be compared with our concept of ethics with its concern for reasons, e.g., "Each client has the moral right to determine what will be done with his/her person . . ." The Interpretive Statements are currently being revised.

Ethical codes have proliferated among the many professions.[54] The variety is perhaps not as great as it seems, for many of the newer codes are modeled after others. The Canadian Nurses' Association follows the ICN code, though the Order of Nurses of Quebec has developed its own and Province groups are developing their own.[55]

Roles and Responsibilities

The Greek philosopher Heraclitus said that the only constant is change itself. We cannot even step into the same river twice. By the time we put our second foot in, the river has changed. Change is part of modern life, as shown in the history of the ANA code. The role of the nurse continues to change. This change includes role variation from an employee (most nurses work in hospitals or for other employers—physicians, schools, companies) to completely independent practitioners, such as some nurse-midwives. There are nurses, like people in general, who view their work as simply a job to earn money or to have something to do. Others consider themselves professionals in the fullest sense of that term. This concept has several ramifications, which we will discuss in Chapter Four.

One aspect of professionalism is accepting responsibility for one's actions. The new nurse is one who is fully accountable, even when carrying out the orders of his or her employer. While the old concept of obedience to the physician is still very much in evidence in our cultural structures, hospital hierarchies, and so on, the emphasis now is on intelligent obedience, which may mean disobedience or refusal to obey when the physician is impaired, incompetent, or simply wrong.

The law has been slow to recognize this independent professional status. In 1973, a Michigan court decision said that a nurse is prohibited from exercising independent judgment. This is a two-edged sword, for it relieved the nurse of a malpractice judgment even as it denied nursing independent professional status. On the other hand, when nurses and other personnel refused to work with a brain surgeon, he sued because they interfered with his making a living. He could not tell the left half of the brain from the right half unless it was pointed out to him. In this case, the nursing and other personnel were upheld in their independent judgment. If a physician is under the influence of alcohol or drugs, or if in ignorance he or she prescribes the wrong medication, nurses can be held liable for obeying incorrect physician orders.

In the widely publicized trial of the Nazi, Adolf Eichmann, Eichmann claimed that in murdering Jews he was only carrying out orders. Thus, he should not be held responsible. The Israeli court disagreed, and he was sentenced to death. The excuse that "I am only carrying out orders" is becoming less viable in today's changing climate of roles and responsibilities.[56]

Some people want the rights and privileges of professional status, but they do not want the responsibilities of that status. This is reminiscent of the adolescent who wants the privileges of adulthood, such as driving the family car, but wants mother or father to fill the gas tank, pay the insurance, and so on. There is, of course, no real adulthood until the rights are balanced with the acceptance of and the exercise of commensurate responsibility. While this ethical concept is widely ignored in today's climate of permissibility, it remains of crucial importance to professional life, nursing and other types, by way of yet another principle that equates professional and ethical. Unprofes-

sional conduct is unethical conduct, by definition. The content of the professional conduct, i.e., the moral standards, the "shoulds" and the "oughts" are
spelled out in terms of codes, ethics in general, religion, society, the changing
roles and responsibilities that we currently see in process in today's culture.[57]

Duties and Obligations

The Greek *deontais*, translated "duty," originally meant obedience to rules.
But doing one's duty might mean disobedience, as noted in the nurse's obligation to care for the patient if the system or other health care providers are
doing harm (maleficence) instead of following the principle of doing good
(beneficence). Joseph Fletcher thus describes duty as meaning "to do what is
best in the situation." This is to be "responsive to obligation."[58] In general
then, one might say that duty is more specific and obligation is more general.
In practice, the two terms are often used interchangeably, as are morals and
ethics.

Carney considers duty to be one of three types of normative judgments in
theological and philosophical ethics: judgments of value, virtue, and obligation or duty. The first speaks of what is good or bad, whereas the second
refers to the qualities of a person that are commendable or reprehensible
(moral character). The obligations or duties answer the question, "What
morally ought to be done?"[59]

Some speak of ordinary duties. Pope Pius XII suggested that we are obligated to use ordinary but not extraordinary means to save lives or treat
illnesses.[60] We may use extraordinary means but we are not obligated to do
so. In the famous case of Karen Ann Quinlan, the family and their priest saw
the resuscitator as extraordinary and asked that it be removed. The physicians
saw it as ordinary and refused to do so. What is ordinary may be a matter of
interpretation.

Some speak of an absolute duty, that is, a duty that overrides all other
ordinary duties. These ordinary duties are sometimes called "prima facie" (on
the face of) duties. This term, however, is also used in different ways.[61] One
meaning is the obvious in relation to the situation, e.g., nurses have a duty to
care for the sick. The ANA code adds that this duty is to be carried out
without regard to "social or economic status, personal attributes, or the nature of the health problems" (Table 1-1).

Still another way of looking at these concerns is to speak of obligation
and supererogation—above and beyond the call of duty. The distinction is
sometimes hard to maintain, but it can be illustrated by the duty to care for a
patient. A patient has a right to the care he or she has contracted for from the
physician, the nurse, the hospital. Sympathy or empathy, however, is not
something that can be demanded. While we know it can contribute to the
recovery of health or the maintenance of health, it is not actually a part of the
paycheck. In the view of some, at least, this makes sympathy supererogatory.[62]

Kohlberg cites the Judeo-Christian concept of *agape*, Greek for love or charity, as supererogation. It is nonexclusive and extended to all, including enemies. It is gracious and extended without regard for merit. Some see this as the description of nursing. It is certainly appropriate for modern nursing from the battlefield to the hospital. It is certainly consistent with the ANA code. This is consistent too with Beauchamp's observation that while "do no harm" is clearly a duty, some philosophers see doing good as a virtue rather than a duty. Thus doing good is supererogatory. Nursing then is supererogatory, demanding a generosity in the moral life that goes beyond duty.[63]

Rights and Privileges

The language of duty is very old. From time immemorial, people have had duties—to God(s), king, tribe, family, church, nation, school, employer, patient, self. The language of "rights" is relatively new as ethics go. While the concepts are older, the language is only several centuries old. Richard Tuck says a Dominican theologian, Silvestre M. de Prierio, wrote of property and rights in 1515.[64] However, the real growth of rights is a post-World War II phenomenon. The ANA code says, "The nurse safeguards the client's right to privacy. . . ." The Interpretive Statements refer to moral and legal rights. There are now several Patient's Bills of Rights, codes such as that of the American Hospital Association, several individual hospitals, and the Pregnant Patient's Bill of Rights.[65]

There is considerable discussion now in the ethics literature about a right to health or a right to health care or a right to equal access to health care. The first has been called absurd because it is so often beyond our control. It has also been noted that much health is within our control. Whenever the American people want better health, they can have it by eating less, by drinking less or not at all, by slowing down on the highway, by not smoking.[66]

However, the United Nations Universal Declaration of Human Rights (1948) says, "Everyone has a right to a standard of living adequate for the health and well-being of himself and his family, including . . . medical care. . . ." This was expanded in the UN International Covenant on Economic, Social, and Cultural Rights (1966) with the recognition of "the right of everyone to the enjoyment of the highest attainable standard of physical and mental health."[67] Bentley Glass has asked, "Is it not equally a right of every person to be born physically and mentally sound, capable of developing into a mature individual?"[68] The right to health care has been noted by the American Medical Society.[69]

The equal access to health care is a matter of equity or distributive justice or the allocation of scarce resources. These principles are part of deontology, as explained in Chapter Two. The whole area of rights has been divided in various ways. The so-called natural rights led Jeremy Bentham (1748-1832) to scoff, "Natural rights is simple nonsense . . , nonsense on stilts." Critics hold rights to be neither self-evident nor inalienable. Some see "rights" as merely self-interest. Others, such as John Locke (1632-1704), talked about the right to life, liberty, and property. The American Declaration of Independence (1776) speaks of "unalienable rights to life, liberty and the pursuit of happiness." The French Declaration of the Rights of Man and of Citizens (1789) speaks of "natural, imprescriptible and inalienable rights . . . liberty, property, security and resistance of oppression." Hugo Grotius gave (1670) the now classic definition: "A right is a moral quality of a person entitling him justly to possess or to perform something." Carl Wellman has suggested "a right is a claim or sphere of decision that is, or ought to be, respected by other individuals and protected by society."

In addition to these natural rights, there is the category of human rights that includes the right to work, the right to privacy, the right to autonomy. Some of these are considered ethical principles. There are legal rights and moral rights, which sometimes overlap and sometimes differ.[70] This overlap and difference are regular features of the relationship between law and morality.[71] Americans are noted for the tendency to write their morals into laws.

Nurses also have rights though more on paper than in practice, more future than present. These include human rights to respect, freedom, equality, and such professional rights as the right to set standards of excellence in nurse practice acts, participation in policy affecting nursing, professional autonomy. Some suggest nursing rights are not an end in themselves but a means to better patient care. We would suggest they are both—nurses have a right to be treated decently, but yes, where nursing standards are high, patients do get better care.[72]

Rights are often matched with duties: where there is a duty, there is a right. There are times at least when one can say that a right is what someone else owes to the individual, whereas a duty is what the individual owes the other(s). One might have a right to help in time of need and someone has a duty to help. This is a positive right or an entitlement. There are negative rights, such as the right to be left alone or the right to privacy. In health care, one might have a right to care, and one might have the right to refuse care. It is noteworthy that while rights are sometimes seen as absolute, they are often limited. One has a right to swing one's arms, but the right ends where someone else's nose begins.[73]

However, rights and duties are not automatically or necessarily matched. One may have a right, for example, a legal right to an abortion. It does not follow that someone else has the duty to provide it. There is considerable controversy over such combinations. Duties may exist without regard to others. One has a duty to stop for a red light whether or not there is another car or person in sight. One may have a right that is impossible to fulfill, such as a right to food, but if there is no food in a time of famine, the right is an empty one, at least at the moment. Glass's observation about the right to be born physically and mentally sound may not mean much, though it has important consequences for maternal nutrition or when defects are discoverable in utero and they can be corrected through fetal treatment or eliminated through abortion.

Abortion is a source of major controversy in our time. Nurses have an obligation or duty to care for patients. They do not, by law (the Senator Frank Church amendment) have a duty to assist in an abortion when it is against their own moral standards. Conversely, a nurse may approve of abortion but not have the right to impose one on a patient or require someone to provide the procedure. The ANA code agrees with the nurse's right not to assist in a procedure with which he or she does not agree but states that the nurse will provide care until substitute care can be arranged, though the better process is to declare such a standard in advance. Thus abortion, under limited circumstances, may be a right, but if there is no one available to perform the abortion, it takes on the nature of privilege, a lesser category in moral theory.

This lesser category has been defined as a benefit, advantage, or immunity given to a person by someone else.[74] Privilege can be illustrated by the state-granted privilege of a driver's license. If the individual does not live by the law, the license can be taken away. Similarly, a license to practice nursing or medicine may be revoked under certain circumstances. What is more controversial is whether a person's right to health care can be revoked, e.g., when through deleterious habits, such as substance abuse, the person "brings it on himself." Hans Jonas claims that freedom of inquiry is a social privilege.[75] Thus research, including nursing research, is a privilege rather than a right. Some, however, might claim a stronger role for research, perhaps even claim it as a right, if health care is to improve and if health care providers are to be able to do what society expects of them.

CONCLUSIONS

Our concern in this chapter has been more a matter of definitions than of substantive discussion. Much has been written about many of the concepts noted. Each can be considered in as much detail as the reader wishes by pursuing the relevant literature. Some are considered further in the following chapters. By way of summary, we reiterate the distinction of ethics as the reasons for the moral shoulds and should nots, the ultimate reasons of metaethics as beyond the ethical why, and bioethics as life ethics, which has become a discipline focused on health care.

By these definitions, the ethical codes might be more accurately called moral codes, though the interchangeable use of morals and ethics make it correct to continue to call them codes of ethics in common usage. They remain general rather than specific guidelines to roles and responsibilities, duties and obligations, rights and privileges, which continue to change though the concepts remain as constants in our current concern with nursing ethics.

NOTES

1. Quoted by *Reader's Digest* 122 (732):140, April 1983.
2. Borowitz, E.B. "Lessons for our society from the days of awe." *Harvard Divinity Bulletin* XII (2): 4–6, December 1982–January 1983.
3. Alastair MacIntyre says that every modern moral philosopher is against everyone but himself (to which we can now add a few "herselves"). "Why is the search for the foundations of ethics so frustrating?" *The Hastings Center Report* 9 (4):16–22, August 1979. The *Report* is cited hereafter as HCR. The variety reflected in these thoughts should not obscure broad areas of agreement among moral philosophers and theologians.
4. Note that in and of itself, this may be neither good nor bad. There are many different kinds of authority—head nurse, hospital, police, government, school, religion, employer, expert. In ethics, there are those with expertise in ethics and those who consider themselves authorities in ethics. Besides individuals, one can note group authority in ethics, such as one's professional group, one's peer group, or the community. Consensus ethics reflect group authority unless the group is led by an individual who determines the ethics.
5. Lawrence Kohlberg (see Chapter Three) claims that children and adolescents are natural philosophers concerned with justice. Teachers too must be so concerned. We extend this to teachers at all levels—undergraduate, graduate, clinical instructors, anyone in a position to be a model for others. The concern includes parents, nurses, physicians, hospital administrators, ad infinitum. Kohlberg notes the "hidden curriculum" that exists in schools and, we would add, in homes and hospitals. Values are being taught, consciously or unconsciously, overtly or covertly. He, and we, prefer to have these values out in the open where they can be honestly and rationally considered in an open democratic fashion. Otherwise, it is a subtle or blatant form of indoctrination. However, as we discuss in Chapter Three, one cannot work with people at a lower stage of moral development as though they had already reached the highest stage. Kohlberg, L. *Essays on Moral Development. Vol. One. The Philosophy of Moral Development.* San Francisco: Harper & Row, 1981, pp. ix–xxv, 1–28, especially pp. 18–23. On the "hidden curriculum," cf. Jackson, P.W. *Life in the Classroom.* New York: Holt, Rinehart, and Winston, 1968. Cf. further Rosenzweig, L. "Kohlberg in the classroom: moral education models." In Munsey, B. (ed.) *Moral Development, Moral Education, and Kohlberg.* Birmingham, AL: Religious Education Press, 1980, pp. 359–380, especially p. 359. Macdonald, J.B. "A look at the Kohlberg curriculum framework for moral education." In Munsey, pp. 381–400, especially p. 395.
6. Beauchamp, T.L., and Childress, J.F. *Principles of Biomedical Ethics,* 2nd ed. New York: Oxford University Press, 1983. Jonsen, A.R., Siegler, M., and Winslade, W.J. *Clinical Ethics.* New York: Macmillan, 1982.
7. Moral education has been tried in a variety of forms. The philosophers' claim to having the answers or being able to supply them is one approach. The method of teaching moral rules has been used by science and state, church and school. While it has a bad press or is in disrepute today, it has a long history of accomplishment. It may be making a comeback. An explanation for its success is readily at hand in the moral development theories of Piaget and Kohlberg. See Kohlberg's Stage 4 in Chapter Three. Kohlberg notes that conventionally virtuous behavior is easy to teach. The Thomas Jefferson Research Center in Pasadena, CA, has done this in over 9000 classrooms in 31 states of the United States. Moral education in

Kohlberg's system has the goal of developing the organizational structures, the problem-solving strategies, to analyze, interpret, and make decisions. As we will see in Chapter Three, he has spent years developing this "better questions" approach to teach moral rules. Rest, J.R. "Developmental psychology and value education." In Munsey, pp. 101–129. Kohlberg, L. "Education for justice." In *Essays*, pp. 29–41, and, "Educating for a just society: An updated and revised statement." In Munsey, pp. 455–470. Goble, F. *Thomas Jefferson Research Center Newsletter*. No. 205:3, June 1983, and 207:1, September 1983. He quotes (p. 2) Herbert Spencer's 1851 *Social Statistics*, "Education has for its object the formation of character."

8. Henry D. Aiken noted four "Levels of moral discourse." In his *Reason and Conduct*. New York: Knopf, 1962, pp. 65–87. The expressive "Great!" is an emotional response. The moral rules level approximates our use of "moral" while his ethical and postethical levels approximate our use of ethics and metaethics. For the ethics–morality distinction used here, cf. also Barry, V. *Moral Aspects of Health Care*. Belmont, CA: Wadsworth, 1982, p. 5. Taylor, P.W. *Principles of Ethics*, 3rd ed. Belmont, CA: Dickinson, 1978. Lucille F. Newman relates morals to judgments, values to the cultural framework, and ethics to socially derived generalizations. "Medical ethics, history of. I. Primitive societies." *Encyclopedia of Bioethics* 2:876–880, 1978. The latter work is cited hereafter as EB. John Ladd notes the varying viewpoints in his "The task of ethics." EB 1:400–407, 1978.

9. The social nature of morality is often noted. Some see society as the source of ethics. Consensus ethics reflects the group. "Moral values are evaluations of action believed by members of a given society to be 'right'." Berkowitz, L. *Development of Motives and Values in a Child*. New York: Basic Books, 1964, p. 44. This view is sometimes called "cultural moral relativism." Kohlberg notes it is the view of ethics practiced in the Soviet Union to build loyalty to the government. "Stages of moral development as a basis for moral education." In Munsey, pp. 15–98. It was the ethics of Nazi Germany. Arendt, H. *The Life of the Mind. Thinking.* New York: Harcourt Brace Jovanovich, 1978, Vol. 1. She noted Adolf Eichmann's mindless adherence to the code.

   Others believe morality is the given of nature—see Natural Law in Chapter Two. Some believe God is the source of morality, perhaps through the laws of nature which God created, perhaps by direct revelation, perhaps through angels or people like Moses or the Prophets. Still others believe the individual is the source—the moral law within, human nature, through reason, by interpretation of nature, the Bible, and so on. A pluralistic approach might acknowledge all of these and more or some combination. For Kohlberg's nonrelativist moral development, see Chapter Three.

10. Margot Joan Fromer emphasizes rationality in ethics to the exclusion of emotionality. *Ethical Issues in Sexuality and Reproduction*. St. Louis: C.V. Mosby, 1983, pp. 1–2. This is perhaps necessary, given the emotionality of her subject. Her position, however, is not unique. Shirley Maurice and Louise Warrich describe ethical principles as emotionless derivations from facts, natural law, evaluations that in turn derive from reason, responsibility, choice, and conscience. Morals, they say, are externally imposed by religion and culture. "Ethics in professional nursing practice." *Journal of Obstetrical, Gynecological, and Neonatal Nursing* 8 (6):327–329, November–December, 1979. Cf. further Aiken. "Moral reasoning." In his *Reason and Conduct*, pp. 88–111.

   On the other hand, Michael A. Guillen suggests that while we like to think of ourselves as rational beings, "we have no clear understanding of what rational really means." "Behavior by the numbers." *Psychology Today* 17 (11):77-78, November 1983. If we did not feel something was important, we would not bother with it. For the relationship of feelings and reason, cf. Midgley, M. *Heart and Mind: The Varieties of Moral Experience.* New York: St. Martin's Press, 1981, and Emmet, D. *The Moral Prism.* New York: Macmillan, 1979. Daniel Callahan claims that "feeling and sentiment are rarely absent from a well-ordered moral life." They reinforce convictions, warn us when values are threatened, and alert us to consequences. "If they are not always reliable guides, their absence is even more hazardous, as anyone who has dealt with a sociopath is painfully aware." "On feeding the dying," HCR 13 (5):22, October 1983. Feeling plays a major role in the ethics of intuitionism, as in Moore, G.E. *Principia Ethica.* Cambridge: University Press, 1903. Cf. Chapter Two, where intuitionism is discussed as Kurt Baier's third category in the deontological approach to ethics. Part of the problem here is that emotional responses may motivate our better selves or they may cloud our judgment. Misperceptions, for example, may trigger strong emotions. James R. Rest notes the strong role of emotionality. It may precede cognitive operations. Empathy is a strong factor in morality. Empathy has been observed in infants, so it may need very little cognitive development.

The works of Piaget, Kohlberg, Rest (see Chapter Three), and others, however, show that moral judgment and moral development are cognitive rather than affective processes. Rest, J.R. "A psychologist looks at the teaching of ethics." HCR 12 (1):29-36, February 1982, and, "Developmental psychology and value education." In Munsey, p. 115. It is perhaps a bit premature to insist too strongly that ethics is strictly a rational study. However, it is quite clear that the area of our concern is not mere emotionality either. Kohlberg objects strenuously to the view that morality is simply arbitrary, emotional, and irrational. He proposes human ethical values that are universal and not relative, a moral development that is not relative, a moral development that is not culture bound but is transcultural. He notes however, a congruence between the cognitive and affective, i.e., a cognitive Stage 6 person is also likely to be affective Stage 6. Cf. Chapter Three, and his "Stages of moral development as a basis for moral education." In Munsey, pp. 23-37.

On religion, cf. further Chapter Two, on moral theology. Here we can note Frederick S. Carney's differentiation of everyday religious morality requiring a minimum of reflection and theological ethics as a theoretical activity of criticism and reflection. Cf. his "Ethics." EB 1:429-437, 1978. B.F. Skinner discounts reason and feeling both. "Origins of a behaviorist." *Psychology Today* 17 (9):22-33, September 1983.

11. Ladd, J. "The task of ethics." EB 1:400-407, 1978.
12. Bernard Rosen says normative ethics provide a device for moral judgments that apply to actions, states of affairs, and such. "Moral dilemmas and their treatments." In Munsey, pp. 232-265. Israela Ettenberg Aron says normative ethics discusses substantive moral issues—concrete or abstract, hypothetical or real. Metaethics is the discussion of ethical discussion itself. Cf. "Moral education: the formalist tradition and the deweyan alternative." In Munsey, pp. 401-426, especially p. 405.
13. Aiken, H.D. "Levels of moral discourse." In his *Reason and Conduct*, p. 70.
14. Kohlberg, L. "From is to ought." In his *Essays*, pp. 101-189, especially p. 175.

Socrates is famous for many things including the Socratic method. He asked questions, and when he received an answer, asked yet another. He pushed the intermediate answers toward an ultimate one or ones.

15. Cotroneo, M. "Nursing ethics: A contextual approach." *Newsletter.* Society of the Alumni of the School of Nursing, University of Pennsylvania. Spring, 1984, p. 13.

16. There are many ideas or things that have served as ultimates for human beings. Science, money, sex, the good, pleasure, one's job, the state, the family, the party, the company, one's profession, the Bible, a teacher, parental commands, society, human nature—these are but a few examples. Some apparent ultimates, such as scientific or religious authority, may be intermediate since they derive their authority from some further source that is the real ultimate. As Socrates found out, people frequently mistake an intermediate for the ultimate. In monotheistic religions, such as Judaism, Christianity, and Islam, it is idolatry to believe in any ultimate beside God.

    Kohlberg has suggested that relativists are moving from conventional to postconventional levels of moral development. Their relativity presupposes valid universal principles. In moral development (see Chapter Four), the relativists are Stage 4 and one half, regressed to Stage 2. Kohlberg, L. "Preface." p. xix, and "From is to ought." p. 130, in *Essays.*

17. Beauchamp, T.L. "Ethical theory and bioethics." In Beauchamp, T.L., and Walters, L. *Contemporary Issues in Bioethics,* 2nd ed. Belmont, CA: Wadsworth, 1982, pp. 1–43. Abelson, R. *Ethics and Metaethics.* New York: St. Martin's Press, 1963.

18. John Dewey said morals have to do with all activity with alternative possibilities. Every and any act is within the scope of morals. *Human Nature and Conduct.* New York: Modern Library, 1930 (original 1922). Quoted by Aron, I.E. "Moral Education." In Munsey, p. 415.

19. Carlton, W. *"In Our Professional Opinion . . .": The Primacy of Clinical Judgment Over Moral Choice.* Notre Dame: University of Notre Dame Press, 1978.

20. Barzun, J. "The professions under siege." *Harper's Magazine* 257 (1541):61–68, October 1978.

21. James Rest speaks of "morality as an ensemble of processes rather than a single, unitary process" in "A psychologist looks at the teaching of ethics." HCR 12 (1):29–36, February 1982. Aiken explores the metaethical question of "Why be moral?" He answers in terms of the moral agent who in the end chooses to be, in "Levels of moral discourse." In *Reason and Conduct,* pp. 83–87.

22. Kollemorten, I., et al. "Ethical aspects of decision-making." *Journal of Medical Ethics* 17 (2):67–69, June 1981, define a significant ethical problem as one "which makes the decision-maker or other members of the staff consider the ethical implications. An ethical problem is also considered important when the decision-maker is in no doubt how to act relative to his or her norms, if he or she at the same time assumes that other clinicians might make a different decision under the same circumstances."

    An interesting example of significance/trivia is the overwhelming concern for the autonomy of convicts on the part of some ethicists who express no concern whatsoever for the autonomy, or any other rights, of the victims. Convicts are the only group in this country who have a right to health care by legal court order. The courts have not yet seen fit to order health care for the victims of crime, nor tor that matter, anyone else. Some see this as bizarre, whereas others see that proper health care for convicts is very important. For a discussion of the issues, see Dubler, N.N. "Jail and prison health care standards: a determination of need without reference to want or desire." In Bayer, R., Caplan, A.L., and Daniels, N. (eds.) *In Search of Equity*. New York and London: Plenum Press, 1983, pp. 69–94. The problem extends to other fields as well. Panos D. Bardis notes "Similarly, the typical sociologist's heart bleeds for the criminal, although it remains apathetic when it comes to the helpless victim." Cf. his "History of sociology." *Social Science* 51 (4):213–245, Autumn 1976.

23. Quoted by Kubler-Ross, E. *Questions and Answers on Death and Dying*. New York: Macmillan, 1974, p. 75.

24. Regan, T., and Singer, P. (eds.) *Animal Rights and Human Obligations*. Englewood Cliffs, NJ: Prentice-Hall, 1976. Singer, P. "Life. I. The value of life." EB 2:822–829, 1978.

25. It is part of Hinduism, Buddhism, and Jainism. The concept has been made famous by Mahatma Gandhi and Albert Schweitzer. For the latter, cf. *Civilization and Ethics, Vol. 2: The Philosophy of Civilization, rev.* London: A. & A. Black, 1946. For Gandhi, cf. Seshagiri Rao, K.L. *Mahatma Gandhi and Comparative Religion*. Delhi: Motilal Banarsidass, 1978.

26. Stone, C.D. "Should trees have standing?—Toward legal rights for natural objects." *Southern California Law Review* 45:450–501, 1972.

27. Epstein, S.S. "Environmental ethics. I. Environmental health and human disease." EB 1:379–388, 1978. Shrader-Frechette, K.S. *Environmental Ethics*. Pacific Grove, CA: Boxwood, 1981.

28. Our thanks to Marsh Pontiac and Datsun, Ardmore, PA, for sharing the Code. The ten-point Code calls for the maintenance of "high standards of business ethics and integrity."

29. Gary Marotta claims that Thomas Percival introduced the phrase "medical ethics" in 1803 in his Code of Ethics. "The enlightenment and bioethics." In Bandman, E.L., and Bandman, B. (eds.) *Bioethics and Human Rights*. Boston: Little, Brown, 1978, pp. 62–65. Richard B. Brandt suggests that separate moral codes are justified for physicians, lawyers, children, bishops, university students, and presumably any other group. Presumably that includes nursing! "The real and alleged problems of utilitarianism." HCR 13 (2):37–43, April 1983. Danner Clouser, K. "Bioethics." EB 1:115–127, 1978.

30. Curtin, L. "Autonomy, accountability and nursing practice." *Topics in Clinical Nursing* 4 (1):5–14, especially p. 10, April 1982.

31. Davis, A.J., and Aroskar, M.A. *Ethical Dilemmas and Nursing Practice*, 2nd ed. Norwalk, CT: Appleton-Century-Crofts, 1983, p. 3. Kohlberg suggests one needs to know but action requires a second phase sense of responsibility and will. "The relations between moral judgment and moral action." *The Psychology of Moral Development. Essays in Moral Development, Vol. 2.* New York: Harper & Row, in press. James Rest makes a similar observation, noting at least seven intervening variables, such as ego, situation, other values. Moral judgment, however, is a major factor in real life decision making as shown by over 100 studies. Rest, J. "Developmental psychology and value education." In Munsey, pp. 119–123, and, "A psychologist looks at the teaching of ethics." HCR 12 (1):32, February 1982. Kohlberg, L. "From is to ought." In *Essays*, pp. 183–189, claims "maturity of moral thought should predict to maturity of moral action." The Aristotle quote is

by Kohlberg, L. "Indoctrination versus relativity in value education." In *Essays*, pp. 6–28, especially p. 9. The Socratic-Platonic "to know is to do" is quoted by Kohlberg, L. "Education for justice: a modern statement of the Socratic view." In *Essays*, pp. 29–48, especially p. 30. See further discussion in Chapter Three.

32. Davis and Aroskar, p. 4.

33. Potter, V.R. "Bioethics: the science of survival." *Perspectives in Biology and Medicine* 14:127–153, 1970, and *Bioethics: Bridge to the Future*. Englewood Cliffs, NJ: Prentice-Hall, 1971.

34. Reich, W.T. "Foreword." EB 1:xvxxii, 1978.

35. Clouser, H.D. "Bioethics." EB 1:120, 1978.

36. EB general editor, Warren T. Reich noted 1500 publications a year in English alone. "Foreword," EB 1:xvi, 1978.

37. We agree with this more general use, as does Reich, E.B., p. xix, 1978. In practice, however, most works in bioethics refer to physicians and rarely or not at all to health care providers, such as nurses, except those specifically written as texts in nursing ethics. A delightful exception is Barry's *Moral Aspects of Health Care*. The narrowness of this view becomes obvious if one stops to realize that over 75 percent of health care providers are nurses. Usually, however, it is physicians who have the power, and the bioethicists are presumably talking to power rather than numbers of providers.

38. Reich, W.T. "Foreword." EB 1:xv, 1978. Davis and Aroskar, pp. ix, 4, 27. Barry, *Moral Aspects of Health Care*, pp. 6–9, lists five reasons. These include advances in medical sciences, the consumer movement, malpractice suits, court-ordered treatment, and the Nuremberg Code. The latter gave a special impetus to the concept of informed consent.

39. Shetland, M.L. "The responsibility of the professional school for preparing nurses for ethical, moral, and humanistic practice." *Nursing Forum* 8:17–22, 1969. Stanley, T. "Nursing." EB 3:1138–1146, 1978. Jonsen, A.R., Jameton, A.L., and Lynch, A. "Medical ethics, history of: North America in the twentieth century." EB 3:992–1004, 1978.

40. Flexner, A. *Medical Education in the United States and Canada*. New York: Carnegie Foundation for the Advancement of Teaching, Bulletin No. 4, 1910.

41. Jonsen, Jameton, and Lynch. "Medical ethics, history of: North America in the twentieth century." p. 993.

42. The President's Commission for the Study of Ethical Problems in Medicine and Biomedical and Behavioral Research (Morris B. Abrams, Chairman). *Making Health Care Decisions. Volume One: Report*. Washington, D.C.: US Government Printing Office, 1982, pp. 145–149.

43. Munhall, P. "Ethical juxtapositions in nursing research." *Topics in Clinical Nursing* 4 (1):66–73, April 1982. Her concern is that nursing research that focuses on a scientific statistical research methodology contradicts this traditional nursing philosophy. A participant observer scientific method is more appropriate. This methodology is common in the social sciences, such as anthropology and sociology.

44. Jonsen, Jameton, Lynch, "Medical ethics, history of: North America in the twentieth century." p. 996. Leake, C.D. (ed.) *Percival's Medical Ethics*. Baltimore: Williams & Wilkins, 1927.

45. Fletcher, J. *Morals and Medicine*. Princeton, NJ: Princeton University Press, 1954.

46. Jakobovits, I. *Jewish Medical Ethics*. New York: Bloch, 1962, rev. 1975. Rosner, F

Modern Medicine and Jewish Law. New York: Yeshiva University, 1972.

47. Jonsen, Jameton, Lynch. "Medical ethics, history of: North America in the twentieth century." p. 996.

48. The development of dialysis was, of course, much more complicated than this simplified sketch. See, for example, Caplan, A.L. "How should values count in the allocation of new technologies in health care?" In Bayer et al. (eds.) *In Search of Equity*, pp. 95–124. Alexander, S. "They decide who lives, who dies." *Life Magazine*, 1962, reprinted in Hunt, R., and Arras, J. *Ethical Issues in Modern Medicine.* Palo Alto, CA: Mayfield, 1977, pp. 409–424. Donald Robinson documents millions of dollars in overcharges and other financial abuses that account for part of the cost of the dialysis program. "Kidney dialysis: a taxpayers' nightmare." *Reader's Digest* 121 (726):149–152, October 1982.

49. Strong, C. "The tiniest newborns." HCR 13 (1):14–19, February 1983. Zuelzer, W.W. "Relationship to pediatrics." In Moore, T.D. (ed.) *Ethical Dilemmas in Current Obstetric and Newborn Care.* Columbus, OH: Ross Laboratories, 1973, pp. 16–20.

50. *Hippocrates: The Theory and Practice of Medicine.* New York: Philosophical Library, 1964. "Appendix. Section I. Oath of Hippocrates." EB 4:1731. Konold, D. "Codes of medical ethics. I. History." EB 1:162–171. Edelstein, L. "The Hippocratic Oath: text, translation and interpretation." *Bulletin of the History of Medicine*, Suppl. 1:1–64, 1943. Veatch, R.M. "Codes of medical ethics. II. Ethical analysis." EB 1:172–180. Basham, A.L. "Hinduism." EB 2:661–667, 1978.

51. Leake, C. *Percival's Medical Ethics.* Baltimore: Williams & Wilkins, 1927.

52. Mohr, J.C. *Abortion in America.* New York: Oxford University Press, 1978. Brandt, A.M. "The ways and means of American medicine." HCR 13 (3):41–43, June 1983. This is a review of Starr, P. *The Social Transformation of American Medicine.* New York: Basic Books, 1983, which emphasizes the insecure profession's rise to power by limiting competition and giving their membership legitimacy.

53. EB 4:1789–1799, 1978.

54. Chalk, R., Frankel, M.S., and Chafer, S.B. *AAAS Professional Ethics Project: Professional Ethics Activities in the Scientific and Engineering Societies.* Washington, D.C.: AAAS, 1980.

55. Jonsen, Jameton, Lynch. "Medical ethics, history of: North America in the twentieth century." p. 995.

56. Nadelson, C.C., and Notman, M.T. "Women and biomedicine. II. Women as health professionals." EB 4:1713–1720, 1978. It has been suggested that nurses and physicians are not independent professionals but interdependent. This focuses on intercollegiality rather than giving and taking orders.

57. The distinction between form and content is an old one. Immanuel Kant (1724–1804) represents a deontological perspective on ethics and will be discussed in Chapter Two. Here we note the interesting observation that Kant's concept of moral law could be put forth theoretically only in form and not in content. Ethical theory can decide in advance on how one should make an act of will to be moral but not on the "what." The what is another matter. Bole, T.J., III, and Schumacher, M. "Obligation and supererogation." EB 3:1147–1152, 1978.

58. Fletcher, J. "Ethics. vs. situation ethics." EB 1:421–429, 1978.

59. Carney, F.S. "Ethics." EB 1:429, 1978.

60. "The prolongation of life." *The Pope Speaks* 4:393–398, 1958.

61. Ladd, J. "The task of ethics." EB 1:405, 1978.
62. Bole and Schumaker. "Obligation and supererogation." EB 3:1152, 1978.
63. Kohlberg, L., and Power, C. "Moral development, religious thinking, and the question of a seventh stage." In *Essays*, pp. 311–372, especially pp. 347–352. Beauchamp, T.L. "Ethical theory and bioethics." p. 29. An alternative view is that professional responsibility goes beyond the duty of ordinary citizens. Thus the "generosity demanded" is not supererogatory but simply professional duty. Personal communication, Dr. Warren G. Thompson.
64. Tuck, R. *Natural Rights: Their Origin and Development.* New York: Cambridge University Press, 1979.
65. Annas, G.J. *The Rights of Hospital Patients.* New York: Avon, 1975. The AHA, 840 North Lake Shore Drive, Chicago, IL 60611. Committee on Patient's Rights, Box 1900, NY, NY 10001. The emphasis is on rights rather than responsibilities, thus reflecting current cultural trends. However, if these rights are to be realities, responsibilities remain for both patients and providers. The Bills of Rights have not gone uncriticized. The AHA Bill was created by the AHA rather than patients. There is an element of paternalism in an organization gratuitously granting to patients what they already have. Gaylin, W. "The patient's bill of rights." *Saturday Review of the Sciences* 1 (2):22, February 24, 1973.
66. Daniels, N. "Health care needs and distributive justice." In *In Search of Equity,* pp. 1–41, especially p. 35. Personal communication, Dr. Warren G. Thompson.
67. Quoted by Jonsen, A.R. "Health care. III. Right to health care services." EB 2:623–630, 1978. The United Methodist Church Health and Welfare Ministries has taken as its focus "Health for All by the Year 2000." *United Methodist Reporter* 130 (22):4, November 1983. Many religious groups have been concerned with health and illness care over the centuries.
68. Quoted by Macklin, R. "Rights. II. Rights in bioethics." EB 4:1507–1516, 1978.
69. Jonsen. "Health care. III. Right to health care services." p. 624.
70. Jonsen. "Health care. III. Right to health care services." p. 624. Beauchamp, T. "Ethical theory and bioethics." pp. 34–37. Golding, M.P. "The concept of rights: a historical sketch." In Bandman and Bandman (eds.) *Bioethics and Human Rights.* Wellman, C. *Morals and Ethics.* Glenview, IL: Scott, Foresman, 1975, p. 252. Barry, *Moral Aspects of Health Care,* p. 11.
71. On nursing law and ethics, see such works as Kelly, L.Y. *Dimensions of Professional Nursing.* New York: Macmillan, 1980. Fenner, K.M. *Ethics and Law in Nursing.* New York: Van Nostrand, 1980. Fiesta, J. *The Law and Liability: A Guide for Nurses.* New York: Wiley, 1983.
72. Fagin, C.M. "Nurses' rights." *American Journal of Nursing* 75:82–85, January 1975. Davis and Aroskar, p. 86.
73. Barry, *Moral Aspects of Health Care.* p. 11. Beauchamp. "Ethical theory and bioethics." p. 37, lists four limits on liberty. The first one of no harm to others is universally accepted, he says. Widely acknowledged might be more accurate. The other three are more controversial. Paternalism restricts another's liberty to prevent self-harm. Laws (legal moralism) restrict immoral behavior. The offense principle justifies restricting offensive behavior.
74. Davis and Aroskar, p. 69.
75. Jonas, H. "Freedom of scientific inquiry and the public interest." HCR 6:15–17, August 1976.

The aim of science is to seek the simplest explanation of complex facts. We are apt to fall into the error of thinking that the facts are simple because simplicity is the goal of our quest. The guiding motto in the life of every natural philosopher should be, "Seek simplicity and distrust it."

—Alfred North Whitehead[1]

Knowledge rests not upon truth alone, but upon error also.

—Carl Gustav Jung[2]

CHAPTER 2
Ethical Systems: Right And Wrong

Tom L. Beauchamp has suggested that philosophy is primarily concerned with criticism and justification. In ethics, the latter concern is to justify some moral point of view.[3] Human beings appear to be capable of almost infinite rationalization—finding reasons to justify anything one chooses to do, but Beauchamp goes on to note that not all reasons are good reasons and not all good reasons are sufficient justification. What constitutes good and sufficient is part of the whole problem. Somewhere during the process, one comes to a moral judgment, which Beauchamp describes as a decision, verdict, or conclusion about a particular action or character trait.[4]

Decision making is the main concern of this book.

Beauchamp talks about levels of justification. Judgments or decisions are justified by moral rules (the oughts/ought nots discussed in Chapter One), which in turn are justified by moral principles that are more general and more fundamental than the rules. His example is the rule that it is wrong to deceive patients. Deception violates the principle of autonomy, to which we would add truth-telling. The principles are in turn justified by ethical theories that we call systems, to which we now turn.

In classic philosophical ethical theories or systems, there are two primary systems—utilitarianism and deontology. The dichotomy was introduced by Charles D. Broad in 1930. He considered it an improvement of Sidgwick's trichotomy of intuitionism, egoism, and utilitarianism.[5] The word deontology comes from the Greek *deon* meaning "rule, principle," or, more accurately, "binding duty." The word was introduced by the founder of utilitarianism, Jeremy Bentham.[6] While the two philosophical systems are often opposed, as though they were contradictory or mutually exclusive, this recent history and utilitarian Bentham's use of the term suggest otherwise. They may be seen as implying two different systems of ethics or as complementary approaches.

Utilitarianism focuses on utility. Thus this system might be a one principle approach to ethics. The principle of utility is often interpreted in other terms, such as the good, which could mean there are several principles in the utilitarian approach. While the two systems are discussed separately, the line between them is not rigid. One suspects there are very few pure deontologists (consequences are irrelevant) or utilitarians (no principles), just as there are few pure relativists.

We also discuss here the approach of natural law, which some see as a third system, whereas others see it as a combination of the other two because it considers both purpose and principle. Much of the content of morals and ethics comes from religion, which is frequently the source of human motivation as well. Prior to the rise of modern secular philosophy, virtually all of ethics came from religion because most of the philosophers were themselves theologians or men of religion.[7] Women philosophers and theologians have been relatively rare until recent times. In part, they have adopted the systems and categories at hand, and in part they are developing new approaches. The impact of these may be felt in years to come.

UTILITARIANISM OR TELEOLOGY: THE BOTTOM LINE

Utilitarianism generally refers to utility. Teleology comes from the Greek word *telos* which means "end," or "the consequences," or in today's vernacular, "the bottom line." Consequentialism is another term for this system of ethics. The words tend to be used interchangeably, though Kurt Baier suggests the concept of the teleological is the larger concept of which utilitarianism is a part. The other parts are ethical egoism ("I am the law," as one politician put it), ethical elitism (the "best" people), and ethical parochialism (what is best for my group is what is ethical). The fourth category is ethical universalism, which is concerned with all humanity. Baier presents utilitarianism as belonging to this fourth type.[8] Others use the words in the opposite sense, with utilitarianism as the more inclusive category. Egoism is also considered a separate category or system of ethics at times.

Utilitarianism is often summarized in two aphorisms. One is "the greatest good for the greatest number." At first glance it sounds very democratic— majority rule and so on. Others suggest that minorities, such as the French-speaking people of Canada or the blacks of the United States or the Jews of Germany, have rights that cannot be rightfully ignored, suggesting that there is some other basis for deciding what is right, which we will come back to in considering deontology. As the other three categories of Baier's teleological approach suggest, there are other determinants of who constitutes the greatest number. A famous American boxer declared, "I am the greatest!" The "greatest" may be the person in power. Health care systems tend to be organized in a hierarchy. One person may be in command, or a group may be in charge. The elite may be those in power or those with the most money or the greatest social status or Nietzsche's superman, from which the Nazi regime derived inspiration for its Aryan superiority.

The greatest may be my group—my family, my political party, my religion, my association, my profession. Under such circumstances, there is a very peculiar twist on democracy. Women, who may be a majority in numbers, become oppressed by the dominant power of the males. The blacks of South Africa are a huge majority, but the tiny white minority rules for the greatest good for the greatest number, which means themselves. Nurses represent the largest number of health care providers in the health care system but rarely have a significant voice in how the system is managed. The numerical minority of whatever color, race, religion, political persuasion, national background are at risk in a system in which the "greatest" represents those in power without any ethical creed other than their own good, even when that good is paternalistically described as caring for society.[9] Having said all that, it remains the opinion of at least some observers that utilitarianism is the dominant ethic of American society.[10]

"The greatest good for the greatest number" may be the ethical stance behind health care policy. In some ways, maybe it has to be. Policy is a broad sweep for the public good. It would be impossible to have a public policy that considered every individual. Patricia L. Munhall, however, has suggested that for this reason the individual is jeopardized in a utilitarian ethical framework.[11]

The second aphorism is that "the end justifies the means." The means are merely the expedient—do whatever you want, and it's all right as long as your final goal or purpose is good. This approach has a bad press these days, in part because of the Nazi holocaust that used the efficient bureaucracy of a modern nation as the means to eliminate huge numbers of people the Nazis did not want, such as gypsies, the handicapped, Jews, and any opponents of the regime. In spite of the bad press, this approach remains a dominant one. The end purpose in health care may be to restore health or to preserve life, no matter how much or who it hurts. A good end is presented as the justification of any means at hand.

The end purpose has varied enormously with various thinkers. The roots of this approach are perhaps as old as humanity. Epicurus (341–270 BC) has been called a utilitarian because he saw the law as simply a matter of that which is expedient.[12] Why should anyone be good? The end purpose varies across a wide spectrum from the good as an abstract end in itself without further definition to obeying God. Other ends are to find satisfaction, to fulfill one's personality, happiness, friendship, love, knowledge, relationships of trust, fairness, justice. In some ways, these end purposes are ultimates, and we are into metaethics here. In some ways, these ends sound like the principles to be considered under deontology. One aspect that makes them different is the concern to maximize the good, happiness, and so on. That was the position of the founders of modern utilitarianism, Jeremy Bentham (1748–1832) and John S. Mill (1806–1873).[13]

The good was a matter of pleasure, familiar to today's world through the work of Sigmund Freud (1857–1939), who believed humans were concerned with maximizing pleasure and minimizing pain.[14] The pleasure may be any one of the items mentioned earlier and many more, such as reading a book or doing a crossword puzzle.[15]

Utilitarians in general have not agreed on what constitutes the good or the end purpose. In health care, one might see health as the good and pain as the illness. One notes, however, that this may be a very narrow view related to physical health and pain. It may also be a broader view that includes mental and emotional health or simply a sense of well-being.

Some distinguish a hedonistic utilitarianism from a pluralistic utilitarianism.[16] The former focuses on pleasure, which for Bentham was individual whereas for Mill it was more social. The pluralistic variety considers the various satisfactions, preferences, and desires noted here that might, however, be simply different interpretations of the good. Some interpreters make a distinction between subjective and objective good. The three forms of egoism might be seen as subjective. The objective would have a broader base of agreement in society as a whole or for humanity as a whole, i.e., some form of universalism.

We need to note also the views of the sum of the good and the concept of net good. In the former, individual happiness or moments of unhappiness do not count. What matters is the bottom line: Does the total good outweigh the bad? Thus, if health care causes pain, it may be acceptable if the final outcome is improved health or the saving of life. The net, similarly, is a balance of the good. The belief is that the good and the bad can be measured and calculated. One subtracts the bad from the good. If the net is good, it is acceptable. While opponents of utilitarianism do not think this utilitarian calculus is possible, one notes that most people at one time or another weigh the good and the bad consequences of various lines of action. Dilemmas may be solved in this way at times. We are frequently faced with a choice between two goods or two evils. The utilitarian calculus is the basis of the cost-benefit analysis so widespread in government, business, and health care. Cost may be financial, but it may also be a matter of learning, time, energy, human suffering, discrimination, and justice.[17]

There are two major divisions of utilitarianism: rule utilitarianism and act utilitarianism. The latter considers each act on its own merits. Act utilitarianism may not weigh every single act. Rules of thumb may guide the daily routine. The rules are not absolute, and the real test is the utility or the final consequences.

Situational Ethics

One of the best-known forms of act utilitarianism is called "situational ethics." The situation determines whether the act is good. The Episcopal clergyman Dr. Joseph Fletcher is perhaps the best-known of the situational-ists.[18] He is not the only one, of course, or even the only clergyperson. He cites Paul Tillich, Dietrich Bonhoeffer, Paul Lehmann, J.A.T. Robinson, James Pike, and Helmut Thielecke, among others. Fletcher determines the utility or the good in terms of love. For any given act, he asks what is the most loving thing to do or what is the least loving or the most unloving line of action. This has been called "Agapism" from the Greek word for divine love or unselfish love. Mill put this in terms of the Golden Rule presented by Jesus of Nazareth: "To do as you would be done by, and to love your neighbor as yourself, constitute the ideal perfection of utilitarian morality."[19] The issues of bioethics—abortion, terminal care, allocation of scarce resources—are not seen as good or bad in themselves. Each situation determines, in terms of consequences based on love, what is the good or the bad. The net gain in human happiness is what is important regardless of any religious or cultural standard of right or wrong.

Rule Utilitarianism

This second major division continues to hold to the bottom line. The difference from act utilitarianism is that past experience reveals that certain rules have greater utility for maximizing the good. Richard B. Brandt holds that this is the real position of J.S. Mill. As noted earlier, he cites Epicurus' attitude toward law in this regard. Richard Cumberland in 1672 presented a theory of action based on rule utilitarianism. Bishop Berkeley in 1712 distinguished two forms of utilitarianism and opted for this second one, which he presented in terms of God's moral laws. God selected these laws because in his benevolence he wants happiness for humanity and these laws will maximize it. It is not in people's long-range interest to violate his laws. Thus, we have both positive and negative reasons for obeying the rules.[20]

A true utilitarian does not see the rules as valid in and of themselves. They are the means to the end purpose of utility, happiness, the good. A nontheistic source of these rules is one's own experience, and thus it is an individualistic rule utilitarianism. However, the source of the rules might also be society or the larger culture. Consensus ethics suggests that whatever people in general believe is right is, and vice versa. Brandt suggests that the morality of society is the source of the individual conscience, or vice versa, the morality of society is the collective conscience of the individuals. We find it in the colloquial "whatever is best for everyone or for most people." Individually, it may be whatever is best for the patient. The utilitarian principle is that the rules are valid if they bring the optimal utility, the best consequences, whatever that may be.

DEONTOLOGY: THE PRINCIPLED WAY

Simply put, deontology is the ethical approach of principles or rules. "Principles" can be defined in several ways. Kohlberg calls a moral principle "a mode of choosing that is universal, a rule of choosing that we want all people to adopt always in all situations." He also notes that mature principles are neither rules (means) nor values (ends) but guides to integrate all the morally relevant elements in concrete situations.[21]

A strict or pure deontologist insists on the ethical absoluteness of the principles regardless of the consequences. Immanuel Kant (1724–1804) insisted on telling the truth no matter who it hurt.[22] As noted earlier, there are probably very few absolute deontologists, for most people are aware of consequences. One criticism of deontologists is that they covertly appeal to consequences.[23]

Of course, one could make consequences a principle. The utility of the utilitarians can be considered a principle. The scientific rule of paucity (that theory is best which most simply explains the most) suggests that such a one-principle approach has value. Other one-principle approaches include Kant himself with his categorical imperative (see later), Joseph Fletcher and his theory of love (noted earlier as an act utilitarianism), and John Rawls with his theory of justice (which might also be considered as utility). Beauchamp calls such one-principle deontology "monistic deontology."[24]

In the other direction, one can note Beauchamp's "pluralistic deontology." There is no theoretical limit on the number of principles in the deontological system. George H. Kieffer lists examples of principles that include several already noted—love, justice, truth-telling, benevolence, reduction of pain, equality, individual rights, fraternal charity (the Golden Rule, listed above as Mill's fulfillment of utility), honesty, the law of double effect. The last has also been included as part of the utilitarian calculus—if the primary intent is good and the good outweighs the bad, an evil side effect can be tolerated.[25]

While the number is theoretically unlimited, many principles can be grouped together under a few headings. In addition and as part of this grouping, relatively few principles can be seen or used as including most of the concerns in bioethics. Beauchamp and James F. Childress present four of these—autonomy, nonmaleficence, beneficence, and justice.[26] Under the first, they include autonomy, informed consent, refusal of treatment, and suicide. Some include truth-telling, privacy, confidentiality, and other principles here. Some consider autonomy the highest of all principles.[27] Under the second, they include nonmaleficence, the principle of double effect, euthanasia, means of treatment, and proxy decision makers. *Primum non nocere*, "above all, do no harm," is one of the most widely quoted principles. It is often easier to agree on no harm than on positive benefit. Some philosophers argue that we have a duty not to harm, whereas doing good is above and beyond duty—supererogation. The role of health care providers, however, often requires positive acts of beneficence. Both the ICN and ANA codes of ethics require doing good as well as avoiding harm. Conflict between autonomy and beneficence/nonmaleficence is one of the main controversies in bioethics.[28]

Beauchamp and Childress' third category, beneficence, includes beneficence, cost-benefit (see utilitarianism, earlier) and paternalism, and justice includes the various concepts of justice, allocation of resources, and fairness. In addition, however, Beauchamp and Childress include a chapter on professional/patient relationships that includes veracity, confidentiality and privacy, faithfulness, and conflicts between contracts and roles. It is of some interest that veracity or truthfulness is virtually absent from health care codes.[29]

A final chapter covers ideals, virtues and character, and conscientious actions noted earlier as part of moral judgment. Their general headings, then, might be considered ultimates to the subheading "intermediate answers" to the philosophical "Why?" The general headings themselves, however, may be intermediate to yet higher metaethical principles.

Divine Command

Baier has suggested a fourfold division of the deontologic approach to ethics that reflects the sources of the rules. The first of these is the Judeo-Christian tradition, to which one might add religious tradition in general.[30]

Religious tradition is sometimes called the "divine command theory of ethics." The religion of Islam means submission, and a Muslim is one who submits. So Jews or Christians following the dictates of their faith submit to the will of God, regardless of consequences. It was noted earlier, however, that Bishop Berkeley saw the will of God in terms of a rule utilitarianism. Perhaps it would be more accurate to say "regardless of the immediate consequences." Difficulties arise in all religions as in all philosophies, all sciences, all the disciplines, or all the ways of life when it comes to interpretation. The will of God is often said to be in the Bible or the Koran or the Vedas or the Laws of Manu or the Analects of Confucius, and so on. The Ten Commandments are a well-known example of divine rules. However, entire libraries are filled with commentaries on what these rules mean. The Jewish Talmud in one version is 63 volumes long. Scientific paucity functions here, too, for there have been a number of attempts to summarize it all, such as Rabbi Hillel's "Do not do unto others that which is hurtful to thyself. That is the whole of the Law. The rest is commentary." The Golden or Silver Rule is part of all the major religious traditions of the world. Following the will of God may not be so simple.

Kant

Baier's second category or paradigm of deontology is Immanuel Kant, for whom he suggests four subcategories. The first of these is Kant's belief that moral reasons override all other reasons for doing anything. This imperative to duty is called the "categorical (no exceptions) imperative."[31] It has been compared to the Golden Rule but is independent of any personal desires. Every rational being is unconditionally required to obey the universal laws that have their source in nature. These are discoverable through reason. This universal is reminiscent of utilitarianism, and, indeed, one way to understand universality is in terms of "What would happen if. . . ." "If I do this, and everyone else does this, what will be the result? If I do not do this, and everyone else refrains from doing this, what will be the result?"

But again, perhaps one needs to say the universal laws are to be obeyed regardless of immediate or particular consequences. This is Kant's second point (in Baier's outline). It is this principled view that keeps Kant in the deontological system of ethics rather than the utilitarian. Kant's theories can be compatible with monotheistic religion, for the universal laws to which we submit may be seen as the laws of God. Religionists would not all agree, however, on Kant's absolutism, since there are those who see the human will as working together with God (synergism).

Kant went on to insist that the will to which one submits is not that of another person but one's own. This third point leaves out religious authorities and could leave out God unless one wills to be in tune with the religious leader or with the divine love, as in Fletcher's act utilitarianism.

Baier's fourth emphasis in Kant's thought are today's ethical principles. Baier sees these as incompatible with the Judeo-Christian tradition. However, many in the latter tradition would argue that Kant's liberal values are the epitome of the faith. These values presumably represent the universal laws of nature. Theists in turn see these laws as the laws of God. These values include autonomy, freedom, dignity, self-respect, and respect for individual rights. Historically, one could note that in Kant's day these were not part of either religion or culture. They are more prominent today but frequently (most of the time?) are more honored in promise than in practice. Kant was clearly ahead of his time and ours.

It is out of these values, however, that we get one of the most widely disseminated concepts in bioethics. Human beings are an end in themselves and are never to be used as a means to some other or someone else's ends. Some see this as a later formulation of the categorical imperative. Like informed consent, which might be seen as derived from it, this concept was thoroughly violated by Nazi physicians in their so-called experiments. The Nuremberg trials of Nazi war criminals gave this dignity of human beings, this concept of self-determination, a powerful impulse that some (but not all) think puts limits on using human subjects in research, medical and otherwise. Others argue that Kant only meant that the individual should not be used exclusively for another's ends.

Munhall's objection to utilitarianism was listed earlier. In turn, she sees deontology as an ethical system that is compatible with the philosophy of nursing that focuses on the individual patient rather than statistical studies of groups of people.[32]

Intuitionism

Baier's third category is intuitionism, which some see as an entirely separate approach to ethics. He cites the Oxford Intuitionists, such as Harold A.

Prichard (1871–1947) and W. David Ross as deontologists who reject absolutism.[33] Consequences are considered, and the intuitionists may be utilitarians in this sense. Bernard Gert claims that the utilitarian intuitionists do not think that we intuit rules of conduct so much as we intuit consequences, sometimes to the point where it can be figured out mathematically, i.e., the utilitarian calculus of cost-benefit.[34] However, intuitionists consider the past as well as the future. The rightness or wrongness of an action is a matter of its intrinsic nature, that is, it is right or wrong in itself. The group name, however, comes from the idea that we intuit the right or wrong. We simply know it. A number, perhaps many, nurses and health care providers are included in this group.[35]

One response to the question, "Why study ethics?" is: "It is no big deal. We already know what is right and wrong." One can recognize the truth in this by considering again the Socratic method, which was concerned with the truth within or, more accurately, drawing or leading out that truth. "Education" comes from *eduo*, "to lead out." This is the guiding function of one form of philosophy noted earlier—asking questions rather than giving answers. This process, of course, is quite different from the sophomoritis "know it all" that is sometimes implied in the response "We already know. . . ." One might note several comparative kinds of study here. The naturalness of this is part of natural law. The concept relates to conscience, which modern thought suggests is not natural but part of our training.[36]

The work of Piaget, Kohlberg, and others suggests that moral development is indeed a part of human nature, though the content varies from one culture to another and among subcultures and even within such groups as nurses. What one intuits then might upon investigation turn out to be a natural moral development, what one has acquired from culture (consensus ethics) or childhood or the voice of the divine. All this is not to say that intuition is wrong but that it might be worth looking to see (ethics) if the inherited, acquired, or divine concept is adequate to the present situation.[37]

The point of this view is that the intuition did not come out of either thin air or genetic makeup. One might note further that Western culture has tended to look condescendingly upon women's intuition, while this emotional aspect has been regularly if not systematically trained out of males in favor of the rational or so-called objective approach. Newer studies have shown that objective science, including health care science, is not really so objective after all, and once again we might consider examining the values hidden behind nursing and other sciences. Having said that, it must also be said that in a crisis, a routine moment, or any other situation where there is no time for thoughtful reflection or no apparent need for it, most of us tend to respond out of our intuition, the vernacular "gut reaction."

Transactional Analysis (TA) is a theory of personality and therapy that has been tested transculturally. TA suggests that human beings have three ego states, colloquially called the Parent, the Adult, and the Child (capitalized to distinguish ego state from biology). The Parent is the Critical and the Nurturing part, which is so prominent in health care. When people are sick or hurt, they tend to be in the Child ego state, whereas caregivers tend to be in the Parent. The Adult is the machinelike, factual, data-processing, problem-solving part of the human personality that is in touch with reality. The Child is the emotional part in both its Free Child aspect, freely, naturally expressing the scared, sad, mad, glad aspects of life, and in its Adapted state, trying to do what will please the Parent in order to continue to receive attention and care. It is the Adapted Child that says, "Yes, Nurse" and then spits out the pill when the nurse leaves the room.

A third part of the Child is colloquially called the "Little Professor." This is where intuition comes in. It is not unusual for a chronological child to know what adult hang-ups prevent adults from seeing or knowing. The intuition, male or female, can be seen as a valuable, indeed a very important, aspect of human nature. The nearby emotionality may cloud the intuitional judgment, but paired with the Adult in touch with reality, the intuition can be checked out for accuracy. My gut tells me something is going on. My Adult can check out the reality. Likewise, the value system, a Parent function, can be combined with Adult reality to determine the adequacy or appropriateness of the values. All three ego states working together form the integrated Adult in touch with reality, in touch with realistic values, including moral or ethical values, in touch with the intuitions and the feelings of the child. If one asks (the Golden Rule) what kind of nurse would you want taking care of you or yours, one might very well answer, "One who knows what he or she is doing and who does it with sympathy (feeling) and the belief that the patient is worth the care." Intuition combined with reality and an understanding of values may be an optimal combination.[38]

Classical Contract Theory

Baier's fourth paradigm involves classical contract theory. The rules come from promises and contracts, especially the social contract, in other words, our mutual relationships. Earlier thinkers like Thomas Hobbes (1588–1697), John Locke, and Jean Jacques Rousseau focused on political contracts. Their thought is important background to the American and French Revolutions, the Declaration of Independence, and similar situations. Modern ethicists focus rather on principles, such as justice, cited earlier in the work of John Rawls. Justice was also cited for its utility, and there is a social utility or consequentialism involved. We are to live, without personal advantage (individual consequences), according to the values that are best for society. It may not be surprising that his values resemble those of Kant, though there is an emphasis on the just allocation of resources as maximizing the good of society. The right to health care discussed earlier is an example of the principle of justice. There are different ways to interpret justice, and some ask if health care is available to everyone, to those in need, to those who deserve it, or on some other basis?[39]

Rawls' theory, like all theory, has received both positive and negative critiques. Baier notes that this combination of teleology and principles "is considered by many moral philosophers in the United States and Great Britain to be the best now available." Another perspective is that Rawls' perspective is abstract and dehumanized. He thinks choices should be made through a "veil of ignorance" so that the same decision is made for everyone. Others suggest that human beings are all different. To be human, one needs to consider real human beings with an ethic of responsibility and care.[40]

Rawls himself insists that justice should favor the disadvantaged. If one really chose through a "veil of ignorance," this could not be done. Some consider the "veil of ignorance" so much nonsense. In health care, one might hesitate at receiving abstract care. Indeed, the system is already too dehumanized as it is. Still, justice or equity seems a desirable ethic. Women, for example, might be said to deserve treatment equal to males.

Just as utilitarianism can be divided into act and rule utilitarianism, so can deontology. Rule deontology is what has been described and is by far the most prominent and most widely accepted. The subdivision into monistic theory (one principle) and pluralistic theory (many principles) was noted earlier. Act deontology relies upon the individual who judges each situation in its uniqueness. There are no promises to fulfill—the only rule is individual judgment or discretion. This perspective does not have a strong appeal among ethicists today.[41] We note here again the sometimes vague lines separating the various theories or systems.

NATURAL LAW: DOES IS MEAN OUGHT?

The law of nature is an old concept often applied to moral law and ethics. Natural law has several different meanings. Aristotle recognized particular laws but thought there was also a universal law of nature that is higher than the particular. In Sophocles' *Antigone,* the heroine buried her brother though it was against the law of the land. Aristotle called her "just" because she acted according to the law of nature.[42]

The Jewish Pharisee Paul wrote in *Romans* 2:15, "When Gentiles who do not know the law [of Moses] are led by nature to do what the law commands, . . . they show that what the law requires is written in their hearts." Thomas Aquinas is said to have put Western Christian theology on an Aristotelian base. That included natural law. It also included the idea that when a manmade law contradicts a natural law, it is not really a law. This was more recently reiterated by Martin Luther King, Jr., in his 1965 "Letter from a Birmingham Jail." A second major idea included in natural law is that nature intended a specific purpose or end for everything.[43]

Natural law can be theistic or nontheistic. Those who believe in a creator God see nature as God's creation, and hence the laws of nature are the laws of God. Others might see nature rather than God as the ultimate.[44] In turn, the law of nature or natural law is interpreted as carrying moral requirements or as containing moral laws. The implication of Paul's statement and the basic theory is that all rational people know this law by intuition or by reason, without revelation from God. For creationists, God put the law into his creatures—wrote the law on the human heart (*Jeremiah* 31:31). Some such concept may be in the minds of health care providers who claim that everyone knows what is right and wrong.

Critics have pointed out a number of problems. One is the impersonal nature of natural law which seems to deny the dignity of the individual. A mechanistic law is not the love so central to the Judeo-Christian and other religious traditions. Further, the critics say, non-Western cultures do not reveal all the same moral laws.[45] Probably the greater problem was the work of David Hume and G.E. Moore on the naturalistic fallacy, that "is" means "ought," that values can be extracted from facts.[46]

An illustration of this problem is the high infant mortality rate in some parts of the world. There are places where it reaches 70 percent. This is the way it is. Is this the way it ought to be? Many say "No," though if one compares human beings to frogs, one can say that Mother Nature in her wisdom produces far more offspring than necessary in order that some might survive long enough to reproduce and keep the species going. In some cultures, a couple produce as many children as possible in order to have someone take care of them in their old age or in order to have a son who will live long enough to do them the proper honors at and after their death. This is the way it is. Is this the way it ought to be? Health care providers now have an enormous and highly sophisticated technology at their disposal. There "is" a great deal that can now be done in health and illness care. Because we can do it, should we? Some say "Yes," and others say "No." Because we have the nuclear power to destroy the world, should we use it? Most say "No," unless someone else does it first, when, of course, it may be too late.

While the naturalistic fallacy is generally assumed "solved," i.e., "is" does not mean "ought," there has been some reassessment of this concern in recent years. We now see, for example, that there is no such thing as value-free facts, and we might rather try to understand what the values are than to waste time denying the existence of the values. Phillipa Foote has suggested that morality has content that is influenced by facts. Wellman suggests that it is possible but implausible that the facts have nothing to do with bioethics. The question is the relationship.[47]

Rita J. Payton thinks bioethics is vital and dynamic rather than static. Morality is determined within the context of the action. She believes the fact–value distinction, the is–ought relationship, is not an absolute distinction. Greater knowledge and advances in technology increase our choices in health care, and ethical decisions mean making choices. Facts and values influence each other. "What was moral at one point in our history of understanding could now be immoral because of a change in our base of knowledge."[48] "Time maketh ancient good uncouth," as James Russell Lowell put it in his poem, "The Present Crisis." Similarly, what was once immoral may now be seen as moral.

To this reassessment of is–ought we might add three other dimensions of natural morality. D'Arcy notes that Darwinian evolution questioned the eternal unchanging aspects of natural law, whereas the concept of chance destroyed the purpose or the end of nature. But what evolutionary biology took away was given back in the rise of social Darwinism in the concept of evolutionary ethics, which tried to get moral rules from facts of nature. J.T. Hobhouse (1906) published four stages of moral evolution from taboos to principles of justice based on equal rights.[49] Society is evolving to a higher plane.[50]

On a biological scale, higher life has greater value for some. The some, of course, are humans, and it is not surprising that they see humans as the highest form of life and as having the highest value. Others, as noted earlier, suggest that animal life, and indeed all of life, has value and has rights. Carl Wellman suggests that the human rights affirmed in medical ethics are the traditional rights under a new name.[51]

To evolutionary ethics as a form of natural law one could add the resurgence of sociobiology. One example goes all the way down to the genetic level, postulating an altruistic gene and a selfish gene. M.L. Hoffman claims that empathic reactivity is a primary human mechanism. H.J. Eysenck considers variable conditionality as the key in moral motivation.[52]

This approach could be seen as a variant on the old nature–nurture controversy. Are we good or bad by nature (natural law) or by training (cultural ethics)? The argument goes back at least to the time of Socrates. In Plato's *Meno* we read, "Can you tell me, Socrates, whether virtue is acquired by teaching or by practice; if neither by teaching nor practice, then whether it comes to man by nature or in what other way?" Aristotle said we become good by doing good actions. There are those who think the question remains unanswered.

Our third dimension of natural law context is the work of Piaget, Kohlberg, and Rest in moral development, which we discuss in more detail in Chapter Three. The development is natural. Checked transculturally, it is a human phenomenon. However, the speed and the distance of this development are heavily influenced and perhaps determined by the environment. To them the nature–nurture question is answered, "Both." Common sense might agree.[53]

Natural law has had an enormous influence through the Roman Catholic Church and through naturalistic philosophers. Protestantism at least initially rejected natural law. The early Reformers did not think the human reason capable of moral thought. Original Sin from the fall of Adam and Eve in the Garden of Eden and man's rebellion against God have impaired the human reason. According to this view, only revelation from God gives moral guidance.[54]

This did not stop the interpretation of the Bible, even as natural law has been interpreted. One of the most influential interpretations has been the concept of an end purpose. Laws, of course, suggest a deontological approach. The end purpose suggests a utilitarian approach. In bioethics, natural law is a factor in debates over contraception, artificial insemination, abortion, organ transplants, euthanasia, test tube babies, surrogate mothers, and other issues. There has been a major resurgence of natural law in health care in recent years. This has ranged from an emphasis upon natural birth to the use of vitamins to such natural remedies as herbs and extracts.[55]

One example of the end purpose concept is that the sexual organs have reproduction as their only purpose, and anything that interferes with this end is unnatural and, hence, wrong. In recent times, sexuality has been seen by some or many as having other purposes. Love may be an end in itself, and/or the requirement "to be fruitful and multiply" applies to the species rather than to the individual. Commentators as early as Augustine and St. John Chrysostom suggested that humanity has accomplished the "fill the earth" part and its time to stop. Some have pushed the natural law end and noted all of health care, and not just artificial insemination, is "unnatural" and, by that standard, wrong. Joseph Fletcher has countered with the suggestion that if anything is "unnatural," it will not work.[56] The early promoters of contraception noted that cutting the fingernails or the hair and indeed all of civilization is "unnatural." On the other hand, natural law proponents have suggested that the law is species specific and the fact that dogs and cockroaches do not build hospitals or do transplants is irrelevant.

One of the major concerns remains the question of interpretation. On what basis does one decide what the end is and what is natural. Here we can note that the rhythm method of birth control is accepted in official Roman Catholic and other circles because it is natural. When Roman Catholic Dr. John Rock helped develop the pill, he hoped it would be seen as natural in its control of the menstrual cycle. More and more Roman Catholic moral theologians in recent years have suggested that sexual intercourse has as a secondary purpose, and perhaps even the primary purpose, the expression of love, and that it is not just a matter of reproduction. They note that even Aquinas allowed sexual intercourse to the infertile (during pregnancy, normal infertility, postmenopausal infertility). Very few accept Aquinas' dictum that rape and incest are lesser offenses than masturbation because the former put the seed where it belongs.[57]

MORAL THEOLOGY: RELIGION AS SOURCE AND REASON

The Greek word *theos* means "god," and technically, theology means the study of god. In practice, it has come to mean the study of religion. In the broad sense, religion does not necessarily involve a god or God. Southern or Theraveda Buddhism believes in a spiritual life but not God in the usual sense. Secular humanism has been recognized by the United States Supreme Court as a religion. Marxism and secularism are religions as much as the traditional religions; that is, they involve faith commitments with ultimate values (gods).

The belief systems of nontheistic religions may be far more elaborate than those of theistic ones. Others, however, prefer to call nontheistic traditions ideologies or worldviews rather than religions, thus restricting the scope of theological ethics.

A further restriction must also be noted. Each religion, such as Hinduism, or the many religious traditions of the world, can be studied for its theological ethics. A comparative religious ethics can, in turn, study a number of these ethics. Currently the United States alone has 900 different Christian groups and 600 non-Christian groups.[58] Nurses are finding this variety among health care providers and among patients. In the Western world, however, virtually all the theological ethics applied to health care has involved the two traditions of Judaism and Christianity. The latter is usually divided between two of its main branches, Roman Catholicism and Protestantism, though Eastern Orthodoxy and other Christianities are becoming more prominent today. There is an enormous diversity under the umbrella of theological ethics, though it is doubtful if the diversity is any greater than that under philosophical ethics or many other umbrellas. As with philosophical ethics and other umbrellas, the diversity can be grasped by grouping diversities into broad categories.

To this diversity, Frederick S. Carney adds yet another—the distinction between ordinary everyday religious morality, which involves a minimum of reflection, and the theoretical reflection, which is the essence of theological ethics. This is the distinction noted earlier of morals as the shoulds and oughts of life, whereas ethics asks "Why?" or for the reasons behind the shoulds. Frequently, though not always, moral theologians or theological ethicists are a part of a religious tradition, and, therefore, the ordinary morality may be their morality as well, even as they also try to step back from their involvement and objectively consider the ethical reasons.[59]

Since very few patients and health care providers are moral theologians, most of them are concerned with the everyday variety of religious morality. As the study of ethics expands among nurses, physicians, and others, this will change, as it should if the equation professional and ethical is correct. The current study of bioethics is heavily oriented to the philosophical rather than the theological, even in theological schools and in schools sponsored by religious groups. Presumably, the philosophical perspective is more acceptable as being more neutral among the diversities of religion and in the face of the growing secularism of society. Public opinion polls, however, suggest that most people (over 90 percent) still believe in God. It is said that in wartime there are no atheists in the foxholes. People often have a heightened sense of religion in the face of danger, death, or illness. This is true for nurses, too, who share a religious perspective.

Hospital chaplaincies have been developed to meet the spiritual needs of patients and staffs. Most of the first hospitals and many of today's hospitals were established by religious groups. The relationship of health care and religion has been a close one over the centuries, a closeness that has been obscured by the increasing numbers of hospitals established by or financed by government and other private groups. The relationship of religion and ethics is also obscured, in part by the current emphasis on secular philosophy and in part by those who reject religion (i.e., traditional religion) but continue to believe in and practice morality or ethics. At one time, and for some people still, religion and morality were absolutely interrelated—no religion, no morality.[60] Others see religion as one source of morality. There may be many sources.[61]

To deny the relationship or to pretend there is none is to be out of touch with reality, or it is to push one's own faith as the only reality. Religion has a moral dimension. At the same time, morality can be considered independently of religion. We suggest that the distinction can and perhaps must be made but without absolutizing or exaggerating it. Most philosophers of the past were also men of religion. Western Christianity interwove its faith with Plato's philosophy and others. In the Middle Ages, Plato was replaced by Aristotle. On the other hand, it is hardly surprising to find a secular philosopher claiming that in morality we must do the loving thing, as in the Jewish and Christian commandments to love our neighbor. Historically, philosophy and religion have influenced each other, even as today health care influences bioethics, and bioethics influences health care. In some religious traditions, such as Buddhism, there is no real distinction between philosophy and religion. So there are times when there is no distinction between health care and ethics. Good health care is ethical care, and vice versa.

With some exceptions, a basic theistic belief is that God has a purpose for the world and for people. His will must be obeyed. Some claim this as an end in itself (metaethics as an ultimate), whereas others claim rewards for obedience and punishment for disobedience (utilitarians and Freudians—the pleasure-pain principle). Thus God is a source of morality and a motivation for moral behavior. Jesus of Nazareth said, "Not all who say, 'Lord, Lord' will enter the Kingdom of Heaven but he that doeth the will of my heavenly Father." This will is known through the natural law discussed earlier. It is known by revelation: God speaks to people like Moses or he speaks through an angel like Gabriel, who revealed God's wisdom to Muhammad the Prophet. The Bible, the Koran, and other religious scriptures are interpreted as being or showing the will of God. The New Testament quotes Jesus as saying, "Care for the sick." Health care providers can think of themselves as carrying out the will of God. As noted earlier, some theists claim God created the human mind and expects us to use our reason—on our own as mature adults or working with God to accomplish his will or in interpretation.

Like the nurses' codes of ethics, however, natural law, the Bible, or other forms of the will of God do not always reveal the details of what to do in each and every situation. We interpret the ethical principles and apply them to the moral action. The Golden Rule is an example of the problem this presents. On the one hand, it has been said that the Golden Rule is a minimalist ethic. "Do unto others as you would have others do unto you" is only the beginning, the bedrock of ethics in a complex world that requires a far more sophisticated ethic. On the other hand, it has been pointed out that most people do not come up to the

Golden Rule's standard. They are ethical troglodytes, underground cave dwellers who have not come up to the bedrock minimum. This point of view says people normally try to hurt back those who hurt them or, failing that, take out their negative feelings on others, frequently innocent others. The health care hierarchy is one example. The top dog does in the underdog, who happens to be top dog to some other underdog. Physicians over nurses, or nurses over other nurses, or RNs over LPNs. While some health care providers are busily perverting the Rule by doing unto others as others have done unto them,[62] the patients are deprived of the best or more adequate health care. However, even following the Golden Rule does not always answer detailed questions in today's health care dilemmas. Interpretation is the order of the day, whether principles are religious or secular. Theoretically, however, religion provides a strong motivation for carrying out that interpretation and carrying it into practice. The ancient Hebrew prophets thundered, "Thus sayeth the Lord . . ." and their thunder continues to reverbrate unto this day.

CONCLUSION

As pointed out earlier, people may function with some combination of the various approaches to morality or ethics. As in natural law, people may be concerned with both ends and means, both the consequences and the rules or principles. Payton has called this "bioethical pluralism."[63] Nurses, like people in general, are frequently if not normally using some aspects of several systems of ethics. To relate to this bioethical pluralism, Payton offers a pluralistic decision-making model, discussed in Chapter Five.

There is value in knowing the various systems. Health care should be concerned with the whole person. On the other hand, if the health problem is liver trouble, one had best know something about the liver if one is going to provide care. Particular knowledge is essential even as we are concerned with the whole picture. That picture contains various perspectives and diverse standards. Individual nurses and health care providers might stand more fully in one tradition rather than another even as they try to understand and appreciate the other(s).

NOTES

1. Quoted by Johanson, D., and Edey, M. *Lucy.* New York: Warner Books, 1981, p. 136
2. Quoted by Johanson and Edey. *Lucy,* p. 220.
3. Beauchamp, T.L. "Ethical theory and bioethics." In Beauchamp, T.L., and Walters, L. (eds.) *Contemporary Issues in Bioethics,* 2nd ed. Belmont, CA: Wadsworth, 1982, pp. 1-43. Lawrence Kohlberg says philosophical theory is the analysis of and justification of normative ideas like truth and justice. "Moral stages and the aims of

education." In *Essays on Moral Development. Volume One. The Philosophy of Moral Development.* San Francisco: Harper & Row, 1981, pp. 1-5. Israela E. Aron claims that one problem with the formalist approach lies in the preoccupation with justification in contrast to the decision making itself. She sees Kohlberg as claiming that the decision making is equivalent to justification. She claims they are different. In real life, we need help making decisions rather than justifying ourselves after the fact. Cf. "Moral education: the formalist tradition and the deweyan alternative." In Munsey, B. (ed.) *Moral Development, Moral Education, and Kohlberg.* Birmingham, AL: Religious Education Press, 1980, pp. 401-426, especially p. 407.

4. James Rest describes moral judgments as reflecting basic natural growth. This is, of course, in line with his perspectives on moral development. He specifically notes that moral judgment is not a matter of mastering tricks of argument. "A psychologist looks at the teaching of ethics." *Hastings Center Report* (HCR) 12 (1):29-36, February 1982. In contrast, a recent university workshop in bioethics turned out to be an exercise in arguing. The best arguer is the most ethical according to the leaders.

5. Broad, C.D. *Five Types of Ethical Theory.* New York: Harcourt, Brace, 1930. Cited by Baier, K. "Ethics. III. Deontological theories." *Encyclopedia of Bioethics* (EB) 1:413-417, 1978. Sidgwick, H. *The Methods of Ethics,* 7th ed. London: Macmillan, 1907. Intuitionism may be considered under deontology, while the other two are part of the teleological (consequences) approach to ethics.

6. Bentham, J. *Deontology.* London: Longman, 1934. Cited by Baier, "Ethics. III. Deontological theories," p. 413, and Emmet, D. *The Moral Prism.* London: Macmillan, 1979, p. 5. Beauchamp, "Ethical theory and bioethics," p. 19.

7. We are speaking here primarily of Western tradition, but a similar statement could be made about other traditions. Ashby, P.H. *Modern Trends in Hinduism.* New York: Columbia University Press, 1974, p. 13. In Hinduism, there is no major or clear distinction between philosophy and theology.

8. Baier, K. "Teleological theories." EB 1:417-421, 1978.

9. This of course is common in all walks of life and not just the health care system. A federal official has said, "What is good for General Motors is good for America."

10. Brandt, R. B. "The real and alleged problems of utilitarianism." HCR 13 (2):37-43, April 1983.

11. Munhall, P.L. "Ethical juxtapositions in nursing research." *Topics in Clinical Nursing* 4 (1):66-73, April 1982. She suggests the same for science with its concern for statistics and a narrow focus that ignores the whole picture or the whole person. The deontological approach can consider the individual.

12. Brandt, "The real and alleged problems of utilitarianism," p. 38.

13. Bentham, J. *Introduction to the Principles of Morals and Legislation.* New York: Humanities Press, 1970 (original 1780). Mill, J.S. *On Liberty.* London: J.W. Parker, 1859. Kohlberg notes that in the study of moral development he has directed, "we have never encountered a live human being who made moral judgments in terms of principle in this sense" of maximization of happiness. Kohlberg's stages of development begin with Stage 1, and Stage 6 is the highest. Bentham was Stage 2. Kohlberg, L. "From is to ought." In Kohlberg, L. *Essays on Moral Development.* San Francisco: Harper & Row, 1981, pp. 101-189, especially p. 174. Henry D. Aiken noted also that to a person faced with a real problem, principles of utility and Kant's categorical imperative are "empty." But Mill was aware of this. For particular actions, we turn to what Mill called secondary rules rather than to the greatest happiness principle. It is again our distinction between the moral oughts and the

ethical reason why. Aiken, H.D. "Levels of moral discourse." In his *Reason and Conduct*. New York: Knopf, 1962, pp. 65-87.

14. Freud, S. *Civilization and Its Discontents*. New York: Norton, 1962. This of course is not as good as it might sound, for some people find pleasure in pain. The sadist and some types of neurotics seek pain, perhaps because it helps relieve their guilt. Freud himself does not seem to have maximized pleasure and avoided pain. A distinction between what we preach and practice is, of course, common to many humans. In Kohlberg's stages, Freud was Stage 2. The greater problem, however, is that human beings are not the simplistic machines Freud envisioned, a problem that has become prominent in health care, where a patient has become an interesting liver rather than a human being.

15. Hare, R.M. "Ethics. VI. Utilitarianism." EB 1:424-429, 1978.

16. Beauchamp, "Ethical theory and bioethics," pp. 13-19. Brandt, "Real and alleged problems of utilitarianism," p. 40. Hare, "Ethics. VI. Utilitarianism," pp. 424-429.

17. Pernick, M.S. "The calculus of suffering in nineteenth century surgery." HCR 13 (2):26-36, April 1983.

18. Fletcher, J. *Situation Ethics*. Philadelphia: Westminster, 1966. Fletcher, J. "Ethics V. Situation ethics." EB 1:421-424, 1978.

19. Quoted by Fletcher, "Ethics. V. Situation ethics," p. 422, from Mill, J.S. *Essential Works*. NY: Bantam Books, 1961, p. 204.

20. Brandt, "Real and alleged problems of utilitarianism," p. 38.

21. Kohlberg, L. "Education for justice," pp. 29-48, and, "From is to ought," pp. 174-175, in *Essays*.

22. Kohlberg sees this totality of principle as chilling as the utilitarian Bolshevik letting ten million Kulaks starve for the greater happiness of the unborn greater number. "Stages of moral development as a basis for moral education." In Munsey B. (ed.) *Moral Development, Moral Education, and Kohlberg*. Birmingham, AL: Religious Education Press, 1980, p. 61. Beauchamp, "Ethical theory and bioethics," p. 25.

23. Beauchamp, "Ethical theory and bioethics," p. 25.

24. Rawls, J. *A Theory of Justice*. Cambridge: Harvard University Press, 1971. So too Kohlberg, "Education for justice," p. 39. Beauchamp, "Ethical theory and bioethics," p. 20.

25. Beauchamp, "Ethical theory and bioethics," p. 20. Kieffer, G.H. *Bioethics*. Reading, MA: Addison-Wesley, 1979, pp. 61-62.

26. Beauchamp, T.L., and Childress, J.F. *Principles of Biomedical Ethics*. 2nd ed. New York: Oxford, 1983. The two middle terms are two sides of the same coin. The Hippocratic oath urges doing good or at least no harm. Beauchamp, "Ethical theory and bioethics," p. 26, lists three main principles in this way.

27. Beauchamp, "Ethical theory and bioethics," pp. 27-28.

28. Beauchamp, "Ethical theory and bioethics," pp. 28-30.

29. Bok. S. *Lying: Moral Choice in Public and Private Life*. New York: Pantheon, 1978, pp. 221-222.

30. Baier, "Ethics. III. Deontological theories," pp. 413-417.

31. Kohlberg notes here as with utilitarian maximization of happiness, "we have never encountered a live human being who made moral judgments in terms of principle in this sense." "From is to ought," p. 174. Aiken, however, notes that Kant was not offering a rule of conduct but a formula for testing rules of conduct. "Levels of moral discourse," p. 82.

32. Munhall, "Ethical juxtapositions in nursing research," p. 69.

33. Baier, "Ethics. III. Deontological theories," p. 415. Prichard, H.A. *Moral Obligations.* Oxford: Clarendon Press, 1968. Ross, W.D. *The Foundations of Ethics.* Oxford: Clarendon, 1939.

34. Gert, B. "Ethics. VIII. Objectivism in ethics." EB 1:438-442, 1978. He cites Sidgwick, *The Methods of Ethics,* and Moore, G.E. *Principia Ethica.* Cambridge: University Press, 1903.

35. R.M. Hare claims "a great number of present-day philosophers (perhaps the majority) become crypto-intuitionists when they descend to discuss practical issues. . . . This often amounts to a mere appeal to received opinion . . . and thus comes close to . . . ethical relativism or subjectivism." The dividing line between this subjectivism "and intuitionism is often invisibly narrow." Hare, R.M. "Ethics. X. Nondescriptivism." EB 1:447-450, 1978. Beauchamp, "Ethical theory and bioethics," p. 25, suggests that pluralistic deontologists slip into intuitionism when asked which duty has priority. We are supposed to simply "know." Marvin W. Berkowitz cites data that suggest that nurses are intuitionists. "The role of discussion in ethics training." *Topics in Clinical Nursing* 4 (1):33-48, April 1982. Sigmund Freud considered himself a very moral man who subscribed to the "very excellent maxim of" F.Th. Vischer, "What is moral is self-evident." He did not understand why he and his six children were thoroughly decent human beings while other people are brutal and untrustworthy. One might consider him, among other things, an intuitionist. Cf. Jones, E. *The Life and Work of Sigmund Freud,* ed. and abridged by Trilling, L., and Marcus, S. New York: Basic Books, 1961.

36. "Conscience is a conditioned avoidance reaction to certain classes of acts or situation." Eysenck, H.J. *Handbook of Abnormal Psychology.* New York: Basic Books, 1961. Others see conscience as Parent values instilled in our Parent ego state. Still others see conscience as given by God in our creation, as the voice of God within— "the still small voice"—or as a nonsupernatural part of human nature.

37. By way of humorous aside, one can note an old story that is also relevant to the question of interpretation noted earlier. A young man went to theological school, but it soon turned out he had little aptitude for study. He explained to his professor, however, that he had been cultivating his father's cornfield when he looked up into the sky and saw written in the clouds the letters "P.C." He believed that God had spoken to him to "Preach Christ." The professor suggested that actually the letters meant "Plow Corn."

38. Berne, E. *Transactional Analysis in Psychotherapy.* New York: Grove Press, 1961. Harris, T.A. *I'm OK—You're OK.* Old Tappan, NJ: Revel, 1967.

39. Rawls, *A Theory of Justice.* Beauchamp, "Ethical theory and bioethics," p. 31.

40. Gilligan, C. "Moral development." In Chickering, A.W., et al. (eds.) *The Modern American College.* San Francisco: Jossey-Bass, 1981, pp. 139-157.

41. Beauchamp, "Ethical theory and bioethics," p. 20.

42. Aristotle. *Rhetoric,* BC. 330 B.C. Quoted by D'Arcy, E. "Natural law." EB 3:1131-1137, 1978.

43. The King letter is quoted by Kohlberg, p. 319, in "Moral development, religious thinking, and the question of a seventh stage." In *Essays,* pp. 311-372. Aquinas, T. *Summa Theologiae* (1266–1274), I-II, 94,6, and 95,2, Suppl. 65,1. Quoted by D'Arcy, "Natural law," p. 1132.

44. Note that some people believe in God but not necessarily a creator. Some writers

distinguish between the natural and supernatural, whereas others claim that if one ascribes a kind of personified purpose to nature, it becomes supernatural or at least metaphysical. Mother Nature or Mother Earth has been equated to the ancient female fertility goddess(es) without the formal worship of ancient times. Kohlberg cites numerous examples of natural law proponents who are theistic (mono-, pan-, poly-) and nontheistic. "Moral development, religious thinking, and the question of a seventh stage." D'Arcy, "Natural law," p. 1134.

45. Kohlberg lists several dozen universal norms, such as life, property, truth, affiliation, sex, authority, law, contract, civil rights, religion, conscience, punishment. There are 29 basic moral categories, concepts, or principles used in all cultures. "From is to ought," pp. 117, 126. D'Arcy points out the rather widespread human preferences, such as life over death, pleasure before pain, health to illness, knowledge to ignorance, love and affection to hatred or being ignored.

46. D'Arcy, "Natural law," pp. 1135-1137. Hume, *A Treatise of Human Nature.* ed by Selby-Bigge, L.A. London: Oxford University Press, 1888 (original 1739). Moore, *Principia Ethica.* Wellman, C. "Ethics. IX. Naturalism." EB 1:442-447, 1978. Hudson, W.D. (ed.) *The Is-Ought Question.* London: Macmillan, 1969. Kohlberg relates the naturalistic fallacy to the psychologist's fallacy: What is good for organizing psychological data is good for purposes of education. He cites B.F. Skinner as an example of this. To Kohlberg, because psychologists can go "beyond freedom and dignity," it does not follow that they should. Indeed, freedom and dignity are the starting point for psychology and education. We could add, "and for health care and research." Kohlberg, "Preface," pp. ix-xxv, "From is to ought," pp. 101-189, and "Moral development, religious thinking, and the question of a seventh stage," pp. 317-321, 345-347, in *Essays.* Skinner, B.F. *Beyond Freedom and Dignity.* New York: Knopf, 1971.

47. D'Arcy, "Natural law," p. 1135. Foote, P. (ed.) *Theories of Ethics.* London: Oxford, 1967, pp. 83-100. Wellman, "Ethics. IX. Naturalism," p. 445. Veatch, R.M. *Value-Freedom in Science and Technology;* Missoula: Scholars Press, 1976.

48. Payton, R.J. "Pluralistic ethical decision making." *Clinical and Scientific Sessions 1979.* Kansas City: American Nurses' Association, 1979, pp. 9-16.

49. Hoff, C. "Immoral and moral uses of animals." *New England Journal of Medicine* 302 (2):115-118, January 10, 1980. Reprinted in Beauchamp and Walters, *Contemporary Issues in Bioethics,* 2nd ed., pp. 576-580. D'Arcy, "Natural law," p. 1134. Savodnik, I. "Biology, philosophy of." EB 1:127-132, 1978. Huxley, J.S. *Evolutionary Ethics.* London: Oxford University Press, 1943. Flew, A.G.N. *Evolutionary Ethics.* NY: St. Martin's, 1967. Canfield, J.V. (ed.) *Purpose in Nature.* Englewood Cliffs, NJ: Prentice-Hall, 1966. Hobhouse, J.T. *Morals in Evolution: A Study in Comparative Ethics.* New York: Holt, 1923 (original 1906). Quoted by Kohlberg as paralleling his stage theory, "From is to ought," p. 128.

50. This optimistic view was shattered by the Nazi horrors. Germany was one of the most advanced of modern nations: advanced technologically—barbarian ethics. The advanced technology was put in the service of the latter.

51. See the earlier discussion on Singer, Hindu thought, environmental ethics, human rights and natural rights, and the Declaration of Independence (Chapter One, p. 6-7, 15-16). Wellman, "Ethics. IX. Naturalism," p. 447.

52. Savodnik, "Biology, philosophy of," p. 132. Wilson, E.O. *Sociobiology: The New Synthesis.* Cambridge: Harvard University Press, 1975. Rest, "A psychologist looks

at the teaching of ethics," p. 33. Hoffman, M.L. "Empathy, role-taking, guilt, and the development of altruistic motives." In Lickona, T. (ed.) *Moral Development and Behavior.* New York: Holt, Rinehart, and Winston, 1976. Eysenck, H.J. "The biology of morality." In Lickona, pp.108-123.

53. Kohlberg considers some forms of the naturalistic fallacy genuine fallacies and others not. In opposition to the blanket condemnation, he thinks the oughts and the is's should be aware of one another. "From is to ought," p. 105. For transcultural data, see pp. 115 and 123; p. 128, Kohlberg's parallel with Hobhouse, was cited earlier.

54. John Calvin thought that all persons of sound reason could know the second half of the Ten Commandments, but Jews and Christians know the divine will. Wallwork, E. "Morality, religion, and Kohlberg's theory." In Munsey, p. 286.

55. Grisez, G.G. *Contraception and the Natural Law.* Milwaukee; Bruce, 1964. Noonan, J.T., Jr. "Contraception." EB 1:204-216, 1978. Pope Paul VI. "Humanae vitae (human life)," *Catholic Mind* pp. 35-48, September 1968. *Homeopathic Medical Index;* Philadelphia: Boericke & Tafel. (no date). Boericke, G.W. *Homeopathy.* Philadelphia: Boericke & Tafel (no date). Holmes, H.B., Hoskins, B.B., and Gross, M. *Birth Control and Controlling Birth: Women-Centered Perspectives* and *The Custom-Made Child?: Women-Centered Perspectives.* Clifton, NJ: Humana Press, 1981. Illich, I. *Medical Nemesis: The Expropriation of Health.* New York: Pantheon Books, 1976.

56. Fletcher, *Situation Ethics.*

57. Aquinas. *Evil* 15.2. "Whether all sex acts are mortal sins." *Questions Disputatae,* 7th ed., 5 vols. Rome: Marietti, 1942.

58. Carney, F.S. "Ethics. VII. Theological ethics." EB 1:429-437, 1978.

59. Wallwork, "Morality, religion, and Kohlberg's theory." In Munsey, pp. 269-297. Wallwork says, "most Americans believe morality to be dependent on religion, in some sense."

60. Kohlberg has found a consistent, universal moral development common to people without regard to religion. It is similar for Buddhists, Hindus, Muslims, Christians, Jews, and others. It is common to atheists, secularists, humanists, communists, and so on. Thus, he sees moral development as independent of religion. At the same time, he recognizes the traditional relationship. He offers an interesting suggestion. Religion answers the metaethical questions, such as "Why be moral?" or "Why live?" Cf. his "Moral and religious education and the public schools: a developmental view," pp. 294-305, and "Moral stages and problems beyond justice," pp. 307-310, and "Moral development, religious thinking, and the question of a seventh stage," p. 321, all in *Essays.*

61. Kohlberg sees this as Stage 2 in moral development, typical of 10-year-olds. He sees the Golden Rule as the heart of ethics, which is recognized as the core of morality in almost every culture and religion. It is the principle behind Rawls' theory of justice. However, it can be interpreted selfishly—do unto others so that they will be nice to you (Stage 2)—or in the sense of reciprocal vengeance just noted or in the sense of mutual affectionate concern (Stage 3), whereas the sense of justice is Stage 6, and in the sense of completely altruistic love, it is beyond justice—a speculated Stage 7. "From is to ought," pp. 149-150; "Introduction," p. xxxii; "Moral stages and the idea of justice," p. 100.

62. Payton, "Pluralistic ethical decision making," p. 11.

63. Payton, "Pluralistic ethical decision making," pp. 12-13.

*Healthy activity demands a goal, a sense of something worth doing . . .
mental illness begins when [people] are deprived of something to look for-
ward to.*

—Colin Wilson

Truth is within ourselves.

—Robert Browning

There comes a time in life when a person must rise above principle.[1]

CHAPTER 3

Moral Development: How People Grow

Some people, like Freud and the intuitionists, think that morality just "is." Others, as indicated earlier, think that morality comes from God or from nature. It is something given to human beings. This is often seen as a complete package handed down by God or by Mother Nature. To be moral comes with human nature. It is a matter of being human. A variant on this is that morality is something that grows or develops. It is a given part of human nature but it is not fully complete from the beginning of life. The newborn infant does not have a complete concept of morality or ethics in its neonate brain—or in its emotional perspective if one thinks morality is a matter of feeling. The basic structure is there, perhaps like the ability to learn to talk, but it develops out of interaction with the environment, again not unlike the development of language. In this view, morality is natural, and we have here a variant of the natural law approach to morality and ethics. The reasoning process of ethics, the eternal "Why?" of the philosopher, is a major element in the natural moral development. To be sure, this is the way we are, but the focus in this third position is on what we have become, or better, what we are becoming.

JEAN PIAGET'S INTELLECTUAL AND MORAL STAGES

Piaget (1896–1980) was a malacologist (malacology is the study of mollusks) who turned to psychology. He became interested in how children think and realized that it is different from adult thinking. This was not a matter of information or of understanding the information but a different perspective. As he studied the way children think, he came to believe that there is not just one different perspective. There are four of them. His theory of cognitive development has been tested and retested. It continues to be debated, denied, refined. Many accept his theory and many do not.[2]

We begin, according to Piaget, with the sensory-motor period, in which infants are learning to coordinate muscles and movements and developing the senses in relation to themselves and their world. The pre-concrete period follows with the concrete period after that. In the third period we think in terms of concrete, specific things. If someone mentions table, we think of a table. In the formal operations period, we think in the abstract. Table becomes an abstract symbol for tables. About half of the adult American population reaches this stage of reasoning.[3]

This intellectual or cognitive development is transcultural. Piagetians have worked in many countries and climates to show it is not simply a Western phenomenon. The sequence is invariable, but the chronological development is not, nor is there any inevitability that people will reach the formal operations period, though most seem to reach the concrete. There is at least an element of bias here, however, for we do view the formal or abstract in different ways. Just a few years before his death Piaget admitted that mechanics and others are not necessarily plateaued at the concrete operations period, but he suggested that the teen-age developmental period may be vocationally specific. The mechanic may have a different way of thinking in the abstract than the lawyer, who may think differently than the logician.

The invariability of the sequence and the transcultural nature of the intellectual development suggest that the development is innate. It is the natural development of human nature, as noted under natural law earlier. The differences in chronological development could be a difference in individual development, but subsequent studies show that this is, in fact, influenced by the environment, including one's work, as just noted for mechanics and lawyers. Piaget rejected both the total genetic determinism of Gesell (nature) and the total environmentalism (nurture) of Skinner, Pavlov, and other behaviorists. "Piaget's position is neither hereditarian nor environmentalistic; it is both. It is interactionist."[4]

Piaget worked with a theory of equilibrium. The child assimilates the environment to itself or accommodates itself to the environment. The small child sees a ball. It wants the ball. That "want" puts it out of equilibrium with its environment. The ball is lying on a sweater and the child pulls the sweater toward itself and gets the ball. The child changes the environment. On the other hand, the child might crawl over to the ball. The child changes itself to get the ball. Getting the ball reestablishes the equilibrium. In real life, equilibrium does not last long, so life is a continuous give and take, a continuous assimilation–accommodation. The "enriched" environment is a familiar concept in child and animal psychology. By enriching the environment, the child is stimulated to respond and develop accordingly.

While Piaget's primary focus was on cognitive development, he did not deny the affective or feeling dimension of life. He considered the two inseparable for "all interaction with the environment involves both a structuring and evaluation. . . . we cannot reason, even in pure mathematics, without experiencing certain feelings, and conversely, no affect can exist without a minimum of understanding or of discrimination."[5]

Within 10 years, Piaget had applied his procedures to the question of how people develop morally. He found that children develop through a two-stage process. Assimilation and accommodation continue. Children up to 12 or 13 were given two similar stories. One story focused on the quantity of wrong, while the other represented intent. The child's choice represents an objective idea of responsibility or a subjective one. Young children were concerned with external authority in determining what should be done, while older children (from 10 to 11) were more concerned for cooperative, mutually beneficial arrangements. Another way of putting it is to speak of constraint and cooperation. The first stage is heteronomous, concerned with rules. The second is autonomous, concerned with mutual respect.[6]

LAWRENCE KOHLBERG'S SIX STAGES

Piaget's work inspired Lawrence Kohlberg to further investigation. Kohlberg's doctoral dissertation (1958) was an attempt to check Piaget's data, to extend them through adolescence, and to extend the data of stage growth to the concept of taking the role of others in the social environment. Kohlberg expanded Piaget's construct to six stages instead of two. The six can be considered as concepts of how people cooperate with one another. The six are grouped under three broader rubrics borrowed from John Dewey: the preconventional level of moral development, the conventional, and the postconventional or principled level. Judgments of right and wrong are assumed to be external to the judger in the first two levels. There are two stages in each level.[7]

The Preconventional Level

Children up to about 10 are usually in the preconventional level.[8] It is preconventional because societal norms are not the real basis for what children do. They tend to be responsive to cultural rules and the labels of good and bad, but these are interpreted in terms of the physical consequences of punishment and reward or the physical power of the rulers who pronounce the rules and labels. The similarity to Freud's pleasure/pain syndrome is obvious. Selfish or self-centered would be the common language here. This is the level of hedonism. While children may be "well behaved," Kohlberg notes the capacity for cruelty that is sometimes tragic, as in William Golding's *Lord of the Flies*,[9] and sometimes comic, as in the character of Lucy in Charles Schultz's "Peanuts" cartoon strip.

The preconventional Stage 1 is the "punishment and obedience" stage. The child obeys without regard to the human meaning or value of the consequences but only in response to the punishment or reward. Literal obedience to rules and authority and not doing physical harm is what is right. "Obey for obedience's sake." The point of view is egocentric without considering the interests of others. It would perhaps be more accurate to say that the individual in this stage simply does not recognize or know that the interest of others is any different than one's own. Earlier we cited examples of politicians ("I am the Law") and businessmen ("What's good for my company is what is good for America.") with this kind of thinking. It is not uncommon in health care. It appears in the fairly widespread view that we had best do what we are told or we will lose our jobs. It is not unusual that the "best interests of the patient" just happen to be the best interests of the practitioner.

The preconventional Stage 2 is technically called the instrumental relativist orientation, noted earlier in comments on relativism in ethics. Expedient or prudent might be more common words for this stage. This is the time of "You scratch my back and I'll scratch yours." It is well known in politics, business, and health care. Right action here is a concern with what satisfies one's own needs. "It's my life isn't it?" is one perspective of this stage.[10] The needs of others might incidently be satisfied but that is not the point at this stage. Fairness, reciprocity, and equality are here, but they are interpreted in terms of "What's in it for No. 1?"[11] The rules are followed in terms of one's own interests, not out of loyalty, gratitude, justice, or consideration for others. Fair deals are all right in terms of concrete exchange because we live in a world where we do our thing and let others do theirs. The perspective is individualistic but with the awareness that others have their self-interests that need to be integrated to maintain goodwill in order to get what one wants.

Mahon and Fowler have called persons in this stage pragmatically opportunistic. The one philosophy that originated on American soil is the philosophy of pragmatism. They note that reciprocity also includes retaliation, a tit-for-tat relationship, an eye-for-an-eye perspective well known in the nursing hierarchy. This perspective was noted earlier as the perversion of the Golden Rule: "Do unto others as others have done unto you," rather than the original, "Do unto others as you would have others do unto you."[12] Note that self-seeking gain or revenge is often covert, hidden under other reasons. Mahon and Fowler offer as an example the nurse with a demanding older patient. The orders read, "Seconal h.s., repeat x 1." The nurse has given the first seconal and now she gives the second, though it is equivocally necessary, because the patient keeps leaning on the light and the nurse is tired of answering all those little complaints, and "Besides, a second one was ordered p.r.n."[13]

We could add here the concept of patient advocate. Nurses who promote this role out of genuine concern for the patient would be Stage 5. Some nurses promote the role of patient advocate to give nursing an issue in its rise to power. Using others as a means to one's own ends is Stage 2.[14]

The Conventional Level

The conventional level is called conformist—maintaining the expectations and the rules of family, group, society, or nation. This is seen as valuable in its own right, and the process is not simply one of maintenance but active support and justification. Note that, like Kant, this is without regard to consequences of pain or pleasure, at least the immediate and obvious consequences. The loyalty here is not simply an expression of one's own feelings. It is demanded of others. This is the realm of consensus ethics. Mahon and Fowler describe it as maintaining the status quo, well known in health care research grant proposals, which must maintain what is acceptable.[15] Do not rock the boat is an axiom for many times and places. As the societal nature of the conventional level indicates, most of the people in society are at this level. Here again there are two stages.

Stage 3 is one of interpersonal concordance—the "good girl, nice boy" perspective. The individual attempts to conform to the stereotype of what the majority call "natural" behavior. The right means being good, being concerned for others, being loyal and keeping trust with others, following the rules and expectations. Mutual relationships are important. Love, affection, friendship, shared feelings, agreements, and expectations take precedent over self-interest. The Golden Rule means putting oneself in the other person's shoes. For the first time, the motive behind one's behavior is important if not crucial. "She means well" may be used to excuse or overlook nonconformity. Sincerity is an important standard. The social pressure to conform is commonly known as peer pressure.[16]

Stage 4 is the law and order stage, which Kohlberg calls the society maintaining orientation. This is the stage of civic responsibility. The right is doing one's duty, respecting authority, obeying the law, maintaining the social order—society, the group, the institution—as an end in itself. One lives by one's defined role, and individual concerns are considered in terms of one's place in the system. The reason for doing what is right is a matter of conscience or the consequences in terms of "What if everyone did it?" This can be seen as the universal question asked by Kant as noted earlier, though "consequences" gives this a utilitarian ring, as does the belief that social chaos will result if we do not obey the law. Kohlberg's key issue of justice is seen as equivalent to law and order. If you have the latter, you have justice according to people at Stage 4.

Mahon and Fowler suggest the difference between Stages 3 and 4 is the conformity to persons in Stage 3 and the conformity to rules in Stage 4. Violations are punished by official sanctions, such as jail or exclusion, rather than personal physical punishment. They cite the old familiar "Because the doctor told us to" (or not to) as an example of Stage 3 among nurses. Do your job and fulfill your expected role.

One might note the interesting theory that societies themselves develop. What is conventional in a given society might be seen as part of its moral development. Societies have approved slavery, for example, and later came to see it as wrong. Many societies have considered abortion wrong, whereas today many societies accept abortion, at least in some circumstances. This approach assumes society is something other than the sum of its individual members. Robert Sinsheimer wrote about "controlled evolution" and said "perhaps a society, like an organism, must follow a developmental program . . . in orderly sequence."[17]

The Intermediate Level

Among the more recent refinements of the stage theory is a transitional level sometimes called Stage 4½. About 20 percent of college youth show these characteristics. It is postconventional but not yet principled. Choices are personal and subjective. "If it feels good, do it." Conscience, duty, the morally right are seen as arbitrary, relative. Persons in this transition may think of themselves as beyond or above law and morality. They may raise the metaethical question, "Why be moral?" The person sees himself as standing outside of society as an individual making his own decisions, though he may be merely an adolescent rebelling against parental authority. The regression to Stage 2 was noted earlier in what, in some cases, is colloquially called "sophomoritis," with apologies to the rest of the sophomores. Kohlberg notes that people usually move on to Stage 5, but they may become fixated here.[18]

The Postconventional Level

The postconventional level is also called the principled level. Kohlberg estimated that about 25 percent of society reaches this level. Here is a major movement to autonomous moral principles with validity apart from people or groups and apart from the individual's identification with the group. Moral decisions come from rights, values, or principles that all (or potentially all) can agree on to create a society concerned with fairness and beneficence. This level is postconventional because it is in a sense beyond society or convention, but it differs from Stage 4½ in this concern for moral principles on a universal scale. This is the official philosophical level in moral development. Here is the philosophical "Why?" The earlier stages simply recognize existing social groupings and institutions. Davis and Aroskar suggest that a full-fledged discussion in moral philosophy develops when we go beyond the stage of obedience to traditional rules and combine these rules with ethical reasoning. Kohlberg's key issue of justice at the postconventional level has the purpose of law and order as the maintenance of justice rather than the other way around. Governments are formed to protect the equal rights of citizens rather than citizens being formed to protect the government. Another way of putting it is to see Stage 4 as maintaining laws already existing while Stage 5 is concerned with creating laws to ensure justice.[19]

The first of the two stages is Stage 5. Kohlberg estimated that about 15 to 20 percent of society reach this stage.[20] It is called the social contract stage. General individual rights and standards have been critically examined and agreed upon by the whole society, perhaps by a formal vote. The group reaches for consensus even as it acknowledges individual differences. Law is acknowledged, but instead of a frozen or fixated rule, it is a rational consideration open to change for social utility. The motive for obeying the law is the social contract for the good of all. The contracts include legal contracts and promises, but the concept goes back to the social contract envisioned by Hobbes, Rawls, and others as noted earlier. This stage acknowledges pluralism—people hold a variety of views that should be upheld in the interest of impartiality. But note that this view itself is not relative or impartial. "The greatest good for the greatest number" is part of this perspective as the basis for the rational calculation of utility, i.e., this is a utilitarian ethic, but it is a rule utilitarianism. The rules are not an end in themselves but serve the higher purpose of the social contract. People are not made for the rules. The rules are made for the people. This is the stage of the founders of the United States. It is the official morality of the United States government, with its concern for nonrelative rights, such as life, liberty, and the pursuit of happiness. As such, Kohlberg notes, it is not unexpected that the Supreme Court decisions sometimes make some people very angry. Most people are in Stages 3 and 4, whereas the Court is more often at Stage 5, responsive to "evolving standards of justice" rather than to common opinion. Kohlberg cites the Gallup Poll in which Americans looked at the Bill of Rights without a label to tell what it was. A majority voted against it.[21]

Mahon and Fowler note that it is not until people reach Stage 5 that they realize there are mutually exclusive, competing rights and values in moral conflicts. Their example is a nurse caught between the two loyalties to the physician and to the family. The physician has not told the family the patient's diagnosis. The family asks the nurse what the problem is. The hospital guidelines say she should support the physician. The nurse gives an evasive answer that supports the physician's ability but later in talking with other staff, she decides to talk with the physician to see if it can all be straightened out. The family has a right to know the patient's status and it is not right to string them along. The hospital and physician claim is the stronger in this nurse's opinion, but the deception is wrong, so she decides to try to change the physician's mind.

Stage 6 is the deontological universal ethical principle stage. The stage is presented in terms of Socrates or the early Plato in which virtue is one and the one is justice. In more pluralistic terms, this stage is concerned with self-chosen ethical principles that have logical comprehensiveness, universality, and consistency. These ethical principles are abstract, e.g., Kant's categorical imperative, rather than specific concrete rules. These principles are universal principles of justice, reciprocity, and equality of human rights, and respect for the dignity of human beings as individuals. By universal, Kohlberg means principles that all humanity should follow. Particular laws or rules are valid when they rest on or are derived from these universals. Aristotle's view of Antigone's action in burying her dead brother so his spirit could rest in peace is such an example. It was against the law to bury him because he was judged a traitor. She obeyed a higher law which Aristotle called "natural law." The universal laws are not just opinions or merely values that someone has recognized. The respect for persons comes from the principle that people are ends in themselves and not a means to someone else's purpose, as with Kant's later formulation of his categorical imperative.

Mahon and Fowler note that because of the universality of the principles, a person's life at this stage has a greater consistency or congruence than is found in earlier stages. There is a breadth and depth and coherence in a person's philosophy of life. There is duty here, but it exists within the realm of these principles rather than being defined legalistically. Their example is a nurse researcher who finds an ideal patient. However, he is comatose. His family and physician give their consent, but in the end, the nurse decides not to use this patient for research. The patient cannot give his own consent and to use him would make him a means, an instrument, rather than an end in himself. The researcher would violate his dignity as a person.

In 1978, Kohlberg wrote "Justice and reversibility: the claim to adequacy of a highest moral stage," discussing Rawls' theory of justice as justification for his Stage 6. In 1979 and 1980, Kohlberg published essays denying there is such a thing as Stage 6.[22] Perhaps it would be more accurate to say it was a restatement of the liberal social contract, and it merged with Stage 5. Earlier, however, he wrote about an American male named Jim who reached Stage 6 at the age of 24, and one named Richard who reached Stage 6 at age 25.[23] Even in the latest article cited, he talks about Socrates and Martin Luther King, Jr., as Stage 6 and Aristotle and John Dewey as Stage 5 personalities.[24] The "Preface" of *Essays*, published in 1981, lists six stages. Stage 6 is "universal ethical principles."[25] The introduction to Part One of this 1981 volume says the descriptions of the six moral stages "are outdated where they refer to young adolescent data as examples of Stage 6, which later work (reported in Volume Two) treats as a rare stage of adult development." In "Development as the aim of education: the Dewey view" (1972), he and Mayer suggested that about 5 percent of the American population reach this stage. The confusion comes from an appeal to the sacredness of human life, which is already present in Stage 4, and other changes in scoring methods. In "Moral stages and the idea of justice," he says longitudinal studies confirm Stage 5. Stage 6 examples are historical figures or people with extensive philosophical training. Perhaps Stage 6 is less an attained psychological reality than a direction. We might rather call it an ideal.[26]

Variables in Moral Development

There are several things to consider about Kohlberg's theory. He describes moral development, so we have the descriptive ethics mentioned in Chapter One. But Kohlberg also prescribes—he wants people to develop to the higher stages rather than become fixated or frozen at a lower stage. While nurses have developed to lower stages, his concern, and that of many if not most ethicists of nursing, would be for nurses to "come up higher." It would hardly be surprising to find most nurses at the conventional level where most people in general are. The ANA Codes, however, like the US Constitution, are postconventional. Thus at least some and perhaps many nurses have developed to the postconventional level. The prescriptive ethicist would urge all nurses to grow and develop their moral understanding and actions to this level.

One might note further that the same bottom line might be reached at several stages. That is, the final decision might be the same in different stages. Henry David Thoreau (1817–1862) did not pay taxes as a matter of principle (Stage 6). Millions fail to pay today for their own advantage (Stage 2). It is the reasoning that is different. It is the moral agent concept noted earlier, though the decision maker is in dialogue with the situation and the other person(s) involved. As persons develop to higher stages, they are also in touch with the ethical principles and the moral rules that apply to the situation and the persons involved.

One might note too that the move to or through stages is not normally precipitous, with a person in one stage one day and the next one the next day. It took about 5 years on the average for one of Kohlberg's subjects to move one stage.[27] On the average, only about half of a subject's responses to Kohlberg's questions are in the subject's predominant stage. There is already some reasoning in the next stage. While we move on through stages, we do not lose the earlier stages, though Kohlberg claims earlier stage reasoning gets used less and less as one moves to later stages. While most people are in the conventional Stages 3 and 4, some reach Stage 5. Earlier, Kohlberg claimed a relatively small percentage of people reach Stage 6.

Education is directly related to the development from one stage to another. High school graduates with no more formal education tend to stay at the stage they were in at the time of graduation. Tested later in life, they tend to be where they were at graduation. The same is true for college graduates and so on.[28] Kohlberg's experimental work with education shows that persons understand the next higher stage from their predominant one, but they do not understand two stages higher. If the student or the class is at a Stage 3 level of development, one might try to help them move to a Stage 4 level. The primary method is discussion through a Socratic style dialogue. Mahon and Fowler note that in their group discussions in ethics rounds, there were people in all stages, so the next level was usually present in the discussion.[29]

Kohlberg himself at one time thought he would help people move to Stage 6. By 1976, he had retrenched to helping people achieve a Stage 5 level of moral development, the level of the US Constitution. More recently, he retrenched to Stage 4, the stage of civic responsibility. He thought this could be acquired by participatory democracy, which is Stage 5. He recognizes the Catch 22 in this—one cannot participate in Stage 5 democracy if one has not arrived at Stage 5, and most people have not developed to that stage. His own theory says that students and teachers are at Stage 3 or lower and do not know what he is talking about at Stage 5. Research shows that most high school students reason at Stages 2 and 3 with some Stage 4 thought in older students, whereas most teachers probably reason at Stages 3 and 4, i.e., where most of the population reasons. Only those who have already reached Stage 3 will understand Kohlberg's call upward to Stage 4. It is of interest to note that bioethicists are working with reasoning at Stages 5 and 6. If they are talking to people more than one stage earlier, they are speaking into the wind.[30]

Moral Development as Universal

Kohlberg has studied two different educational ideologies that he finds common in our culture and that he finds objectionable. One is cultural transmission, which he sees as indoctrination with the values held by those in power. It is external to the person and imposed. It is most well known today through the work of B.F. Skinner. Kohlberg notes this as the system in use in the Soviet Union. It is widespread in the American educational system. It represents the cultural relativism preached by many social scientists who look at externals rather than meaning. It is the ideology of health care education. The other ideology is the romantic, which sees the child as developing from within. This is the position of A.S. Neill, famous for his school, Summerhill, though Neill's real ethic is also relativism.

The progressivism of John Dewey and the moral development of Piaget and Kohlberg are interactional, a concept that goes back to Socrates and Plato and, more recently, Hegel. There is an interaction between the within and the without, between the internal development and the external stimulus of society. In Piaget's terms, differences between the internal and external cause disequilibrium. The interaction is to restore equilibrium. Kohlberg is concerned with a democratic ideal that considers both the rights of the child and the rights of others, in terms of justice.[31]

While many or most social scientists consider morality relative—each society has its own rules—Kohlberg presents moral development as universal. The social scientists have looked at externals without asking what the various customs mean. He cites many universals, such as society itself, government, law, family, morality itself. By universal here, he means common to all humanity, common to different classes and different cultures. Within the concept of morality, he lists several dozen universal aspects of morality, such as rights, duties, love, respect, justice, life, property, authority, truth. The epitome of all is justice, the concept of that rare Stage 6. The stages themselves are common to all humanity, though people as a whole may not get beyond the conventional level of Stages 3 and 4. What remains relative in his system are personal values and opinions.[32] Alternately, one might turn to our earlier distinction of morals and ethics. The shoulds and should nots vary within and between cultures, but there are many ethical principles that are universal.

Earlier we noted the contrast between the rational and the emotional or feeling perspective on morality. Kohlberg rejects completely the theory that morality is merely an irrational emotionality. He claims that the cognitive and affective go hand in hand. They are different aspects of, or perspectives on, the same mental events. All mental events have both aspects. This is in contrast to the question about whether states of cognition or states of affect are more influential in moral judgment. They are both there. Fear, pleasure, honor and dishonor, community respect and self-respect, and religion are but a few of the motivations for the various stages. However, while on the one hand he notes that the presence of strong emotion in no way reduces the cognitive component of moral judgment, he also notes that the sentiment that enters into moral judgment is a development of structures with a heavy cognitive component. It would seem that his own emphasis is on the cognitive, following Piaget's understanding of cognitive or intellectual development.

This cognitive development is necessary for moral judgment (see the correlation of moral judgment and formal education). For example, Stage 5 presupposes Piaget's formal operations stage of intellectual development. However, cognitive development is not sufficient for moral behavior. Low cognitive development means a lower stage of moral judgment, but high cognitive development does not automatically mean high moral development. Something more is needed for this, and something more is needed for moral behavior. Moral dilemmas or challenge (disequilibrium) is needed for moral development. Moral behavior needs something more, such as will power. Kohlberg, however, does not see moral judgment and moral behavior as being very far apart.[33]

In one sense, moral development is natural. It happens. At the same time, it is clear in Kohlberg's system of thought that later stages are better. The higher stages are of higher value. He notes that if it were simply a matter of later being better, death would be best of all, a conclusion with which he disagrees. The morality of Martin Luther King, Jr., was more adequate than the morality of most people who survive longer. In contrast to the relativist who sees one moral standard as good as another, whether it is murder or cheating in school, Kohlberg suggests that some moral standards are better. There are some reasons for morality that are better than other reasons. Higher stages are supposedly better because here one can do a more thorough job of analyzing, tracing out implications, and integrating the variety of considerations. The higher stage can solve problems the lower stage cannot handle. It is conceptually more adequate. Stage 5 can answer the problems of Stage 4½, whereas Stage 6 can handle problems of Stage 5. The higher includes the lower or earlier stage. In Piagetian terms, the later stages are more equilibrated. People prefer the stage above their own over lower stages because the higher stage represents better equilibrium. The progression from self-centered to society centered to universal principles points to reasons that move from self to society to humanity. The end concept is one of universal principles(s) that are not dependent on any individual or individual society. The progression is reminiscent of evolutionary ethics. Kohlberg does call his system a natural law system. The progression through stages is natural and it is universal and in that sense a law of nature.[34]

Earlier we noted Kohlberg's observations that teaching conventionally virtuous behavior is easy. He is talking about Stages 3 and 4. In the face of rising crime rates, vandalism, juvenile delinquency, the well-known so-called breakdown in public morality, there are those who would be only too happy to have an increase in civic responsibility. That generalization extends into health care. The horror stories of what happens to people caught in the meatgrinder of the health care system are also well known. Kohlberg's concern, however, is a concern with the good, which he understands to be justice. That one virtue contains and epitomizes all the rest. It is the principle that characterizes his stages. His aim is one of understanding that translates into behavior. It is based on the interaction between the internal and external. For him, the cultural transmission approach is inadequate. It is cultural rather than universal. It is imposed rather than drawn out. If the imposition is withdrawn, the original behavior returns. To put it another way, when the external controls of Stages 1 through 4 are removed, there is no reason for moral behavior. If there is no punishment or reward (Stage 1), no advantage to the self to consider others (Stage 2), no personal authority (Stage 3), no external law (Stage 4), there is no reason for moral behavior. People may be externally conformist but internally nothing. The question "Why be moral?" comes out of the Stage 4½ person who has recognized this and responds, "There is no reason to be moral." When that person moves beyond to Stage 5 and 6, the question answers itself from within the person's own growth. The focus in Kohlberg's work is on competencies that transfer to later life and to moral standards of the moral agent himself or herself—Stages 5 and 6. He presents his system as more adequate for a democratic society, which in turn is part of humanity.[35]

One can agree or disagree with Kohlberg's democratic perspective. The proposed concepts of teamwork in health care and the making of team decisions in ethics may be a reflection of the concepts of democracy. At least they are contrasted to a head nurse, physician, hospital administrator, or a philosopher handing down what should be done. A team, of course, could do the same without regard to the patient or the family or the principle of justice, so merely having a team does not ensure justice. One could also note the value of someone knowing the good and being committed to the good. Parents who raise children merely through the imposition of external control should not be surprised if other things happen when the parents are not there to impose that external control. Therefore, one question for the health care system is what happens to the patients and the personnel in that impersonal system when no one is around, i.e., when the light of publicity is turned off? When politicians (including health care providers) control the system on a cost/benefit basis, one might wonder if the cost or the benefit gets the greater emphasis.

There is a greater concern for nursing, however, with Kohlberg's system. The entire field of bioethics has developed in response, at least in part, to the rapid advances in technology and health care procedures. There are those who would suggest that the advance has been so rapid, it has outrun conventional ethics. Kohlberg's concern with the postconventional levels of social contract and justice might offer the higher principles necessary to deal with the new day in which health care now finds itself. Among other things, it may be a way of approaching and utilizing the ANA *Code for Nurses*—not as a set of rules to be blindly followed but as guidelines to be considered in relation to the Interpretive Statements, and the whole to be considered in terms of justice.[36]

JAMES REST'S DEFINING OF THE ISSUES

Kohlberg and Piaget used the subject interview method for acquiring data on moral development. Piaget and his co-workers used two stories with a single variable to focus the subject's attention on one aspect of moral judgment. Kohlberg and associates used a series of stories with an open-ended discussion. The judging of the responses is a bit complicated. In one form of his scoring system, there are 184 scoring categories, though the potential for the six stages is 12,240. Needless to say, the judging requires considerable training. James R. Rest has devised an objective test that can be scored by almost anyone.

The "Defining the Issues Test" (DIT) involves six stories with 12 statements for a total of 72 items. The person doing this questionnaire is asked to rate each statement for its importance in making a decision about the choices in the story. Then the person is asked to rank the top four choices in terms of importance. The statements represent a spectrum in moral development. The way in which the person chooses the most important issues gives a stage score. This information can be used in several ways. The most common usage is to add together the scores from Stages 5 and 6 to give a P score. "P" stands for "principled morality," since these two stages are the universal principle stages in Kohlberg's moral development theory. The two together represent the post-conventional level III.[37]

Thousands of people have filled out the DIT. A large number of experiments have been done with it. People can fake a lower score but cannot fake a higher score. As noted earlier, one understands the stage above one's own but not two stages. That understanding may be vague, whereas the understanding of the lower stages is quite clear. Several items within the questionnaire are nonsense statements with high sounding words to see if a person is responding seriously. While most people are inconsistent to some degree, too much inconsistency (checked by two different measures) also suggests a lack of serious response. These response sheets can be eliminated from data analysis. The reliability of the DIT is now thoroughly established, though there are several cautions. It cannot be used with people younger than 13 to 14 years of age, Piaget's top level. Kohlberg's interview can be used with children as young as 7 to 8. The DIT systematically puts people at developmentally more advanced stages than Kohlberg's interviews. A number of studies show the two "are not equivalent."[38]

Kohlberg uses a Moral Maturity Quotient in addition to his view of the individual's predominant stage. This MMQ involves a weighted average. A person who is 100 percent Stage 2 would have an MMQ of 200. One who is 90 percent Stage 2 and 10 percent Stage 3 would have an MMQ of 210. The MMQ recognizes that people are on a continuum rather than simply in a given stage. The DIT utilizes the P score to yield a figure that shows where one is on the continuum. Studies suggest the average junior high student has a P score or P-Index of 21.9 (note that these are group averages), whereas the average college student has a P-Index of 42.3, staff nurses 46.4, practicing physicians 49.5, moral philosophy and political science doctoral students 65.2.

These figures reflect development over time with additional formal education. Gender is not a factor. The liberal bias noted earlier is reflected in the scores of conservative seminary students, 22.5, and liberal seminary students, 59.8. While Rest claims that these P-Index scores are not equivalent to Kohlberg's stages, he also notes that "the average college student has a hard time distinguishing principled thinking (philosophical thinking at Stages 5 and 6) from gibberish—their P scores on the DIT are substantially less than 50 percent." Since other research suggests we can understand the next stage above our own but not two stages above our own, it would follow that the 42.3 DIT P score represents Stages 3 and 4. The average for adults in general is 40.0, and one would assume they are at the conventional level in moral reasoning. He also uses the figure of 50.0 as the break between conventional and postconventional moral reasoning, i.e., Stage 4 is below 50 and Stage 5 is above 50.[39]

One aspect of Rest's research is of particular interest. It is well known in learning theory that one can recognize things easier than recall them. Many people cannot give directions to a destination but have no difficulty finding it themselves. Children can recognize a triangle or other figure before they can draw one. In moral judgment studies, Rest notes the different types of tasks required in different tests of moral judgment. Kohlberg's free response interview is a recall type of task that involves a spontaneous reaction in which the subject has to interpret the problem and construct or produce a solution. This requires identifying relevant features, imagining consequences for various courses of action, and integrating all this into an answer. A comprehension type task involves understanding. The story and solution are structured for the person who may be able to follow the ideas involved at a higher level than in the spontaneous production task with Kohlberg. A preference test is even easier. The developmental hierarchy of moral judgment may be reflected in these levels of acquisition. Rest suggests we have here the acquisition of new ideas at different points of consolidation. A person may prefer, understand, and use concepts in that order. They may have a preference for a stage in moral development before they understand it. They may understand it before they use it.

There are several implications of these observations. One is that it is ambiguous to say that a person has or does not have a particular concept or that a person is at a certain stage in moral development. We are looking at a spectrum within stage development rather than a clean-cut jump from one stage to another, as noted earlier. Another point is that a person's readiness for change may be indicated by the advance of preference or comprehension beyond the level of use. Alternately, a person may be fixated or frozen at a given stage if his comprehension and preference levels are the same as the level of production.[40]

There are two further aspects of Rest's work that are of significance for our study. One is the positive correlation between artificial or theoretical study and real life situations. The other is the positive correlation between the moral judgment shown on the DIT and what actually happens in terms of behavior or use in real life. As noted earlier, there is a major relationship here, though it is not the whole story. Kohlberg notes a second level of activity involving ego strength or will power. Rest notes at least seven different variables, such as ego, the situation, and other values that intervene between the moral judgment and the action or the actual practice. Shakte Ketefian has used the DIT with her instrument, Judgments About Nursing Decisions (JAND). She found a positive correlation between moral reasoning and nurses' perception of realistic moral behavior. Using the ANA *Code for Nurses* as the standard for behavior, she found a positive correlation between the process of moral reasoning and moral behavior. She found that professionally prepared nurses had higher levels of moral reasoning and behavior than nursing technicians. However, she notes Leah L. Curtin's point that ethical behavior "presupposes an agent who is free of undue coercion in decision making," and the nurse is not always a free agent. She also cites Andrew Jameton's study of the "nurse in the middle" problem where the nurse often has many responsibilities and little authority.[41]

Helen Holmes, in two volumes subtitled *Women-Centered Perspectives*, notes that in health care, there is a difference between the publicly stated moral code and the real values, which range from sheer financial or material greed to power and status to technologic tinkering as opposed to the natural.[42]

The latter is illustrated by the physician who considered it no big deal to deliver a baby vaginally but pridefully noted that it took real skill to deliver one by cesarean section. In health care, if the machinery does not work right, more machinery is brought in, rather than stopping to consider whether the machinery is unnecessary. Some have gone so far as to say that most of the illness today is iatrogenic in violation of the often stated "do good/do no harm" principle carried over since the days of Hippocrates. Thus one could give high stage responses to the stories in Kohlberg or Rest research while practicing by a different set of values that do not necessarily appear in the DIT. However, the earlier implication could still hold that a person's readiness to change may be indicated by the level of understanding, which has outstripped the level of use.

Rest notes the development of new tests concerned with specific professions. Patricia Crisham has developed a Nursing Dilemma Test (NDT) that is comparable to the DIT.[43] She interviewed 130 staff nurses to find 21 recurrent nursing moral dilemmas in real life. These were "grouped according to four underlying ethical issues: deciding the right to know and determining the right to decide, defining and promoting quality of life, maintaining professional and institutional standards, and distributing nursing resources." Six recurrent dilemmas were chosen for study: "newborn with anomalies," "forcing medication" (psychiatric nursing), "adult's request to die," "new nurse orientation" (care of children), "medication error," "terminally ill adult" (right to know in surgical nursing). The final format of the NDT included "three tasks for each of the six dilemmas: deciding what the nurse should do, ranking the moral and practical considerations in order of importance, and indicating the degree of previous involvement with a similar dilemma."[44]

Crisham's NP score parallels the P score on the DIT. The top score for her NP is 66. She also measured practical considerations (PC) across the six dilemmas. The highest score here was 36. The familiarity (F) score reflected previous involvement in ethical dilemmas. An F scale of 6 through 17 represented familiarity, whereas 18 through 30 shows unfamiliarity. Crisham tested 225 people with the NDT, which included the five categories. There were 57 staff nurses, 85 baccalaureate nurses, 10 master's degree nurses, 36 college junior prenurses, and 37 graduate level nonnurses. Of the 152 nurses, 146 (96 percent) indicated familiarity with the dilemmas. PC showed no consistent pattern across groups, but the NP scores reflected education, as does the P score in the DIT. The associate degree group had the lowest NP score while the master's degree nurses had the highest. Those who were familiar with the dilemmas scored higher than those who were not.

Between moral judgment and moral action for nurses, Crisham found that staff nurses listed a number of things. These included distractions and pressures in the hospital setting, such as hospital policy, time constraints, loyalties to the nursing profession, the hospital, and the patient, confusion about the most effective way to use professional knowledge, lack of clarity on responsibilities and authority, contrary expectations from patients, administrators, and peers. She adds such factors as paternalism, discrimination, exploitation, the culture shock experienced by new nurses in the real work situation when they find nursing protocol is not operational in the hospital setting.[45]

PRO AND CON

We have touched on some of the favorable and unfavorable views of moral development and Kohlberg's theories. Here we might note the caution that because of the continuum of development postulated by Rest and acknowledged by Kohlberg, individuals should not be labeled with any particular stage designation. Among other things, it might fixate or freeze them there, giving the thought that that is where they are. The self-fulfilling prophecy may block further development. We might better work with groups or classes to see where the group is on the average and try to arrange discussion a stage higher. In a thoroughly mixed group, as noted by Mahon and Fowler, one might plan for discussion at several stages to help individuals develop.

Kohlberg is emphatic that claims for the superiority of the higher stages are not a system for grading the moral worth of individual people.[46]

A second caution is that the work of Rest, Kohlberg, and others is work in progress. Earlier, we noted Kohlberg's own wondering if Stage 6 is really his imagination. One can expect changes in the developmental theories as time goes on. Others, however, see this as a matter of refinement rather than wholesale changes. Virtually every aspect of Kohlberg's theories has been negatively critiqued.[47]

One major challenge comes from Carol Gilligan. She does not deny the development theory as such. She points to the repeated exclusion of women from critical theory building in psychology (Freud), including moral development (Piaget and Kohlberg). When males become the standard for development, women who differ become deviants. Thus the theorists talk about "human" development when they mean male development. For a complete human developmental picture, Gilligan insists that women be included. One can agree on any of several bases, including Kohlberg's own theories of justice.[48]

The distinction, however, may be one of interpretation as much as it is the theory of moral development. She cites studies in which males were considered Stage 4 and possibly 5 and females were considered Stage 3. What is not clear is whether she made that judgment or Kohlberg made it. She has worked with Kohlberg and presumably knows something of the categories Kohlberg interviewers need to know to decide in which stage a person is at the time of the interview. From our perspective, the females who were concerned with what was best for all were not Stage 3 but Stage 5. For this stage, Kohlberg says one is not to violate the rights of others even where these are not legally protected. Their concern that everyone be helped (as in health care?) sounds like the justice of Stage 6.[49]

Gilligan cites psychological studies suggesting that males must separate from the mother and individuate, whereas females identify with the mother and their concern is continuity and relationship. Their concern is not so much a hierarchy of values as it is a web or network of relationships. This causes them to see both sides of an issue when males often see only one side. She cites studies showing that males are conditioned to achievement and success no matter who is hurt. If they are lucky, they come in their later years to an appreciation of relationship. The unlucky ones die with their sterile dreams. The supreme principle is nonviolence rather than justice. Women do not want anyone to be hurt, says Gilligan. Women are primarily concerned with an ethic of care and responsibility. Gilligan sees the ethic of care and responsibility as sharply different from an ethic of rights out of which Kohlberg derives his theory of justice.

Gilligan's description is false on several counts. Her reference to responsibility and rights represents a higher stage development. Women, like men, have hurt men, women, and children. There are irresponsible women as there are irresponsible men. Gilligan herself cites a number of women who had illegitimate children. This is not usually seen as being responsible. In the past, illegitimacy has been harmful to children. Whether it still harms children is debated, but it at least raises a question about Gilligan's women not hurting or wanting to hurt others. In a similar contrast to Gilligan's observations, one should note that there are women who are concerned for justice. Many women have been involved in the civil rights movement, and rights are a major part of the feminist movement. To suggest that women are not concerned with rights appears to deny both these realities.

We noted earlier our belief that rights and responsibilities are two sides of the same coin. They should not be separated. Our society, however, is far more concerned with rights and frequently prefers to ignore responsibilities (Stage 2). Kohlberg says duties are reciprocal to rights—no duties, no rights; no rights, no duties. Right implies the duty to recognize that right in others. The rights of others limit the rights of the individual. One who violates the rights of others can make no claim to have his or her rights respected. Davis and Aroskar see duties and rights as correlative. One invariably includes the other.[50]

Gilligan's comment on networking is especially interesting. The old-boy network is a well-known phenomenon in male continuity and relationships. Piaget's study of moral development distinguished older children from younger. The older ones were concerned with cooperative, mutually beneficial arrangements. If he worked only with males, as Gilligan claims, this male concern for cooperation removes half of her dichotomy.

Moreover, Kohlberg in writing "Moral stages and the idea of justice" notes that the different stages represent successive modes of taking the role of others in social situations. This reversibility is the Golden Rule—put yourself in the other person's place. This is a matter of relationship. The norm of relationship between people is justice—we add "should be" justice. But Kohlberg goes farther. He speculates on a Stage 7, in which people like Andrea Simpson and Marcus Aurelius feel a sense of connectedness to life, nature, God, ultimate reality. This connectedness is what Gilligan claims women have naturally. Kohlberg's description of stages describes women. The male–female dichotomy does not hold, which does not, of course, preclude a biased interviewer from assigning a lower stage to a female interviewee. However, this is a problem with the interviewer, not Kohlberg's system. One might site also Gilligan's own earlier work on college students whose moral development moved to an ethic of responsibility and care, the official ethic of nursing. She cites no distinction between women and male students.[51]

Similarly, the nonviolent approach to problem solving—so no one gets hurt if possible—is reflective of Stage 6. The primary examples of nonviolence, Mahatma Gandhi and Martin Luther King, Jr., are two of Kohlberg's examples of Stage 6 persons. Gilligan quotes Erik H. Erickson's observation on Gandhi's psychological violence to those close to him. Her women go Gandhi one better in being concerned about all violence.[52]

Kohlberg notes the hierarchy of stages in that a higher stage is more inclusive. The higher includes the lower stages. In a study of women making a decision on abortion, Gilligan noted that their first concern was with survival. They would do what they had to do to keep their husband or boyfriend taking care of them (Stage 2). Through the forced decision-making process, they passed through several stages, including two transitions, and a year later, reflected their understanding of morality as a concern for everyone, including themselves. Survival was still a part of their basic concern, but it was included in a Stage 5 morality reflecting the social contract that recognizes different values but also the commonalities, including the concern for others. When these women added that everyone needed consideration, they were reasoning at a Stage 6 level.[53]

The role taking for moral judgment is related to sympathy[54] for others, says Kohlberg. He goes on to talk about different kinds of justice, such as the absolute and the commutative, which includes mercy. This is the way Gilligan describes the women whom she interviewed. To the degree that women try to live up to the expectations of society, they are at the conventional level of Stages 3 and 4, but when they move beyond, as many of her interviewees did, they are postconventional. Gilligan cautions that we need longitudinal studies of women. Her current research on adolescent and preadolescent girls may add to our understanding.[55] At the same time, we note that her longitudinal study of 1 year of women in crisis showed a jump from Stage 2 to Stage 5. As noted earlier, Kohlberg's subjects (all male) took 5 years or more to move one stage.[56]

It is of course possible that Gilligan's pregnant women were at Stage 5 before they became pregnant but regressed under stress. Alternately, this could be development stimulated by stress, a form of Piaget's disequilibrium. Faced with decisions that could not be assimilated within their then current moral stage of understanding, they accommodated by moving to a higher stage. The reader will recall that "higher" is more inclusive and not necessarily superior in the sense of arrogance. The stress of the abortion decision was a form of the Socratic dialogue. To have the child would do harm. To abort would do harm. Each woman presumably chose what she thought would do the least harm.

Lois Erickson's study cited earlier included 23 high school students. The final number 1 year later was 21. These women took a course in women in literature that involved field work. They interviewed females from grammar school to maturity using Piagetian and Kohlberg type questions and measures. They found that women tend to plateau at Stage 3. Kohlberg ascribes this to the limitations of our society; fewer women then men enter the professions, and so on. This point seems born out by S. Weisbrodt's studies, which show that professional women and women in graduate school attain the higher stages with the same frequency as men of similar background. The 21 students themselves advanced one third of a stage. It was a stable advance that held through the follow-up study.[57]

Of course, as the above makes clear, not all women are at Stage 5 in their moral development. It is worthy of note, however, that the women who were at Stage 2, using men for their survival, separated from the men in moving to Stage 5. Alternately, they moved on from their parents, including their fathers. One of Gilligan's subjects had already separated from her parents at the age of 12. It appears that separation is not limited to males. One might note further that the studies she cites of men maturing to find intimacy and relationship were studies of the elite. She cautions that her studies are not complete and much remains to be done. Perhaps the studies of males she cites are not complete. We need studies of the average male or the poor. One can note, at least anecdotally, that there are males who appreciate their families and other relationships and do not wait until old age for that appreciation. There are males who are both caring and responsible, as there are women who are neither. For both psychological development and moral development, one might say that much remains to be studied for both women and men. Both Kohlberg and Rest repeatedly state that their work is work in process; i.e., much remains to be done.[58]

When this is said, however, we return to our own concern about ethics for nurses. If it is legitimate to have a medical ethics for physicians and a legal ethics for lawyers and a business ethics for business people, it is surely legitimate to have an ethics for nurses. The question remains if there is a nursing ethics that is more than ordinary human ethics applied in the special field of nursing. Nurses have from time to time talked about their profession as a profession of caring. Perhaps Gilligan's ethic of caring speaks to this concern.

NOTES

1. *Detroit Free Press* (July 13, 1983), 11B, quoting *1,001 Logical Laws;* Garden City: Doubleday.
2. Out of Piaget's many books, *The Psychology of the Child,* co-authored with Barbel Inhelder (New York: Basic, 1969) is probably the best introduction to his thought. The finest overall introduction to Piaget available is *The Essential Piaget,* Gruber H.E., and Voneche, J.J. (eds). New York: Basic, 1977. For the continuing debate, see Pines, P. "Can a rock walk?" *Psychology Today* 17 (11):46-54, November 1983. For both appreciation and critique, see Elkind, D., and Flavell, J.H. (eds.) *Studies in Cognitive Development: Essays in Honor of Jean Piaget.* New York: Oxford, 1969.
3. Kohlberg, L., and Mayer, R. "Development as the aim of education: the Dewey view." In Kohlberg, L. *Essays on Moral Development. Vol. One. The Philosophy of Moral Development.* San Francisco: Harper & Row, 1981, pp. 49-96, especially p. 88.
4. Hunt, J.McV. "The impact and limitations of the giant of developmental psychology." In Elkind and Flavell, pp. 3-66, especially p. 11.
5. Piaget, J. *The Psychology of Intelligence.* Paterson, NJ: Littlefield, Adams, 1960 (original 1947), quoted by Hunt, "The impact and limitations of the giant of developmental psychology." In Elkind and Flavell, p. 30.
6. Piaget, J. *The Moral Judgment of the Child.* New York: Free Press, 1965 (original 1932). Rest, J.R. *Development in Judging Moral Issues.* Minneapolis: University of Minnesota Press, 1979, pp. 4-8, and "New approaches in the assessment of moral judgment." In Lickona, T. (ed.) *Moral Development and Behavior.* New York; Holt, Rinehart, & Winston, 1976, pp. 198-218, and, "A psychologist looks at the teaching of ethics." *Hastings Center Report* 12,(1):29-36, February 1982. Gilligan, C. "Moral development." In Chickering, A.W. (ed.) *The Modern American College.* San Francisco: Jossey-Bass, 1981, pp. 139-157. Kohlberg refers to Piaget's three stages, to which Kohlberg added Stages 4, 5 and 6. "Foreword." In Rest, pp. vii-xvi.
7. "Preface," pp. ix-xxv, "Indoctrination versus relativity in value education," pp. 6-28, and, "Appendix: the six stages of moral judgment," pp. 409-412. In *Essays.* Kohlberg, L. "Stages of moral development as a basis for moral education." In Munsey, B. *Moral Development, Moral Education, and Kohlberg.* Birmingham, AL: Religious Education Press, 1980, pp. 15-98. Rest, *Development in Judging Moral Issues,* pp. 7-12, 21-47f, and "A psychologist looks at the teaching of ethics," p. 31. In addition to Dewey and Piaget, Kohlberg notes J.T. Hobhouse (1906), whose social evolution had four stages: (1) taboo and private or group vengeance, (2) ideals of character, (3) social rules and maintenance of social order, and (4) general ethical

principles of justice based on equal rights. Kohlberg relates these to his stages 1, 3, 4, and 5-6, respectively. Hobhouse, J.T. *Morals in Evolution: A study in Comparative Ethics*. New York: Holt, 1923 (original 1906). Cited by Kohlberg, "From is to ought." In *Essays*, pp. 101-189, especially p. 128.

8. Note that ages vary considerably. In "Stages of moral development as a basis for moral education." In Munsey, p. 31, Kohlberg gives an example of a boy in Stage 1 at age 10, Stage 2 at age 13, and Stage 3 at age 16. Another boy is Stage 4 at age 10, Stage 5 at age 20, and Stage 6 at age 24.

9. Golding, W. *Lord of the Flies*. New York: Coward-McCann, 1955.

10. The Stage 2 person means "Yes." From other perspectives, the answer is "No." The religious person sees life as belonging to God. One's life belongs in some sense to one's family of origin, one's spouse and/or children, one's country, society, school, professional group, job, friends, and all the multiple relationships of the ordinary human being. This has been called a powerful argument against autonomy. Actually it is an argument against unlimited autonomy, sometimes called anarchy or narcissism. It is an argument for the interdependence cited earlier.

11. Kohlberg sees Robert Ringer's book, *Looking Out for Number One* (New York: Fawcett Books, 1977) as Stage 2 along with the privatism of youth and the new conservatism of the 1980s. The old conservatism of Senator Goldwater is Stage 4—maintain American society—or Stage 5—a commitment to liberty and democracy threatened by Communism. See "Educating for a just society: an updated and revised statement." In Munsey, pp. 455-470, especially p. 61. From an earlier day, Jeremy Bentham's utilitarianism is Stage 2. Kohlberg, "Stages in moral development as a basis for moral education." In Munsey, p. 67.

12. Kohlberg, "From is to ought." In *Essays*, p. 149.

13. Mahon, K.A., and Fowler, M.D. "Moral development and clinical decision-making." *Nursing Clinics of North America* 14 (1):2-12, March 1979.

14. According to Mohr, J.C. *Abortion in America* (New York: Oxford, 1978), "regular" physicians used abortion as an issue to get rid of the "irregulars" between 1825 and 1875.

15. Loren R. Graham wrote, "If the research is highly unorthodox, it may not receive support even if potential applications are visualizable." "Concerns about science and attempts to regulate inquiry." *Daedalus* 107 (2):1-17, Spring 1978. Coughlin, E.K. "Finding the message in the medium: the rhetoric of scholarly research." *The Chronicle of Higher Education* 27 (7):7-9, April 11, 1984, suggests orthodoxy is the norm. Personal communications suggest that the research must be orthodox.

16. Here the Golden Rule is interpreted as mutual affectionate concern, as noted earlier. Kohlberg, "From is to ought." In *Essays*, pp. 149-150.

17. Sinsheimer, R. "Troubled dawn for genetic engineering." *New Scientist* 68 (971):148-151, October 16, 1975. We noted the various concepts of social evolution earlier under the rubric of social Darwinism.

18. "Sophomoric" is of course a derogatory term. Kohlberg claims most social scientists are hung up in relativism, as are many adolescents, college students, and teachers. It seems to be relatively common in health care as well. Kohlberg, "From is to ought." In *Essays*, pp. 130, 156. V. Lois Erickson worked with 23 high school sophomore women in moral education and found measurable stage change. "Deliberate psychological education for women, from Iphigenia to Antigone." *Counselor Education and Supervision* 14 (4):297-309, June 1975, and, "The development of women: an issue of justice." In Scharf, P. (ed.) *Readings in Moral Education*. Minneapolis:

Winston Press, 1978, pp. 110-123. Quoted by Rosenzweig, L. "Kohlberg in the classroom: moral education models." In Munsey, pp. 359-380.

19. Rest, "A psychologist looks at the teaching of ethics," p. 31. Kohlberg, "Stages of moral development as a basis for moral education." In Munsey, p. 35, and "From is to ought." In *Essays*, pp. 152-156. Davis, A.J., and Aroskar, M.A. *Ethical Dilemmas and Nursing Practice*, 2nd ed. Norwalk, CT: Appleton-Century-Crofts, 1983.

20. Kohlberg, "From is to ought." In *Essays*, pp. 152-156, and "Capital punishment, moral development, and the Constitution." In *Essays*, pp. 243-293, especially p. 252.

21. Kohlberg, "Introduction." In *Essays*, pp. xxvii-xxxv, especially p. xxxiii, "Educating for a just society." p. 457, "Stages of moral development as a basis for moral education." p. 92. In Munsey, and "From is to ought." In *Essays*, pp. 152-156.

22. Kohlberg, "Justice and reversibility: the claim to adequacy of a highest moral stage." In *Essays*, pp. 190-226 (note that *Essays* was published in 1981). "Educating for a just society." In Munsey, pp. 455-470. "Meaning and measurement in moral development." *Heinz Werner Memorial Lecture*. Worcester, MA: Clark University Press, 1979.

23. Kohlberg, "Stages of moral development as a basis for moral education." In Munsey, p. 31. "From is to ought." In *Essays*, p. 120.

24. Kohlberg, "Educating for a just society." In Munsey, p. 466.

25. Kohlberg, "Preface." In *Essays*, p. xxviii.

26. Kohlberg, "Moral stages and the aims of education," pp. 1-5, "From is to ought," p. 122, and "Moral stages and the idea of justice," pp. 97-100, in *Essays*. Alternately, one could say the confusion comes from the inconsistency of publishing as empirically confirmed what was really conjecture or the use of the same word in many different ways. James Rest's research normally suggests people are at a higher stage then does Kohlberg's research. One result is that Rest finds more people at Stage 6. *Development in Judging Moral Issues*, p. 46.

27. Kohlberg, "Stages of moral development as a basis for moral education." In Munsey, p. 31. Rest, "New approaches in the assessment of moral judgment." In Likona, pp. 207-208, and "Developmental psychology and value education." In Munsey, pp. 101-129. Rest, *Development in Judging Moral Issues*, pp. 71, 205, cites Kohlberg data that give an average of 12.3 years to move one stage.

28. One might note here that Kohlberg is working with probabilities and groups. Socrates did not have a Ph.D. and yet he is Kohlberg's premier example of a Stage 6 personality. Nor does it follow that having a Ph.D. or any other degree puts one automatically at any stage of moral development. Many Nazis were well educated. It is rather that advancing education increases one's cognitive abilities, which are also important for moral understanding. Rest, "A psychologist looks at the teaching of ethics," *HCR* p. 32. Gilligan, "Moral development." In Chickering, p. 139.

29. Rest, *Development in Judging Moral Issues*, pp. 73-74, questions these concepts of understanding and intervention. He claims moral development is more complicated than this simple stage theory.

30. Kohlberg, "Educating for a just society." In Munsey, pp. 457-459. Rosenzweig, "Kohlberg in the Classroom." In Munsey, p. 376.

31. Kohlberg and Mayer, "Development as the aim of education." In *Essays*, pp. 49-100, "Stages of moral development as a basis for moral education." In Munsey,

pp. 18–37. Rest, "Developmental psychology and value education." In Munsey, p. 106. Neill, A.S. *Summerhill.* New York: Hart, 1960. Skinner, B.F. *Walden Two.* New York: Macmillan, 1948, and *Beyond Freedom and Dignity.* New York: Knopf, 1971, and "Origins of a behaviorist." *Psychology Today* 17 (9):22–23, September 1983. One of the limitations of democracy is majority rule. If a majority of the voters is at Stage 2, they could vote in a government or a health care system reflecting Stage 2 morality. Kohlberg and Mayer, "Development as the aim of education." In *Essays,* p. 73, says both Skinner and Neill would rather a child "be a happy pig then an unhappy Socrates. We may question, however, whether they have the right to withhold the choice."

32. Kohlberg, "Stages of moral development as a basis for moral education." In Munsey, pp. 92–94. "From is to ought." In *Essays,* pp. 100–189.

33. Kohlberg, "From is to ought." In *Essays,* pp. 155, 183–189. For a discussion of the emotive theory of ethics, see Aiken, H.D. *Reason and Conduct.* New York: Knopf, especially pp. 15ff, 91ff, 114–121. Kohlberg, "Stages of moral development as a basis for moral education." In Munsey, pp. 38–42. Rest, *Development in Judging Moral Issues,* pp. 169–195, 259–261 (on behavior). On page 73, he notes that the requirement of the formal operations stage as a prerequisite to principled moral reasoning is questionable, although on page 207, he acknowledges the prerequisite. Macdonald, J.B. "A look at the Kohlberg curriculum framework for moral education." In Munsey, pp. 381–400, especially p. 388. Kohlberg and Mayer, "Development as the aim of education." In *Essays,* p. 93. Ego development includes self-awareness and awareness of the world.

34. Kohlberg, "Stages of moral development as a basis for moral education." In Munsey, pp. 44, 71. Kohlberg and Mayer, "Development as the aim of education." In *Essays,* p. 85. "The question of a seventh stage." *Essays,* pp. 311–372. In Rest, "Developmental psychology and value education." In Munsey, p. 104. Stage 7 is a theoretical stage associated in part with religion. It is not conventional religion but a level of commitment that goes beyond justice. This is not a higher stage of moral development. It is beyond the highest Stage 6. Martin Luther King, Jr., and Socrates are examples of this. Kohlberg also offers as an example Janusz Korczak, a Warsaw pediatrician who ran orphanages for Christian and Jewish children. He went with his Jewish orphans to their death at the hands of the Nazis. While identifying with his Jewish orphans, his own faith was not traditionally Jewish but a "mystic pantheism." Rest discusses "conceptually more adequate," in *Development in Judging Moral Issues,* pp. 24, 123–124.

35. Kohlberg, "Stages of moral development as a basis for moral education." In Munsey, pp. 15–23. Rest, *Development in Judging Moral Issues,* p. 33, and "Developmental psychology and value education." In Munsey, p. 103. One can note that one of the several things the Stage 4½ person fails to note is that, as a matter of fact, the reasons for being moral are normally present in Stages 1 through 4. What is being sought, often ignorantly, as a "real" reason, is the universal(s) of the postconventional level.

36. Rest, *Development in Judging Moral Issues,* p. 12.

37. Rest, *Development in Judging Moral Issues.* "New approaches in the assessment of moral judgment." In Likona, pp. 198–200. "Developmental psychology and value education." In Munsey, p. 109. A D score rates all 72 items. It is a very complicated measure done by computer program. For the most part, the D score has not shown any particular advantage over the P score.

38. Rest, "Developmental psychology and value education." In Munsey, pp. 109–113.

39. Rest, "A psychologist looks at the teaching of ethics," p. 32, and, "New approaches in the assessment of moral judgments." In Munsey, p. 209, and *Revised Manual for the Defining Issues Test.* Minneapolis: Minnesota Moral Research Projects, 1979, p. 7–15. In *Development in Judging Moral Issues,* p. 165, he cites studies showing that scales of liberalism–conservatism have a nonsignificant correlation with DIT.

40. Rest, "New approaches in the assessment of moral judgments." In Lickona, pp. 201–203. Kohlberg, "Stages of moral development as a basis for moral education." In Munsey, p. 44, notes that people prefer the stage above their own because it represents a better equilibrium. It is more differentiated and integrated.

41. Rest, *Development in Judging Moral Issues,* pp. 169-195. Ketefian, S. "Moral reasoning and moral behavior." *Nursing Research* 30 (3):171-176, May-June 1981. Curtin, L.L. "Nursing ethics: theories and pragmatics." *Nursing Forum* 17 (1):4-11, 1978. Jameton, A. "The nurse: when rules and roles conflict." *HCR* 7:22-23 August 1977.

42. Holmes, H.B., Hoskins, B.B., and Gross, M. (eds.) *Birth Control and Controlling Birth* and *The Custom-Made Child?* Clifton, NJ: Humana Press, 1980.

43. Rest, "A psychologist looks at the teaching of ethics," p. 33. Crisham, P. "Measuring moral judgement in nursing dilemmas." *Nursing Research* 30 (2):104-110, March-April 1981.

44. Crisham, "Measuring moral judgment in nursing dilemmas," p. 106.

45. Crisham, "Measuring moral judgment in nursing dilemmas," p. 110. See also Ketefian, "Moral reasoning and moral behavior," and Kramer, M. *Reality Shock: Why Nurses Leave Nursing.* St. Louis: Mosby, 1974.

46. Kohlberg, "From is to ought." In *Essays,* pp. 169-170. Rosenzweig, "Kohlberg in the classroom: moral education models." In Munsey, p. 374, has noted this danger. Teachers have used IQ scores to label students and to establish positive and negative expectancies. So teachers may use Kohlberg labels to establish the moral worth of students. One can appreciate her observations while noting that the misuse of a theory argues for correction of the misuse rather than rejection of the theory.

47. Rest, "A psychologist looks at the teaching of ethics," p. 35. Kohlberg, "Moral stages and the idea of justice," In *Essays,* pp. 97-100. On critiques, see the Munsey volume, and the literature cited there.

48. Gilligan, C. *In a Different Voice: Psychological Theory and Women's Development.* Cambridge: Harvard University Press, 1982. See the work cited earlier by V. Lois Erickson with high school women in a Kohlberg type program, "Deliberate psychological education for women, from Iphigenia to Antigone," and "The development of women: an issue of justice." Neither the DIT nor Kohlberg's research shows any consistent sex differences. Rest, *Development in Judging Moral Issues,* pp. 122, 250. Rest discusses, pp. 120-124, the charge of sex bias by Holstein, C.B. "Irreversible, stepwise sequence in the development of moral judgment: a longitudinal study of males and females." *Child Development* 47:51-61, 1976. Rest cites 22 studies of the DIT in which 2 showed females with a 6 percent higher score, whereas 20 showed no distinction.

49. Holstein cites studies showing women at Stage 3 and men at Stage 4. Rest notes the variance is small, with women 41 percent at Stage 3 and 39 percent at Stage 4. The males were 22 percent Stage 3 and 43 percent Stage 4. Other studies show no differences.

50. Kohlberg, "From is to ought." In *Essays,* p. 167. McDonald, J.B., "A look at the Kohlberg Curriculum framework for moral education." In Munsey, pp. 392-393. Davis and Aroskar, *Ethical Dilemmas and Nursing Practice,* 2nd ed., p. 5.

51. Kohlberg, "The question of a seventh stage." In *Essays*, p. 356. Gilligan, "Moral development." In Chickering.

52. Gilligan, *In a Different Voice: Psychological Theory and Women's Development*, pp. 103–105. Erickson, E.H. *Gandhi's Truth*. New York: W.W. Norton, 1969.

53. Kohlberg, "From is to ought." In *Essays*, pp. 134, 137, 152–157. Gilligan, *In a Different Voice: Psychological Theory and Women's Development*, pp. 106–127. Gilligan, C., and Belenky, M.F. "A naturalistic study of abortion decisions." In Selman, R., and Yando, R. (eds.) *Clinical-Developmental Psychology*. San Francisco: Jossey-Bass, 1980.

54. James Michael Lee sees role taking as an exercise in empathy. Lee, J.M. "Christian religious education and moral development." In Munsey, pp. 326–355, especially p. 338.

55. Public lecture, University of Pennsylvania, April 7, 1984.

56. Kohlberg, "From is to ought." In *Essays*, pp. 141, 144. Personal communication, Dr. W. G. Thompson. We note here in relation to Freud, an interesting possibility based on Gilligan's work. Freud's misogyny is well known. One of the reasons he considered women inferior is of course his culture. To Freud, women were a mystery. He told Marie Bonaparte that even after 30 years of research into the female soul, he still could not answer the question, "What does a woman want?" This romantic but destructive mythology was also part of his culture and is part of ours today echoed by males on numerous occasions—"I just don't understand women." The cultural influence sounds like Stage 4, but Freud was Stage 2 or 1 in Kohlberg's theory. Fear of punishment (Stage 1) and relating to others to use them (Stage 2) are the basis of his pleasure/pain theory. Human beings (including himself, presumably) function on the pleasure/pain principle—Stage 2. Kohlberg notes that we understand the next higher stage but not two stages above our own. Freud rejected authority (Stage 3) except his own (to his followers, Freud *is* the authority), and considered Stage 4 primitive (Kohlberg, "From is to ought." In *Essays*, p. 151), i.e., he did not understand it. He could not even begin to fathom Stages 5 and 6, where Gilligan's women are. No wonder Freud said he could not understand women! He was Stage 2 and they are Stage 5! James, M. "Cultural scripts: historical events vs. historical interpretation." *Transactional Analysis Journal* 13 (4):217–223, October 1983. Jones, E. *The Life and Work of Sigmund Freud*, edited and abridged by Trilling, L., and Marcus, S. New York: Basic Books, 1961, pp. 375–377. Jones notes here that Freud thought women were nobler and more ethical than men. He also thought of himself as being very moral and as having a sense of justice, whereas other people are brutal and untrustworthy. It was unfathomable to him why he and his six children were thoroughly decent human beings.

57. Erickson, "Deliberate psychological education for women, from Iphigenia to Antigone." Weisbrodt, S. "Moral judgment, sex and parental identification in adults." *Developmental Psychology* 2:396–402, 1970.

58. For additional studies by Gilligan, see "In a different voice: women's conceptions of self and morality." *Harvard Educational Review* 47:481–517, 1977. "Psychoanalytic theory and morality." In Lickona. Gilligan and Murphy, M.J. "Development from adolescence to adulthood: the philosopher and the 'dilemma of the fact'." In Kuhn, D. (ed.) *Intellectual Development Beyond Childhood*. San Francisco: Jossey-Bass, 1979. Gilligan and Kohlberg, "The adolescent as a philosopher: the discovery of the self in a postconventional world." *Daedalus* 100:1051–1086, Fall 1971.

The nurse provides services with respect for human dignity and the unique-
ness of the client unrestricted by considerations of social or economic status,
personal attributes, or the nature of the health problem.

–American Nurses' Association Code for Nurses, 1976[1]

Everything we do, every decision we make and course of action we take is
based on our consciously and unconsciously held beliefs, attitudes, and
values.

–*Diane Uustal, RN*[2]

CHAPTER 4

We are Moral Beings

One of the primary goals of nursing practice is to provide the best care for
each client. It is not always clear what is best for another individual, however. Who defines "best" and how it is defined in the situation involve value
judgments. Values and values clarification play a central role in a text devoted to ethical decision making in health/illness care. They are necessary for
understanding the extent to which a person's beliefs and values influence the
decisions made in health care, whether these decisions are made by patients,
physician, or nurse.

Nurses are involved daily in ethical decisions, decisions about what
should or ought to be done for a given patient. They, therefore, can benefit
from understanding the values and beliefs of patients and other individuals
involved in the ethical dimensions of caring.[3] Nurses often learn how to
understand the patient within the context of family and community. Less
time is spent on examining the value set of those same individuals and how
those values might influence the person's ability to accept or reject health
care. And even less time is spent on examining our own values and those of
our professional colleagues.

New technologies available for use in illness care have created choices
that did not exist a few years ago. These choices often require actions that
touch the very core of our belief systems and challenge previously held
values. Our newness in dealing with the choices created by technology also
warrants attention to the personal and professional values that are placed in
potential conflict.

Nurses are individuals with personal values, beliefs, and attitudes. We come to nursing at an age where many values have been internalized to the point where we no longer question their source. We bring these personal values to the professional role during our education as nurses. The profession of nursing also has a set of values and expects its members to know, understand, and internalize these values. Therefore nurses are also professionals with professional values, beliefs, and attitudes.[4]

As professionals, nurses need to know themselves—what they believe in and value. This self-knowledge contributes to ethical decision making and practice. In an emergency, the decision one makes for patient care often reflects who the nurse is and what is believed and valued in the situation. One danger of the unexamined value system is that our patients may bear the consequences of the professional's imposed values and beliefs without benefit of self-determination or choice.

The maternalistic or paternalistic view in health care implies that it is all right for professionals to impose their values on patients. The professional "knows best." The current scene in ethics, however, emphasizes informed consent and autonomy/self-determination of patients.[5] The health care provider may agree or disagree with the patient's values and choices. When the patient is given full information and declines to comply with the prescribed regimen, the provider may have a different kind of ethical dilemma. The AMA *Principles of Medical Ethics* (Appendix B) is quite clear that physicians may choose whom they serve or accept as a client, except in emergencies. Once a patient has been accepted, however, the patient may not be abandoned, although a patient can be referred to another provider.[6] The ANA *Code for Nurses* (p. 12) also has a provision for transferring care to another nurse when one has a moral disagreement with the client's choice of treatment. However, the largely employed status of nursing makes this more difficult. When possible, e.g., in caring for people whose procedures are scheduled in advance, the transfer of care should be carried out in advance. Professionals, however, do not always have a free hand in deciding who they will or will not care for. The *Code for Nurses* calls for care without discrimination.[7]

Current health care ethics is largely agreed that providers should not impose their own values on their patients who have the capacity to make their own decisions based on full information. The consensus ethic of the President's Commission for the Study of Ethical Problems in Medicine and Biomedical and Behavioral Research stated that the goal of ethical decision making is "shared decision-making based on mutual respect."[8] Respect for others implies understanding of who they are and what they value. Understanding implies knowledge of what values are, which are held inviolate, which are changing or in need of change, and which are in conflict with others. This knowledge of values and their importance in evaluating consequences for individuals will help ensure a final choice in health care based on both cognitive and affective aspects of the situation.

PERSONAL VALUE SET: WHO AM I?

Socrates said, "The unexamined life is not worth living." An inscription at the Delphic Oracle said, "Know thyself." This dictum remains a valid one for today. If nursing is to be ethical, nurses must know ethics. If nurses are going to be ethical, they must know themselves. While ethics is a reflection on morality, the knowing of the self comes from self-reflection. The extrovert may have some difficulty looking within to examine the assumptions by which he or she practices and lives. The introvert supposedly would have an easier time of this, but not necessarily. Sometimes psychotherapy helps one understand the hidden springs of one's beliefs, values, and actions. Sometimes a straight question will help one see where a moral value came from. Such questions include, "Can I live with this?" or "Why does this bother me?" "What would I do (or want done) in this situation?" The important thing to remember is that nurses are persons with personal value sets that influence how they practice the profession of nursing. We need to know what we value in life, in health, during illness, and in death.

We touched on this concern for values in discussing intuitionism. In the three-part personality theory of Transactional Analysis, the value system is preserved in the Parent Ego State. The point of asking about our own values is not to destroy them. It is to examine them honestly to see if they remain adequate for our own time. A given value may have been quite appropriate when we were 3 or 13 or even last year. It may still be appropriate, but, then again, it may need modification or replacement. New duties teach new truths, or vice versa. It is important to add that just because we take time to know our own values, it does not follow that we can impose them on others.

Definitions

Let us begin our discussion of the personal value set with some basic definitions. *Values,* as defined by Simon and Clark, are a set of personal beliefs and attitudes about the truth, beauty, or worth of any thought, object, or behavior.[9] Many philosophers do not agree on an absolute definition of values or valuing. This can be confusing. In this confusion we have found it helpful to use the work of Raths, Harmin, and Simon. They help to clarify values related to personal beliefs and human behavior. They reserve the term "value" for those individual beliefs, attitudes, activities, or feelings that satisfy seven criteria. These criteria are (1) having been freely chosen (no outside pressures forced the choice), (2) having been chosen from among alternatives, (3) having been chosen after due reflection (excludes impulse or highly emotional choices), (4) having been prized and cherished, (5) having been affirmed to others, (6) having been incorporated into actual behavior (lack of putting into practice usually implies a belief or attitude but not a value), and (7) having been repeated in one's life.[10] The distinction between belief and value, which is a belief put into practice, is important. We note its similarity to James Rest's notion that we first prefer a stage of moral development, then understand it, and finally put it into use (see Chapter Three).

Values clarification is a process or way of examining one's life to determine what is meaningful (valued) to the individual. It is a collection of strategies that help one identify significant values that are fixed as well as those that are emerging or changing.[11] Values clarification is best done in groups, as it exposes individuals to a variety of value positions different from one's own. We are often so tied to our own values that we cannot think of an alternate view on the issue. Talking with others who hold alternate values on a given issue can help our understanding of others as well as require that we clearly state our own value preferences. Inherent in group discussion of values is trust and mutual respect for others. Simon and Clark caution that values cannot be truthfully examined or strengthened in an atmosphere of fear or mistrust.[12] The process often involves a deep searching of self and should not be taken lightly.

During values clarification we can discover what values are prized or cherished. This implies that values are organized into a hierarchy and that some are of greater importance than others. Consideration of our value hierarchy helps us to understand what is most important to us. The goal of values clarification is to facilitate ethical decision making through self-understanding and practice in making choices.[13] It is not synonymous with ethical decision making, however.

Where do our values come from? It is commonly accepted that values come from a variety of sources. Early in life, parental, religious, and other authority figures influence our perceptions of what is right and good in behavior or beliefs. Value development comes from life experience, including culture, science, religion and the notion of self-discovery.[14] Hall identifies two primary values. The first is self-value or the notion that I am of worth to significant others. The second is that others are of equal worth. These two primary values are possible only when in relationship to each other. They are also vital in understanding the nature of professional nursing based on relationships with others—both clients and colleagues. Values come, therefore, from association with other people, the environment, and with self. We have already noted that values may not be rigid or fixed. Analysis may determine what is presently appropriate.

One of the most exciting aspects of values clarification may be understanding the source of a particular value. We may then see our capacity to retain a value or change it. Hopefully, either decision will be appropriate for others, the environment, and one's self. In addition, personal self-discovery is the first step toward positive growth. Healthy personality growth can lead to healthy professional practice. Once again we note the relationship of value development and theories of moral development.

There is another definition that is needed before we approach the practical dimensions of exploring one's personal value set. "Axiology" comes from the Greek *axios*, meaning worthy, and *logos*, word or study. Axiology is the science of values.[15] Axiology is important as a science and as a decision tool. Axiology inquires into the nature of values. In this sense it is similar to one of the definitions of metaethics described in Chapter One. Axiology is one of the three most general kinds of inquiry, the other two being metaphysics and epistemology. Bahm posits that national and global crises involve values— more specifically, the misunderstanding of values. Because values may be complex and difficult to understand, they often become accepted as feelings or opinion without understanding. He suggests that when people are equal and decisions are based on votes, the result is determined by which biased (personal) opinion happens to be most prevalent among those voting.[16] This may happen in bioethics when people make decisions based on feelings ("I know best") or so-called clinical judgment ("the doctor/nurse knows best") without understanding the nature of values and the need for moral reasoning. Recognizing and developing axiology is necessary for ethical decision making, both in health care and in society at large.

We offer a final concept for consideration as we approach the discussion of what we value as individuals and as professionals. *Socialization* is the process of instilling values in individuals. Some professionals accept responsibility for socializing their members to the values of the profession. These values are not often clearly articulated nor openly taught in classrooms, however. In fact, we suspect that most professional educators do not even realize they are inculcating values in their teaching and practice.[17] In the professional value section of this chapter we will discuss some of the values of nursing as described in the literature and ANA *Code for Nurses*. Socialization of values usually begins in the home and continues throughout school experiences and in job settings. We cannot escape it. We can, however, become more knowledgeable about what values are being instilled. We can decide whether those values are appropriate. Job satisfaction could increase if people knowingly choose an occupation whose values they can support. This will be discussed further.

Personal Values Exploration

Exploration of values and valuing exercises help one to discover the values held and how we make moral choices in life. There are several excellent texts on values clarification exercises.[18] Only a few exercises will be reviewed here. The importance of such exercises is the awareness of what we personally value in life. The exercises help show how those values may influence the decisions we make as individuals and as professionals.

A beginning to this values exploration is asking "What are the characteristics I like (or dislike) about myself?" "What do I believe in?" Answers to these questions might take the form of ten statements that reflect who you are, ten things you like to do, ten things you like about yourself, and ten things you dislike. The number of statements is not as important as the content of the statements and the analysis of them. This analysis often takes the form of marking the things you prefer. A review of things you dislike about yourself may promote some thoughts about what you may wish to change. These dislikes may also refer to things that turn you off when viewed in others and can help you understand such reactions if they occur.

After some of the initial exercises, you may be ready to list ten values that guide your daily interactions. Often a comparison of lists with a trusted friend or colleague leads to discussion of similarities, differences, and reasons for the items listed. Other exercises that help to elicit personal values for review and analysis are responses to specific ethical concerns. These include such issues as abortion, sanctity of life, euthanasia, informed consent, truth-telling. Remember to distinguish between your attitudes and beliefs (preferences) and what you actually put into daily practice (values).

Henry Aiken[19] described four levels of moral discourse that are helpful in understanding one's growth in understanding values and the valuing process. He listed the first as expressive, referring to such statements as "I hate lying." The second level is the definition of moral rules, such as "Do not tell a lie," or "Always tell the truth." The third level is that of ethical principles, expressed in "Lying is wrong," or "Telling the truth is good." The final level of moral discourse is the postethical. When we begin to explore what we value as individuals, we often find that we express our values as feelings—the expressive level of discourse. As we expand our knowledge and experience with values clarification, we are able to articulate moral rules and then move toward explication of moral principles. One may again see the parallel with stages of moral development discussed in Chapter Three.

As we grow and mature as persons, we can also grow in understanding ourselves. "The end result of values clarification is someone with more awareness, empathy, and insight than a person who has not had this experience."[20] Simon and Clark add that values clarification (knowing oneself) narrows the gap between our words and our actions, as well as promoting a high level of self-actualization.[21] Persons who take the time to know who they are and what they believe are better prepared to care for patients—they are better nurses.

PROFESSIONAL VALUE SET: WHAT IS A GOOD NURSE?

When one expends time and energy to learn what is valued in life, one cannot escape thinking about what one values in the professional role as well. The interaction between personal and professional values in daily nursing practice is a given. Following the line of reasoning of Simon et al. that values need to be acted upon (put into practice) to meet the criterion of being valued, the fact that one values self-determination personally will influence how one works with patients. Steele postulates that congruence of personal and professional values contributes to comfort in carrying out the professional role.[22] While recognizing that persons who are comfortable with their professional role will probably experience greater satisfaction and possibly provide better care for clients, this latter point may not be true. We could list any number of situations where nurses were comfortable with their role to the point of not making waves or standing up for a morally defensible decision. They may be at ease with their role, but they were not necessarily practicing in an ethical manner. They may not have taken the time to examine their personal or professional values either. The comfort was not the comfort of congruence of values.

The lack of congruence between personal and professional values has a positive side. It forces one to look closely at what values are in conflict, determine which is appropriate, and then make a reasoned choice to follow one path. We earlier discussed Piaget's concept of disequilibrium and its motivation to look for more understanding in moral development (Chapter Three). In other words, such dissonance or disequilibrium can contribute to personal and professional moral growth through increased understanding, which brings a new equilibrium. This may mean that one will decide to leave a given job or the profession of nursing if the gap between personal and professional values is too wide. It may also mean that one will decide to change one's view of the nursing situation and become better able to provide needed nursing care.

Definition of Health

Different definitions of health raise different concerns for moral responsibility in nursing practice.[23] One's definition of health affects one's view of what professional nursing is about. Commitment to a concept of health and illness reflects both personal and professional values. We need to understand this relationship even as we strive for greater understanding of health and its influence on nurses and nursing.

We spoke earlier of definitions of health. What kind of nursing results from a definition of health as the absence of illness? How might such a nurse respond when assigned to care for a person who is terminally ill (is not disease free)? Other definitions of health include emotional, social and cultural as well as physiological well-being. Here the nurse is concerned with such things as equity or justice in the allocation of scarce resources, whether this be in hospitals or housing or food. This concern may extend to the well born children who now have little food to eat as well as the seriously ill newborn. Here health care also extends to fighting government subsidy of such drugs as tobacco as well as caring for the person with lung cancer.

A final note is offered on how we personally and professionally value health in relation to our definition of health. We can turn to the conflict of beliefs and values as illustrated by the obese, hypertensive nurse attempting to counsel obese, hypertensive patients on the value of good nutrition and medical care. What message does the client receive? Do actions speak louder than educational efforts? Is the nurse actively promoting the value of individual choice (good or bad) so that scarce resources are used to care for illness caused by bad eating habits? These are difficult questions for all of us and are not readily answered. They do, however, warrant consideration as health care professionals seek to understand not only what they value personally and professionally but also how those values may affect our ability to provide health services.

Views of Health Care

Aroskar and others have discussed the importance of professional nurses examining the values placed on health and illness as well as their role in the delivery system. She lists four mind sets about health care that she suggests may limit or prohibit ethical nursing practice. These views of health care are (1) medical cases or scientific projects with the cure of diseases as the major objective, (2) a commodity in the marketplace to be sold to others, (3) the patient's right to relief from pain or other debilitating condition, and (4) the promotion, maintenance, and restoration of health within a cooperative community.

In the first concept of health care, nurses view themselves as primarily accountable to the physician. Medical values dominate. The nurse is concerned with doing what the physician decides. In the second view, nurses are employees accountable to the employer, the institution. Institutions often function under the utilitarian ethic. Concern for the needs of the individual patient may conflict with the nurse's accountability to the administrative hierarchy. However, the nurse has already made the ethical decision—his or her loyalties lie with the institution.

The third view of health care is that the nurse's primary obligation is to patients and their needs as defined by the patients' themselves. Both institutional and nursing practice would be dictated by patient needs and interests. This view of health care may be an abdication of responsibility by health care professionals. It is also a tempting "out" for the professional when the ethical dilemma is particularly difficult, and the nurse does not want to participate in deciding what should be done. Support of patient autonomy does not require abdication of professional responsibility. A pregnant woman decides to have a vaginal birth no matter what the consequences to the fetus or dangers to herself. A nurse–midwife who merely accepts that position is practicing unethically and without due consideration or respect for the health and well-being of both mother and infant. The ethic of competence requires that the nurse–midwife use that knowledge and experience. If nurses view their role as subordinate to both patient and physician, they may encounter difficulty in implementing a value of autonomy or of promoting health in an illness-dominated system, let alone be able to practice in an ethical manner.

Aroskar suggests that the mind set or view of health care compatible

with ethical nursing practice views "health care as promotion, maintenance and restoration of client well-being in a cooperative community"
where all participants' values are taken into account in decision making.
Both providers and clients have rights and responsibilities in this view of
health care.[24]

Professional Values in Nursing

Nursing is a profession based on caring for others. It espouses its own values
documented in such statements as the ANA *Code for Nurses, Standards of
Practice, Social Policy,* and guidelines for research. These statements are important because they contain a consensus of the profession on what constitutes the professional ethic of nursing. In addition, they speak to what the
public can expect from nurses and nursing.[25]

The *Code for Nurses* (p. 12) offers an ideal view of the ethic of nursing
in this country. It offers general guidelines for the conduct (behavior) of professional nurses.[26] This behavior constitutes the elements of moral responsibility of nurses and nursing to the public. The elements are often referred to
as moral duties or obligations. The 1973 International Council of Nurses
Code for Nurses (Appendix B) offers a more global view of the moral responsibilities of nurses in relation to people (clients), practice, society, co-workers,
and the profession of nursing.[27]

Let us take a closer look at the values espoused in the ANA *Code for
Nurses.* The 11 statements of the *Code for Nurses* are moral in nature, i.e.,
they describe what nurses should and ought to do and to be. The Interpretive
Statements that follow each moral guideline provide some of the reasons why
the nurse should follow the guideline, i.e., the reasons behind the moral
prescription (ethics). The values discussed in the *Code* include respect for
persons, nondiscrimination in providing care, right to privacy, self-
determination/autonomy of clients, informed consent, safeguarding (beneficence) clients' welfare, accountability for judgments and responsible actions,
competence, participation in research, and promoting efforts to meet health
needs of the public. Two of the major ethical concerns in health care are not
clearly addressed in the ANA *Code.* These are truth-telling and the allocation
of scarce resources. Theoretically, they can be assumed under the others, but
they are not specified.

Recently, there has been support for defining the ethic of caring as one
of the central foci of nursing.[28] Caring is a value itself, although some would
break it down into subparts, such as mercy and compassion or respect for
persons. Another view is that of Levine, who proposes that the nursing profession is based on the ethic of competence and the ethic of compassion. Here
we find the suggestion that "proper perspective is maintained when the ethic
of competence grows out of the ethic of compassion as the motivating force
of the nursing profession."[29] Whatever one's view of the ethic of nursing, it is
important to clearly articulate and understand the values involved.

SUMMARY

One could go on and add other values implied or explicit in the profession of nursing, although the main ones have been presented. As one thinks about these professional values, it is helpful to also think of one's personal stand on each of them. The personal and professional value systems of decision makers influence how one presents an ethical dilemma for discussion. Though it is often difficult to separate our personal values from our professional values (being thoroughly socialized and accepting of the role of nurse), it is an important effort as we strive to practice in an ethical manner. Changing values in major social institutions within society—the family, health, education, health care institutions—make the task of ethical nursing practice even more difficult. However, when we understand and accept what we believe and value in nursing, we have clearer direction in what constitutes ethical practice.

Ethical decision making is fostered as all affected persons are willing to share and respect each other's values while searching for a morally justifiable action that is best. The willingness to share values is predicated on knowledge of them. We end as we began this chapter, reinforcing the need and importance of nurses understanding what they value as persons and professionals. Thus, they may contribute openly and knowledgeably to ethical decision making and the moral reasoning process on which it is based.

NOTES

1. American Nurses Association. *Code for Nurses with Interpretive Statements*. Kansas City, MO: American Nurses' Association, 1976.
2. Uustal, D. *Values and Ethics Considerations in Nursing Practice*. South Deerfield, MA: Uustal, 1978, p. 11.
3. Thompson, J.B., and Thompson, H.O. *Ethics in Nursing*. New York: Macmillan, 1981, pp. 3–6. Steele, S., and Harmon, V. *Values Clarification in Nursing*, 2nd ed. Norwalk, CT: Appleton-Century-Crofts, 1983, pp. vii, 6–7. Aroskar, M.A. "Anatomy of an ethical dilemma: the theory." *American Journal of Nursing* 80(4):659, April 1980. Brody, H. *Ethical Decisions in Medicine*. Boston: Little, Brown, 1976, pp. 7, 13.
4. Steele and Harmon, *Values Clarification in Nursing*, pp. 6–7. Kelly, L. *Dimensions of Professional Nursing*, 3rd ed. New York: Macmillan, 1975, pp. 208–220. Coleta, S.S. "Values clarification in nursing: Why?" *AJN* 78 (12):2057, December 1978. Davis, A.J., and Aroskar, M.A. *Ethical Dilemmas and Nursing Practice*, 2nd ed. Norwalk, CT: Appleton-Century-Crofts, 1983, pp. 24–25. Fromer, M.J. *Ethical Issues in Health Care*. St. Louis: Mosby, 1981, pp. 12–14.
5. President's Commission for the Study of Ethical Problems in Medicine and Biomedical and Behavioral Research. *Making Health Care Decisions. Volume One: The Report*. Washington, DC: US Government Printing Office, October 1982.
6. American Medical Association. *Principles of Medical Ethics*, Chicago: AMA House of Delegates, July 1980.

7. ANA, *Code for Nurses with Interpretive Statements*, 1.4, p. 5. Muyskens, J.L. *Moral Problems in Nursing. A Philosophical Investigation.* Totowa, NJ: Rowman and Littlefield, 1982, pp. 168–178.

8. President's Commission, *Making Health Care Decisions. Volume One:* pp. 2–6; *Deciding to Forego Life Sustaining Treatment.* Washington, DC: US Government Printing Office, March 1983, pp. 2–4.

9. Simon, S.B., and Clark, J. *Beginning Values Clarification.* San Diego: Pennant, 1975.

10. Raths, L.E., Harmin, M., and Simon, S.B. *Values and Teaching: Working with Values in the Classroom*, 2nd ed. Columbus: Merrill Publishing Co., 1978, p. 47. Also note critique of values clarification in MacDonald, J.P. "A look at the Kohlberg curriculum and framework for moral education." In Munsey, B. *Moral Development, Moral Education and Kohlberg.* Birmingham, AL: Religious Education Press, 1980, p. 398. Also cf. Rest, J. "Developmental psychology and value education." In Munsey, p. 103.

11. Steele, S.M., and Harmon, V.M. *Values Clarification in Nursing*, pp. 1, 13. Barry, V. *Moral Aspects of Health Care.* Belmont, CA: Wadsworth: 182, pp. 39–42.

12. Simon and Clark, *Beginning Values Clarification.*

13. Steele and Harmon, *Values Clarification in Nursing*, p. 13. Brody, *Ethical Decisions in Medicine*, pp. 15, 294.

14. Hall, B.P. *Value Clarification as a Learning Process.* New York: Paulist Press, 1973. Barry, *Moral Aspects of Health Care*, pp. 23–32.

15. Bahm, A.J. *Axiology: The Science of Values.* Albuquerque: World Books, 1980, p. 5.

16. Bahm, *Axiology: The Science of Values*, p. 10.

17. Note Kohlberg's disagreement with the educational ideology of cultural transmission and socialization of values discussed in Chapter Three.

18. Steele and Harmon, *Values Clarification in Nursing.* Uustal, *Values and Ethics Considerations in Nursing Practice.* Hall, *Value Clarification as a Learning Process.* Simon and Clark, *Beginning Values Clarification.*

19. Aiken, H.D. *Reason and Moral Conduct.* New York: Knopf, 1962.

20. Steele and Harmon, *Values Clarification in Nursing*, p. 15.

21. Simon and Clark, *Beginning Values Clarification.* Brody adds that "we will act better in the long run if we get into the habit of making our values explicit and of being ready to examine our values critically." In *Ethical Decisions in Medicine*, p. 294.

22. Steele and Harmon, *Values Clarification in Nursing*, p. 7.

23. Steele and Harmon, *Values Clarification in Nursing*, pp. 18–22.

24. Aroskar, M.A. "Are nurses' mind sets compatible with ethical nursing practice?" *Topics in Clinical Nursing* 4(1):24, April 1982. Payton, R.J. "Pluralistic ethical decision making." *Clinical and Scientific Sessions 1979.* Kansas City, MO: ANA, 1979, p. 14. Other health care providers agree with the fourth mind set as compatible with ethical health care practice.

25. Fry, S.T. "Dilemmas in community health ethics." *Nursing Outlook* 31(3):177, May–June 1983.

26. ANA, *Code for Nurses.* ANA, *Perspectives on the Code for Nurses.* Kansas City, MO: ANA, 1978.

27. International Council of Nurses, *Code for Nurses Ethical Concepts Applied to Nursing.* Geneva, Switzerland: ICN, 1973.

28. Davis, A.J. "Compassion, suffering, morality: Ethical dilemmas in caring." *Nursing Law and Ethics* 2(5):1–2, 6, 8, May 1981. Carper, B.A. "The ethics of caring." *Advances in Nursing Science* 1(3):11–19, April 1979.

29. Levine, M.E. "Nursing ethics and the ethical nurse." *AJN* 77(5):845, May 1977.

PART II
A Bioethical Decision Model

The essence of this text is the description of a decision model for nurses facing the ethical dimensions of professional practice. The model was developed by the authors and has been successfully used by a variety of health care professionals. It is pluralistic in nature, allowing for differences in personal and professional values and for change over time in one's view of what constitutes ethical practice in health care. The theoretical basis of the model is moral reasoning—a critical inquiry into the ethical dimensions of health care with awareness that one may agree or disagree with others during the process. The ten-step model for decision making represents a *process* rather than a fail-safe formula for choosing the right or best alternative for action.

The simple-minded use of the notions of "right or wrong" is one of the chief obstacles to the progress of understanding.

—*Alfred North Whitehead*

CHAPTER 5
The Decision Model

Decision making in health and illness care ethics ideally is a reasoning process. It ends in the choice of a morally justifiable action to be taken in a given situation. A necessary corollary to making ethical decisions is that the persons involved understand and accept responsibility for the consequences of the action(s) decided upon.

The following description of ethical decision making is concerned with (1) critical inquiry or moral reasoning, (2) decision theory that may be applied in analyzing a situation as well as identifying and selecting alternative actions, (3) elements of moral development and ethical theory that are helpful in identifying the ethical issues in a situation and that may be used in morally justifying a given action, and (4) evaluation of the action taken as well as the process that led to that action. This chapter provides a brief description of each of these and summarizes the theoretical bases of the decision model presented here.

CRITICAL INQUIRY AND REASONED ANALYSIS

It could be redundant to discuss reasoned analysis with health care professionals. After all, do not all clinical judgments demand a reasoned approach? Certainly all decisions in health and illness care should be made after careful analysis and reasoning. In practice, this is not always the case. One of the more obvious situations where reasoned analysis is limited or nonexistent is during an emergency. Reasoning requires time, and time is very limited in an emergency. At these times, response is based on years of training and past exposure to similar emergencies. Reasoning is also limited when individuals, through apathy, boredom, or lack of ambition, provide care by rote with little thought for individual needs and concerns. Neither of these situations provides the optimum for reasoning. However, while action is necessary in emergencies, reflection should come afterward. The second example of unexamined professional practice is unethical. It may be detrimental to the welfare of the patient. It violates the autonomy and dignity of the individual as well as patient rights and professional duties.[1]

Moral reasoning is the critical examination of a situation involving moral or ethical issues by analyzing, weighing, justifying, choosing, and evaluating competing reasons for a given action.[2] Current issues in health and illness care ethics include dilemmas about which responsible persons have varying views. A reasoned approach for deciding what should be done can help provide the best care for the patient. Moral reasoning can help to sort out the goods and harms of alternative actions in patient care. It provides an opportunity to discuss values and determine the moral justification for a chosen action.

Analysis helps the participants to examine a given situation, sort out the ethical issues, and consider possible actions.[3] The weighing function assesses the strengths and weaknesses of alternatives. The justifying aspect of moral reasoning encourages participants to provide sufficient reason based on principles for the alternative actions. Ideally, the selection of a morally justifiable action comes after consideration of the alternatives and weighing the risks/ benefits, goods/harms. One may decide to take no action when proposed actions are seen as unethical. Taking no action is also a decision with ethical components.

It may be that more than one action is morally defensible in a situation. The final choice may consider a hierarchy of values, such as the patient's autonomy or a consensus of participants (team decision making). The final aspect of moral reasoning is evaluation. This means reexamining the choices in relation to the results. Were the results correctly anticipated? Is further consideration necessary? Are there aspects of this situation that may be helpful in other cases or for future reference?

Moral reasoning takes time and effort. It can be time well spent in gaining better care for clients and a more professional practice. Some reasoning can take place even in emergency situations. Reflection after the fact can still have value in future emergencies. How a given professional responds to an emergency situation is probably a combination of personal values, professional expertise, and the condition of the patient. Moral reasoning expands these considerations to include the values of the patient, society, and the larger concerns of religion and philosophy. It avoids the unconscious imposition of one's personal values on others.

There are several reasons why moral reasoning has often been left out of clinical decision making. One has been the professional's lack of awareness that most, if not all, such decisions have an ethical component.[4] The very nature of the patient–professional relationship is moral. Clinical judgment has often been the justification used by physician or nurse to avoid or deny input from patient/client or client family. After all, does not the physician or nurse know what is best for the patient?[5] The reasoning here is that the professional has specialized knowledge by or from education and practice that provides the basis for competent decisions in health and illness care. The patient and family presumably do not have this knowledge or expertise. It is important to note, however, that the physician or nurse may not have any more expertise to make ethical decisions than the client/family.

Brody[6] adds that people trained in science frequently try to solve ethical problems simply by accumulating more and more scientific data (tests, and so on). They ignore the need to make value judgments and think the mere accumulation of data can solve any empirical questions. One can spend days and weeks gathering such data without coming to grips with the need to examine values and make a value judgment. The gathering of data is not wrong, and, indeed, data are necessary for value judgments. However, the ethical dilemma will continue until such valuing takes place.

In recent years, health care professionals have begun to seek assistance in ethical decision making from their philosophical/theological colleagues trained in biomedical ethics.[7] We have once again learned the importance of collaboration as we reach the limits of expertise that any one person can claim. Knowledge in health care continues to expand at a rapid pace, and we often have to work hard just to maintain expertise in a circumscribed area of nursing or medicine. Availability of colleagues with expertise in bioethics, whether or not they are health professionals, is a valuable asset to health care and ethical decision making. Nurses and physicians are improving in their ability and willingness to ask for help with some of the difficult ethical issues in practice. We do not always know what is best for a patient, and yet we are willing to learn.

Health professionals have increasingly recognized the ability of clients to understand their illnesses when time and effort are taken to explain them. An increase in societal mistrust of health professionals (a willingness to question treatment and decisions) and an eagerness to want to know what is wrong and how it can be fixed have lent support to the ethical concepts of self-determination and informed consent in health care.[8] Health care knowledge can be transmitted, and clients can also participate knowledgeably in decisions affecting them. Both parties to such decisions need to recognize the importance of taking responsibility not only for the informed decisions but also for the consequences.[9]

In summary, moral reasoning provides an alternative to intuitionism and casuistry in making ethical decisions in health and illness care.[10] It provides a vehicle for examining how such decisions should be made, including orderly steps so that important details will not be overlooked. It is a process for determining the rightness or wrongness of a proposed action before it is tried out on the patient/client. However, it is important to realize that moral reasoning alone will not automatically produce correct answers to ethical questions and dilemmas.[11] It is a process that helps guide intelligent, responsible human beings toward ethical actions, although the path may be fraught with disagreements, frustrations, and indecision at times.

> *To the rational being only the irrational is unendurable.*
>
> —*Epictetus*

DECISION THEORIES FOR HEALTH PROFESSIONALS

Various decision theories have been proposed for helping professionals make bioethical decisions.[12] This may be a very difficult and confusing area of study. We are examining how people make choices, ethical choices in particular. The various theories explain the process in different ways. An understanding of the theories can, in turn, help to analyze a given situation and find alternatives for action. Health care professionals often think in quantifiable or mathematical terms. Thus, final selection of an alternative may be based on mathematical probabilities. It may also be an intuitive guess, or it may be a reasoned decision for what is best. There are basic concerns raised when looking at decision theories that will help one understand and make ethical decisions in health and illness care. One concern is whether it is possible to quantify ethical concerns in the same way that one might quantify the value of an automobile or a home.[13]

Decision theory has its roots in mathematics. Powerful mathematical tools, such as calculus, were formulated in the late 1600s. Probability theory was developed in the mid-1700s. These tools led many scientists to believe that even human behavior could be explained with mathematics.[14] Recent publications in bioethical decision making include some aspects of probability theory. These are applied to the weighing of values attached to proposed actions. These include cross matrix impact analysis and decision trees that represent a quantitative approach to decision making.[15] Decision trees and algorithms have been helpful to health care professionals in analyzing complex problems in patient care. Many find them helpful in ethical dilemmas as well. Individuals trained in the sciences tend to gravitate toward mathematical (quantifiable) solutions to complex problems whenever possible. We suggest that the nature of bioethical decisions, however, requires a blend of the analytical mind as well as the caring heart.[16]

Janis and Mann[17] provide three prerequisites to true decision making that help in understanding the nature of ethical decisions. They posit that first we have to feel that all obvious choices are risky, which keeps us from simply doing what feels good or right. Then we have to believe that there may be a better choice that is not so obvious so that we take the time to search for alternatives. Finally, we have to have sufficient time to look for the best and most ethical alternative. The time is spent in "vigilant information processing" that includes gathering and analyzing all the available information—the medical facts, the legal and social facts, the moral principles applicable to the situation, and the emotional and personal information relevant to the problem. It is important to note that bioethics often involves making decisions with incomplete information. This is due to the nature of human illness and our responses to it. We still must gather as much information as possible, however. In the end we make the best decision possible with the information available.

Howard Brody developed a model of ethical decision making during the 1970s that has become the foundation for many newer models in this field. This model incorporates moral reasoning, making choices from alternatives, and taking action consistent with either a deontological or utilitarian approach to ethics.[18] People often function out of various ethical systems over time. The pluralistic nature of such decisions calls for a pluralistic decision model.[19]

The model presented in this volume was developed during the late 1970s. It was designed for variety in values, differing ethical systems, and changing views over time as new knowledge and experience are gained. Decision theories helped focus the steps in the model in an orderly manner that fits most closely to the way health care professionals make decisions. Thus it is that one is encouraged to begin with an analysis of the patient situation to determine what ethical issues are present. A key step is to identify the decision(s) needed so that people involved can direct their efforts accordingly. When the ethical issues are identified, one gathers further information that will help clarify the issues as well as the values of the persons involved. Next, one is directed to define alternative actions and potential consequences so that choice can be based on critical reasoning. An important corollary in making an ethical choice is determining who can best make the choice. The model is not dependent on any one individual's deciding—it is designed so that whoever makes the final decision can follow the steps.

RECOGNIZING ETHICAL ISSUES AND DILEMMAS

The third component of decision making in health care ethics is applying ethical theory to patient situations. Ethical theory helps identify the ethical issues. It may also be used to justify a given action. For a detailed discussion of ethical theories see Chapter Two. One way to tell whether one is involved in an ethical decision is to note if the moral statement, "What ought to be done," is present. This can be represented by, "In situation X, person Y ought to do thing Z."[20] The major emphasis in this section is on recognition of an ethical dilemma.

Professional nursing is ethical. When nursing is unethical, it is unprofessional. Professional nursing practice requires the recognition of the ethical dimensions of nursing. In a discussion of the ethical aspects of nursing, someone frequently asks how one knows when one is involved in a question of ethics. In one sense, the response to this inquiry is relatively simple. All professional nursing is ethical. All decisions made with, for, or about patients or clients or other human beings have an ethical dimension.[21] However, the question may be how to identify the ethical dilemmas experienced by nurses and written about in the literature. We begin with these dilemmas while we also offer a note of caution. The lack of a dilemma or conflict in a given situation does not automatically imply that ethical action is planned or being carried out. All participants in the situation may agree on the action, but the action may still be unethical by society's or some other standard.

Criteria for a Dilemma

The nature of moral dilemmas in nursing is closely related to dilemmas in any profession. One might define a dilemma in general as a situation involving a choice between equally satisfactory or unsatisfactory alternatives or a difficult problem that seems to have no satisfactory solution.[22] For purposes of discussion throughout this text, we use the following criteria for defining moral/ethical dilemmas in nursing practice.

AWARENESS OF DIFFERENT OPTIONS. Nursing as a caring profession involves relationships with others—clients, client families, other health workers, and institutions/employers. These relationships entail duties, obligations, and loyalties that may conflict or simply present different options.[23] In an emergency situation as noted earlier, action may be based on personal value systems or a gut reaction.

Different options are a reality in health care. However, the earliest sense of an impending or actual ethical/moral dilemma may be an awareness that something is happening that is inappropriate. It may be an intellectual (cognitive dissonance) or an emotional (affective dissonance) awareness that things do not feel just right. These differences may include various opinions of what should be done and why or conflicts between or among individuals about who should make the decision and on what basis.

NATURE OF ISSUE WITH DIFFERENT OPTIONS. Not all situations that create cognitive or affective dissonance are moral or ethical dilemmas.[24] Therefore, the second criterion for recognizing an ethical dilemma in nursing practice is the determination of whether the dilemma is a matter of moral principle. Moral or ethical dilemmas in nursing may involve balancing principles. It may be the allocation of scarce resources compared with individual client autonomy. There may be differences of opinion on what should or ought to be done. There may be a conflict between personal and professional value systems (Chapter Four). For example, one might believe in client self-determination (autonomy) yet be unwilling to support the client's decision for suicide.

Smith and Davis elaborate on the nature of ethical dilemmas for nurses. They use five categories: (1) conflicts between two ethical principles one holds, (2) conflicts between two possible actions in which there are some reasons for and against the same action, (3) conflicts between a demand for action and the need for time to reflect on a situation not previously encountered, (4) conflicts between two equally unsatisfactory alternatives, and (5) conflicts between one's ethical principles and one's obligations as a nurse.[25]

TWO OR MORE ANSWERS WITH TRUE CHOICE.

TWO OR MORE ANSWERS WITH TRUE CHOICE. In one sense, a dilemma is obvious. We live with dilemmas on a frequent and perhaps daily basis. Shall I wear the blue outfit or the brown one? Shall we have hamburger for supper or macaroni and cheese? Ethical dilemmas involve choices in terms of principles or actions or some related moral concern.[26] The final criterion for recognizing an ethical dilemma, therefore, is the existence of choice between or among alternative actions that are possible and available to participants.

For many people, moral or ethical choices are a matter of hierarchy. We might recognize a lie as wrong, but if it meant saving the life of a friend, many would not hesitate to lie. It is the small wrong for a greater good. In utilitarian terms, the end justifies the means. Sometimes we think we have a choice between only two political candidates. We may not think much of either so we choose the lesser of two evils. When there is a difference in the hierarchy of values involved, some would say we do not have a true dilemma. Most of us, however, would rather have a good candidate for whom to vote, and many people would rather not tell a lie. For some then, such choices remain a dilemma whether it is a true dilemma or not. From this negative perspective, Patricia Crisham calls moral dilemmas "problems with two equally unacceptable alternatives."[27]

Another choice comes between two goods. Again, if there is a hierarchy, some would claim there is no true dilemma. However, if the two goods are equal in weight, we are faced with that true dilemma. Some believe that these true dilemmas are rare. Something in the situation tips the scale and weighs one option heavier than another. As one writer put it, other things being equal, we have a dilemma in choosing between these options.[28] But it is very rare that all things are equal. In an absolutist system of ethics, principles and rules tend to be weighted equally. Dilemmas may arise more often when principles conflict with one another, but even in one-principle systems, it is not always easy to know what to do. Fletcher's situation ethics suggests that the situation will tell us what to do. He suggests that we do the loving thing, a concept in accord with the Judeo–Christian and other religious traditions, but in real life, it is not always crystal clear just what is the loving thing to do.[29]

Physicians have in the past claimed a "therapeutic privilege." The illness is terminal, but they do not want to say that for fear the patient will lose the will to live. So the physician fudges or simply lies to the patient and perhaps to the family as well, or the family may be told the truth, but they do not want the patient to know. Nurses often get caught in the middle of this kind of exchange. Patients may ask the nurse. They suspect they are not being told the truth, or they are afraid to bother the doctor. In times past the nurse was to respond, "You'll have to ask your doctor." Public opinion polls show an enormous change in physician attitudes toward telling terminally ill patients the truth. Where it was once about 85 percent against telling the patient, it is now about 45 percent for telling the patient,[30] but such dilemmas continue. They may be stronger because of the growing recognition that nursing is a profession. Professionals are ethical, which means that nurses have a responsibility to tell the truth. Some nurses do—all too quickly and even brutally. There are other principles, such as mercy and compassion, and there are gentle and harsh ways of telling the truth. Therefore, the dilemma is not simply a blind following of a principle. It is also a matter of how the principle is upheld.

Occasionally such problems reach the literature. Nurse Tuma was asked about alternative methods of treatment, and it was obvious that the physician had not informed the patient about these. The nurse fulfilled the principle of informed consent. She was fired for interfering with the doctor–patient relationship. The literature did not point out that the physician had violated the concept of informed consent, nor did the source suggest that he should have been fired for his unethical/unprofessional conduct and illegal care. The courts sidestepped the issues by claiming the state practice act for nursing was too vague, and, therefore, Nurse Tuma should be reinstated.[31] There are other examples of nurses who chose to keep quiet and keep their jobs. They reasoned that choosing that side of the dilemma allowed them to continue their practice. Thus they might be quietly effective in promoting a more ethical health care system. Davis and Aroskar note that this dilemma raises the very real question, "Can nurses be ethical?"[32] As an absolute, one can say, "No"; that is, nurses cannot be absolutely ethical all the time any more than anyone else can be. We choose what we hope is best in the situation, and then, hopefully, we keep on trying to be ethical or as ethical as possible thereafter.

Patients have a right to know.[33] It is a matter of autonomy, self-determination, informed consent, their right to accept or refuse a given treatment, truthfulness. However, most nurses need their jobs even as most of them also want to practice with integrity and in an ethical way. What is in the best interest of the patient as well as the nurse? To what extent can paternalism or maternalism be exercised by health care providers? When a patient is too ill to participate in her or his care, current ethics calls for the participation of the family in decision making.[34] If the family is not available or in an emergency situation, the health care providers may have to use their best judgment without benefit of knowing what the patient thinks is best. When time permits, the team approach shares that decision making among nurses, physicians, and others.

Whether on a moment's notice, over time, individually, or as a group, nurses are faced with the problem of how to make ethical decisions. How do we make such decisions? The ten-step model presented here is designed to aid in the process of ethical decision making.

EVALUATION OF PROCESS AND OUTCOME

The final component of bioethical decision making involves looking at the results of the choice made. Was the outcome what was intended? People may decide that an alternative should be chosen. The first did not work as planned or the patient's condition changed, and a different decision may now be indicated. In addition, we suggest that one determine whether the moral reasoning process was carried out. Was any knowledge gained from the current problem that may be helpful in future situations?

Evaluation of ethical decisions provides feedback and reinforcement of positive reasoning patterns. Ethical decisions in nursing practice are often difficult. We do not always like the results of the decisions. However, such decisions are a reality, as is responsibility for the consequences of the decisions made. It may be helpful to remember the responsibility. The temptation is to fall prey to the adolescent demands for self-determination without responsibility for one's actions. Being accountable for one's professional practice is central to the provision of good care for clients. The addition of ethical decision making helps to insure that such care will be the best that one can provide.

A BIOETHICAL DECISION MODEL

We developed the decision model (process) that follows using critical inquiry and moral reasoning. Steps One through Seven are part of the analyzing process. Step Eight includes the weighing and justifying processes. Step Nine is the choice, and Step Ten is the evaluation. This model is based on the importance of raising the proper questions for analysis while following a step-by-step reasoning process. It is a process for working through a variety of clinical situations by gathering and analyzing relevant information prior to deciding upon a course of action. This is not a model of decision making that will result in the correct answers by mere mechanical application. We realize that there are differences and varying values in how intelligent, rational people make ethical and moral choices in our pluralistic society. These differences also exist in that microcosm of society, the hospital or other health care setting.

We propose the following model for use in identifying and analyzing the ethical dimensions and dilemmas in nursing practice. The model is theoretically based in ethical systems of thought, stages of moral development, and values clarification. It is practically based on recognition of when one is facing a moral/ethical dilemma or dimension of practice so that the model can be put into action. Each step of the model will be described in detail in the following chapters.

An additional note is offered about the use of this or any other decision model or process in health and illness care ethics. We recognize that how, when, and whether a nurse or any other health care professional uses moral reasoning is related to the time available in a situation. It is also related to the value a person attaches to critical inquiry and bioethical decision making. We mentioned these points earlier in this text, but they bear repeating. As Aroskar has noted, nurses may value critical reasoning differently. Some may decide that reflective thinking prior to taking action is valuable. Others prefer to justify their decisions and actions after the fact.[35]

Our decision model is offered to encourage nurses to critically examine ethical situations at all times, but preferably prior to making a decision when time permits. Even when situations are critically analyzed after the fact, however, the participants can learn. They may be able to rationally determine the appropriate and inappropriate of the past. They may also gain insight that will help them make ethical decisions in the future. Timing in the use of this decision model will reflect the user's value position on moral reasoning. However, the fact that it is used is probably the more important consideration.

Conditions for Use of the Model

The final caveat for the use of the model in this text is the need for understanding the nature of the setting in which it is used. We have used the model for years with groups of professionals, though individual use has also been encouraged. Since the very essence of moral reasoning involves disclosure of one's thought processes and personal values, there are a few conditions that are important to its success. First, all participants in the group are encouraged to be truthful in their responses to each step. In order for such veracity to be supported, an environment of trust, confidentiality, and mutual respect is needed. This means that each member of the discussion group listens carefully to others, tries to understand what is being said, and accepts those statements as representing what the other person believes or values. Confidentiality implies that values and positions shared will be kept within the confines of the discussion group and not shared outside the group without consent. Respect implies acceptance of others but not necessarily agreement with them. In situations of disagreement, respect involves stating that disagreement clearly without implying that the other position is necessarily right or wrong (passing judgment). The nature of moral reasoning encourages discussion. This includes disagreement as well as mutual searching for the reasons behind each individual's beliefs/values so that further understanding of ethical pluralism in our society results. The group works toward possible consensus for decision and action. Individuals need to be aware that, at times, their personal value position may not be the one used to determine action. Once again respect implies that even when I cannot personally support the final choice of action, I will have learned about and understood an alternative perspective.

In the following chapters we present the bioethical decision model developed to facilitate moral reasoning in nursing practice. A list of the ten steps follows:

A Bioethical Decision Model*

Step One	Review the situation to determine health problems, decision needed, ethical components, and key individuals
Step Two	Gather additional information to clarify situation
Step Three	Identify the ethical issues in the situation
Step Four	Define personal and professional moral positions
Step Five	Identify moral positions of key individuals involved
Step Six	Identify value conflicts, if any
Step Seven	Determine who should make the decision
Step Eight	Identify range of actions with anticipated outcomes
Step Nine	Decide on a course of action and carry it out
Step Ten	Evaluate/review results of decision/action

*Thompson, J.B., and Thompson, H.O. Ethics in Nursing. New York: Macmillan, 1981, with permission.

NOTES

1. Francouer, R.T. *An Operational Decision Workbook for Biomedical Ethics.* Madison, NJ: Fairleigh Dickinson University, 1977, 1979, p. 6.
2. Harron, F., Burnside, J., and Beauchamp, T.L. *Health and Human Values: A Guide to Making Your Own Decisions.* New Haven: Yale University Press, 1983, p. 4. Beauchamp, T.L., and Childress, J.F. *Principles of Biomedical Ethics,* 2nd ed. New York: Oxford University Press, 1983, p. 3–6. Howard Brody states that moral reasoning prevents a moral free-for-all by insisting that no one can claim ethical validity for his statements until he has subjected them to rigorous and rational analysis. Brody, H. *Ethical Decisions in Medicine.* Boston: Little, Brown, 1976, p. 16.
3. Brody, *Ethical Decisions in Medicine.* Callahan, D., and Bok, S. *Ethics Teaching in Higher Education.* New York: Plenum Press, 1980, p. 67. Murphy, E.A. "Decision making, medical." EB 1:307, 1978.
4. Thompson, J.B., and Thompson, H.O. *Ethics in Nursing.* New York: Macmillan, 1981, p. 2. Brody, *Ethical Decisions in Medicine,* p. 7. Payton, R. "Pluralistic ethical decision making." *Clinical and Scientific Sessions.* Kansas City: ANA,

1979, p. 11. Fromer, M.J. "Solving ethical dilemmas in nursing practice." *Topics in Clinical Nursing* 4(1):15, April 1982.

5. Carlton, W. *"In Our Professional Opinion . . ." The Primacy of Clinical Judgment Over Moral Choice.* Notre Dame: University of Notre Dame Press, 1978. Murphy, E. A. "Decision making, medical," p. 307. Aroskar, M.A. "Anatomy of an ethical dilemma: The practice." *AJN* 80(4):661, April 1980, states, "Technical expertise cannot be generalized to the moral or ethical dimensions of a situation."

6. Brody, *Ethical Decisions in Medicine*, p. 7.

7. Harron et al., *Health and Human Values*, p. xii. Jonsen, A.R., Siegler, M., and Winslade, W.I. *Clinical Ethics*. New York: Macmillan, 1982.

8. Bandman, E., and Bandman, B. "There is nothing automatic about rights." *AJN* 77 (5):867–872, May 1977. Barry, V. *Moral Aspects of Health Care*. Belmont, CA: Wadsworth, 1982, pp. 164–200. American Hospital Association. *Statement on a Patient's Bill of Rights*. Chicago: AHA, 1972.

9. Callahan and Bok, *Ethics Teaching in Higher Education*, p. 66, note that ethical analysis cannot be separated from a sense of moral obligation. They go on to say that individuals are free to make moral choices but they are also responsible for the choices they make.

10. Brody, *Ethical Decisions in Medicine*, p. 16. Harron et al., *Health and Human Values*, p. xii. Francouer, R.T. *Biomedical Ethics, A Guide to Decision Making*. New York: John Wiley & Sons, 1983, p. 83.

11. Aroskar, M.A. "Anatomy of an ethical dilemma: The theory." *AJN* 80(4):659, April 1980. Harron et al., *Health and Human Values*, p. 4.

12. Hill, P., et al. *Making Decisions: A Multidisciplinary Introduction*. Reading, MA: Addison-Wesley, 1978. Aroskar, "Anatomy of an ethical dilemma: The theory," p. 660. Sigman, P. "Ethical choice in nursing." *Advances in Nursing Science* 1:38–41, April 1979.

13. Tarlov, A.R. "The increasing supply of physicians, the changing structure of the health-services system, and the future practice of medicine." *New England Journal of Medicine* 308 (20):1242, May 1983.

14. Guillen, M.A. "Behavior by the numbers." *Psychology Today* 17 (11):77, November 1983.

15. Francouer, *Biomedical Ethics, A Guide to Decision Making*, pp. 119–137.

16. Midgley, M. *Heart and Mind: The Varieties of Moral Experience*. New York: St. Martin's Press, 1981, p. 12. Callahan and Bok, *Ethics Teaching in Higher Education*, p. 65.

17. Janis, I.L., and Mann, L. *Decision Making: A Psychological Analysis of Conflict, Choice, and Commitment*. New York: Free Press, 1977.

18. Brody, *Ethical Decisions in Medicine*, pp. 11, A2a, A2b.

19. Payton, "Pluralistic ethical decision making," pp. 11–16.

20. Brody, *Ethical Decisions in Medicine*, p. 6.

21. Thompson and Thompson, *Ethics in Nursing*, p. 2. Aroskar, M.A. "Are nurses' mind sets compatible with ethical nursing practice?" *Topics in Clinical Nursing* 4(1):22–23, April 1982.

22. Aroskar, M.A., et al. "ANS open forum: The most pressing ethical problems faced by nurses." *Advances in Nursing Science* 1:89–99, April 1979. Churchill, L. "Ethical issues of a profession in transition." *AJN* 77(5):873–875, May 1977. Fromer, M.J. *Ethical Issues in Health Care*. St. Louis: Mosby, 1981. Curtin, L., and Flaherty, M.J. *Nursing Ethics: Theories and Pragmatics*. Bowie, MD: Brady, 1982.

23. Jameton, A. "The nurse: When roles and rules conflict." *Hastings Center Report (HCR)* 7:22–23, August 1977. Smith, S.J., and Davis, A.J. "Ethical dilemmas: Conflicts among rights, duties and obligations." *AJN* 80(8):1465–1466, August 1980. Murphy, C.P. "Models of the nurse–patient relationship." In Murphy, C.P., Hunter, H. (eds). *Ethical Problems in the Nurse-Patient Relationship*. Boston: Allyn Bacon, 1982. Beauchamp and Childress, *Principles of Biomedical Ethics*, Chap. 8, "Ideals, virtues, and conscientious actions." pp. 255–280. Brock, D.W. "The nurse–patient relation: Some rights and duties." In Spicker, S.F., and Gadow, S. (eds). *Nursing: Images and Ideals*. New York: Springer, 1980, pp. 108–124.

24. Davis, A.J., and Aroskar, M.A. *Ethical Dilemmas and Nursing Practice*, 2nd ed. Norwalk, CT: Appleton-Century-Crofts, 1983, pp. 6–8. Beauchamp and Childress, *Principles of Biomedical Ethics*, p. 14.

25. Smith and Davis, "Ethical dilemmas: Conflicts among rights, duties and obligations," p. 1463–1464.

26. Rosen, B. "Moral dilemmas and their treatment." In Munsey, B. (ed). *Moral Development, Moral Education, and Kohlberg*. Birmingham, AL: Religious Education Press, 1980, pp. 232–265. Davis and Aroskar, *Ethical Dilemmas and Nursing Practice*. Aroskar, "Anatomy of an ethical dilemma: the theory," pp. 658–660.

27. Crisham, P. "Measuring moral judgment in nursing dilemmas." *Nursing Research* 30(2)104–110, March–April 1981.

28. Ladd, J. "Ethics: the task of ethics." *EB* 1:404, 1978.

29. Davis and Aroskar, *Ethical Dilemmas and Nursing Practice*, p. 2.

30. President's Commission, *Making Health Care Decisions*. Vol. II. *Appendices*. Washington, DC: US Government Printing Office, October 1982, p. 223.

31. "Jolene Tuma wins: Court rules practice act did not define unprofessional conduct." *Nursing Outlook* 27:376, June 1979.

32. Davis and Aroskar, *Ethical Dilemmas and Nursing Practice*, p. 54.

33. Kelly, L.Y. "Legal aspects of patient's rights and unethical nursing practice." In Thompson and Thompson, *Ethics in Nursing*, pp. 211–232.

34. President's Commission, *Making Health Care Decisions*. Vol. II, p. 5.

35. Aroskar, "Anatomy of an ethical dilemma: The practice," p. 663.

Technical expertise cannot be generalized to the moral and ethical dimensions of a situation.

Mila A. Aroskar, RN[1]

CHAPTER 6
Step One: Review the Situation

The following case will be reviewed for each of the 10 steps of the decision-making process. It will be considered at the end of each chapter to show how the step just discussed can be applied to a specific case. The same case throughout will give continuity to the ten steps as we move through them. In Appendix A a case will be analyzed as a whole.

BIRTH OF A FAMILY

Case Study

G.W. was the student nurse–midwife caring for Sara, a woman having her first child in a large tertiary care setting. Sara's husband, Tom, was her principal support person. The labor progressed rapidly and Sara was prepared for delivery. Under the supervision of the nurse–midwife instructor, G.W. assisted Sara with the birth of her healthy, 7-pound son. As the infant was born, the circulating nurse stood by with a warm towel to recieve the infant. The midwifery instructor quickly asked Sara if she would like to take her newborn into her arms. Sara's response was a hesitant, "Are you sure it's okay? Can I?" With reassurance from the nurse–midwife, Sara responded with a delighted, "Yes!"

The nurse immediately tried to take the infant away to the warmer but was asked instead to place the warm blanket over the mother and baby and help the parents dry off the infant. She refused and insisted that the infant must be taken to the warmer for heat and suctioning. As the parents lovingly dried their newborn son, the nurse–midwife gently suggested to the nurse that the infant was being kept warm by his mother's body and he was breathing well. The nurse mumbled, "I don't think we are supposed to let mothers have their babies before they are identified. I'll have to check the policies when we finish. I'm new here and don't want to get into trouble."

The way in which a health care situation is presented for discussion and analysis often determines what the final decision will be. Nurses are educated to assess, gather information, decide, and evaluate those situations in daily practice. Nurses and other health professionals are value laden.[2] The way they view the patient and the situation and the data they decide to gather before taking action reflect their values. These may also predetermine what the decision will be.[3]

The goal with the ten-step decision model is to identify, clarify, and, if necessary, change, the individual value orientations of people involved in a situation. This is especially important for the professionals whose power to decide often overrides others and whose decision may not be the best one. The model requires an orderly, step-by-step thought process, with key questions to be asked at each step. The questions are designed to guide participants through moral reasoning. They are to encourage the examination of personal and other values for the actions proposed. That examination includes the reasons for the final choice in the situation.

As noted earlier, it is recommended that the model be used in the order of the steps. It is understood that there is an overlap in many of the areas. Once one is familiar with the process, short cuts in following the steps may be taken. That is done with the understanding, however, that a critical piece of data may be missed in the process. Howard Brody suggests that ethical persons do not use moral reasoning continually. They are prepared to use it anytime when decisions require formal justification. Once a new situation has been critically examined, similar situations may require a lower level of reasoning (cf. Aiken's third level of moral discourse, i.e., moral rules).[4] We are concerned about the use of shortcuts in ethical reasoning. The novice in the field with limited experience in moral reasoning may think incorrectly that a step is not needed. As quoted earlier, technical expertise (nursing, medicine) does not automatically imply expertise in moral or ethical dimensions of health care practice. Many nurses and physicians have not had the opportunity to learn moral reasoning in their professional training.[5] This text generally and this decision model specifically are aimed at increasing the knowledge of and exposure to moral reasoning for health care professionals.

The first step in our decision model is designed to assist nurses and others involved in ethical decision making to gather data for ethical inquiry. It builds upon the first step in the nursing process, that of assessing the situation (a familiar orientation). Then it directs the nurse to specifics in the situation that begin to highlight the ethical components of the case. Patient care situations do not all involve ethical decision making to the same degree because the nature and intensity of the ethical issues vary. However, there is an ethical component in every decision in health and illness care. We welcome you on this exciting journey into critical inquiry and ethical decision making in health and illness care.

WHAT ARE THE HEALTH PROBLEMS IN THE SITUATION?

How one defines health or illness may influence how one identifies the problem(s). For many health care professionals, health is the absence of disease, and even then, there are various shades of gray in defining disease. Many physicians have been schooled in the value of curing disease at all cost, which may even include some treatments or cure efforts that are potentially more damaging than the condition itself.[6] Many nurses claim to support the value of caring as well as curing.[7] However, they define health with equal narrowness as the absence of disease. A quick look at hypertensive, overweight, or smoking health professionals belies a commitment to health in its broadest sense.

Similarly, patients bring a variety of definitions of health to the hospital or health care setting. For many people, health constitutes the ability to get out of bed each day and perform one's job. For others, just being alive is considered a state of health even though physical or mental or emotional capacities are severely limited, and there remain many who define health as broadly as the World Health Organization.[8] That definition includes physical, emotional, intellectual, economic, and social well-being. The definition of illness is also a personal value judgment.[9] It may determine when a person will seek care. Some people seek care for the slightest problem. Others come only when their condition is grave and even terminal. Many people remain somewhere in the middle.

Who Defines Health?

Who defines the health problems in the situation may also determine what decisions are needed. For example, health care providers might define the health problem as gangrene of the foot. To them, this may dictate amputation. The patient's definition of the health problem may be doing what is necessary to maintain the wholeness of the body. That may hold even if death results from lack of amputation. At once we are embroiled in a web of value judgments. These are both personal and professional and require attention as we proceed to structure the situation for analysis. We need to be aware of who defines the problems as well as how they are defined.

Values permeate each of our decision steps. It is important to begin immediately to recognize these before they unconsciously determine the final decision. We can proceed by listing the health problems. They include those identified by patient, nurse, physician, and others involved in the case at hand. This is a beginning step in formulating action alternatives. It is helpful to note when there is disagreement for further discussion in succeeding steps. This initial listing can begin to highlight the ethical components of the situation as well. Disagreements in definition of the health problems often help to clarify early in the decision process why there is an ethical dilemma at a later point.

WHAT DECISION(S) NEEDS TO BE MADE?

Once the health problems are clearly identified and listed, it is possible to more clearly identify the decision(s) needed. Aroskar[10] uses the question, "What is the proposed action(s)?" Such clarity is not always easy or apparent. Earlier, we discussed the gut-level reaction of decision making. Moral reasoning requires more from us. It means investigating and explicitly stating what we value and how we made a decision. The alternative may be to unconsciously impose faulty reasoning or personal preferences on our patients.[11]

When one asks health professionals to define the decision or decisions needed in a patient situation, the response may be negative. The temptation may be to respond from an all-knowing, gut-level, "how dare you question my authority" pose. This may be a cover-up for not knowing what to do and an unwillingness to admit it. It may be an unwillingness to share information.[12] Ethical practice requires resistance to this temptation whatever the reason. The moral reasoning process is an alternative that considers both patients and providers.[13]

Identification of the decisions needed in a specific patient situation involves focusing on what the patient or provider wants or needs. It is a listing of items to be decided upon without passing judgment. Later in the decision process, these items will need to be viewed in the light of what is possible, i.e., what patient needs can be met within the capabilities of providers, setting, and technology. Many times the decision list begins with an open question of what can be done for a patient with the identified health problem(s). We may ask the question of whether a specific treatment or action is indicated or whether no further treatment is indicated. We may be asking whether another form of treatment should be tried because the current one has been ineffective or has unwanted side effects. The final statement of decision reflects the ethical or moral component, "What should be done?"

An example of a decision identified from health problems is whether the terminally ill patient should be resuscitated in the event of cardiopulmonary arrest. This decision statement is phrased in moral language, "Should action Z (resuscitation) be carried out by person Y (nurse or physician) in situation X (this patient who has this terminal illness)?"[14] This type of decision is now easier to recognize as having an ethical component. There have been extensive media coverage and multiple articles on the subject in the past few years.

A more subtle and often missed decision with an ethical component is whether a nurse should spend time with Ms R. She has expressed a need to talk about her illness, but the nurse must tend to the other patients as well. Allocation of professional time and expertise is an ethical decision. That remains true even though it often yields to institutional rules, scheduling patterns, and personal preferences of staff.

One of the problems with identifying what decisions need to be made is that some decisions are clear and others are hidden. Needed decisions must be attended to throughout the ten-step model as new information and insight are gained during moral reasoning. The process of gathering further information, identifying ethical issues, and defining possible actions and consequences may present new decisions for consideration. Add these to your original list. The important thing to remember is that the early identification of decisions or actions needed helps one to begin to structure the situation for ethical analysis. The fact that new decisions are discovered later does not detract from the initial step. This finding serves to reinforce the idea that the process of moral reasoning does assist one in making ethical decisions. It helps to identify the unseen or unconscious elements of a situation, as well as those that appear very obvious.

WHAT ARE THE ETHICAL AND SCIENTIFIC COMPONENTS OF THE DECISION(S)?

All decisions in health and illness care have an ethical component. These components can be clarified by separating the ethical and scientific elements of the case.[15] It is a way for health care providers to learn to identify the ethical dimensions of a clinical situation. This can also help personnel become sensitized to moral dilemmas in clinical practice. The criteria for dilemmas were discussed in Chapter Five.

Listing the scientific components of decisions may reveal some difficulty in separating these from the ethical or moral dimensions of the decision. What form of contraception is best for a 40-year-old woman who smokes two packs of cigarettes a day? One's scientific knowledge base suggests discarding oral contraceptives. The data on oral contraceptives present a risk/benefit ratio. These oral contraceptives cannot be purchased over the counter, so she is dependent on a person with the authority to write prescriptions. Whether she receives the prescription will depend on the willingness of both the woman and the health care provider to take the risk of potential harm in relation to the benefit of not getting pregnant. Initially, this seemed to be a clearly scientific matter. Now it can be seen as also involving moral considerations, such as autonomy, informed consent, accountability, the Hippocratic principles of do good and do no harm. Many situations in health care practice are similar to this—an interface of ethics, science, and even the law (in this case licensing for prescription writing). (Contraception was itself a legal issue for much of human history and remains so in some areas. For numbers of groups, contraception is unethical, as is smoking. The patient in this case presumably does not belong to such groups or at least feels free to seek oral contraceptives. Among other ethical dimensions there is also the question of alternative methods such as a tubal ligation.[16])

Attempts to separate the scientific from the ethical components of the decisions needed help one to clarify the ethical questions. The language of rights, responsibilities, duties, and obligations begins to appear in the ethical questions.[17] The early questions with "should" and "ought" can be further elaborated in an attempt to more clearly focus the discussion that follows. For example, the general question of "What should be done in this situation?" has now become several questions. "Should the patient be allowed to decide for X treatment? What rights do the family, physician, or others have in such a situation? What responsibility does the nurse have to support the patient's decision? What other possible treatments might be indicated for this patient?" This list could continue, but it is probably sufficient to illustrate the value of stating needed decisions as clearly as possible as one begins the analysis of a patient situation.

WHAT INDIVIDUALS ARE INVOLVED/AFFECTED BY THE DECISION(S)?

One of the lessons from decision theory is that as one prepares to make a decision, it is important to identify who is involved or will be affected by the decision to be made.[18] We place this component of critical inquiry early in our decision model in recognition of its importance in the decision process. It is also important to note that by the very consideration of more than one individual we are accepting the societal context of individuals living in relationship to other individuals. It is rare, if ever, that a decision in health care affects only one person. What is more common is that individuals will have greater or lesser involvement or investment in the decision or its consequences. The extent of involvement or investment becomes crucial as we approach Step Seven and the determination of who should make the final choice. At this early phase of situation analysis, however, it is helpful to identify all the persons who should be involved or will be affected by the decision.

The list of individuals always includes the patient and may include family members, physicians, nurses, friends, clergy, social workers, lawyers. When one is involved in the heat of a difficult patient situation, the temptation is to concentrate solely on the patient, immediate family, and primary provider. However, decisions about individuals in the hospital or health setting often affect other patients, the institution, and other staff, as well as society as a whole. There is some disagreement as to how far one might extend the list of participants in a patient care situation. One suggestion is the consideration of larger policy issues at the institutional and societal levels. One may decide to weigh these very lightly or not at all in the final analysis, but ethical reasoning requires their consideration at a conscious level.[19]

An important consideration when deciding which individuals are involved includes recognition of the competence or capacity of each regarding decision making. The first-level decision about who to include is everyone who might have a stake in the outcome as well as being affected by the decision. If the patient is unconscious, one should at least try to understand what that person would prefer. For comatose patients one needs to include someone, therefore, who can speak on behalf of the patient. In the past, physicians held that when patients were unable to speak for themselves (provided they were asked for input), the physician was probably the best one to decide what should be done. Current societal ethics do not unequivocably support the physician as decision maker in such situations.[20]   We discuss this further in Chapter 12.

One final note regarding choice of participants involved in ethical decision making is indicated. Some have suggested that only key individuals in a situation be allowed to participate in the analysis and decision making. It is quickly noted that the definition of "key" carries a value judgment just as do all other components of the decision model. At this early stage, the list should at least be maximized rather than minimized. This allows for expansion of one's ethical thinking to society and policy levels, though not all will be in positions to make those kind of decisions. When the time comes to determine who should make the actual decision, value judgments on key individuals may be indicated. It is easy to see that no one person can speak on behalf of all society. Utilitarian concerns of the world may not help make the decision for one individual today. Once again, we suggest that these larger concerns are important in ethical inquiry. They may or may not influence the decision we are about to make at the moment.

SUMMARY

The first step of the decision model has been concerned with identifying significant components in the situation at hand. Preparing the list of decisions and actors will facilitate each of the following steps in moral reasoning. It has also hopefully expanded the knowledge of participants about what constitutes a situation for analysis. That includes the ethical and scientific components of clinical decisions, value and time considerations, and preparation needed for ethical decision making. Building upon the data compiled in this first step, we are now ready to proceed to Step Two, Gathering Further Information, but before we move to Step Two, this is how Step One might proceed in "Birth of A Family."

THE CASE

What Are the Health Problems in the Situation?

The most obvious health problem defined by the nurse–midwife in this situation was the emotional and psychological element of parent–infant bonding, providing the parents wished to do so. The circulating nurse's definition appears to be support for the infant's transition to extrauterine life, including a clear airway and maintenance of body temperature. The birth itself might be viewed as a health problem if the parents or professionals see pregnancy and birth as an illness or a health problem. The health of the infant is often an unknown until the infant is born and makes the successful transition to air breathing.

What Decision(s) Needs To Be Made?

The initial decision made after the delivery of this infant and a quick assessment of his health status was what to do with the infant. The nurse was waiting to receive him. The midwifery instructor decided to ask Sara if she wanted to hold her son. When Sara said "Yes," the student decided (or simply followed the instructor's direction) to give her the infant. The next decision was how long and under what conditions Sara and Tom could continue to hold their son. The nurse made a decision on whether to leave the infant with the mother or insist on having the child. She left the child but decided on a mild protest. The student decided to let the instructor decide (see Step 5).

What Are the Ethical and Scientific Components of the Decision(s)?

The ethical components include informed choice by professionals and parents, treating parents, infant, and professional colleagues with respect, and consideration of the rights, duties, and obligations of all participants in this birth. The professionals have the duty or obligation to promote health and well-being for Sara, Tom, and their son. They also have a duty to offer patient choice or participation in decisions that are available to them. The nurse–midwife viewed the situation as offering more choices for the parents than the circulating nurse did. However, one might raise the question of whether the nurse–midwife had an obligation to follow hospital policy if it, indeed, said that infants cannot be handed to parents until identified. This policy was not in effect, however, and the new nurse had a responsibility to know those policies as she was oriented to the labor area. One could suggest that the nurse–midwife had a professional responsibility to share this information with her nurse colleague, and vice versa if there was such a policy. If the nurse needed to complete her duties with this couple in order to care for others, the allocation of the scarce resource of her time is an ethical consideration.

The scientific components of the decision to offer Sara her newborn considered the successful transition and healthy status of the infant as well as the need to dry and warm him to prevent hypothermia. The scientific bases for how long Sara might continue to hold her newborn would include ongoing health, breathing and warmth of the infant, and safety of the position on the mother if uncomfortable or painful procedures still remained to be done (e.g., placental delivery, episiotomy repair).

What Individuals Are Involved or Affected by the Decision(s)?

Sara, Tom, the infant, G.W., the midwifery instructor, the student, and the circulating nurse are the most immediate individuals involved in this situation. However, if either or both professionals have responsibilities to care for other individuals in the labor area, these others could also be affected by how long Sara holds the infant and keeps the nurse from identifying, weighing, and treating the infant's eyes (her official duties). Some may also add that all future patients in this setting might be affected by the decision to let Sara hold her infant if they now know it is possible to do so. The nursing supervisor and other nurses on the unit may also be affected by the midwife's decision. They may have to care for the patient(s) waiting for this nurse or spend time dealing with other patients' requests to follow this pattern. The student's future patients will be affected also if she chooses to follow this pattern or does not.

NOTES

1. Aroskar, M.A. "Anatomy of an ethical dilemma: The practice." *AJN* 80(4):661, April 1980.
2. Steele, S., and Harmon, V. *Values Clarification in Nursing,* 2nd ed. Norwalk, CT: Appleton-Century-Crofts, 1983, pp. 6, 7–13. Aroskar, "Anatomy of an ethical dilemma: The theory," p. 659. Fromer, M. *Ethical Issues in Health Care.* St. Louis: Mosby, 1981, p. 15.
3. Aroskar, "Anatomy of an ethical dilemma: The practice," p. 663. Brody, H. *Ethical Decisions in Medicine.* Boston: Little, Brown, 1976, pp. 12–13. Steele and Harmon, *Values Clarification in Nursing,* pp. 13, 20.
4. Brody, *Ethical Decisions in Medicine,* p. 18. One could note, of course, the shortcut that does not leave out steps but moves more quickly through the given step when practice and insight help one see the next step more clearly.
5. Ruddick, W. "What should we teach and test?" *HCR* 13 (3):22, June 1983. Schwartz, W., et al. *American Journal of Medicine* 55:49, October 1973. Barry, V. *Moral Aspects of Health Care.* Belmont, CA: Wadsworth, 1982, p. viii. Callahan, D., and Bok, S. (eds). *Ethics Teaching in Higher Education.* New York: Plenum Press, 1980, p. 299.
6. Berkowitz, M. "The role of discussion in ethics training." *Topics in Clinical Nursing* 4(1):33, April 1982. Illich, I. *Medical Nemesis.* New York: Bantam Books, 1976. Carlton, W. *"In Our Professional Opinion . . .": The Primacy of Clinical*

Judgment Over Moral Choice. Notre Dame: University of Notre Dame Press, 1978, p. 8.

7. Carper, B. "The ethics of caring." *Advances in Nursing Science* 1:11–19, April 1979. Churchill, L. "Ethical issues of a profession in transition." *AJN* 77(5):873, May 1977. McCullough, L. "The code for nurses: A philosophical perspective." *Perspectives on the Code for Nurses*. Kansas City, MO: American Nurses Association, 1976, pp. 40–41.

8. Beauchamp, T.L., and Walters, L. (eds). "World Health Organization: A definition of health." *Contemporary Issues in Bioethics*, 2nd ed. Belmont, CA: Wadsworth, 1982, p. 48.

9. A "definition of illness is [a] personal value judgment." Steele and Harmon, *Values Clarification in Nursing*, p. 21.

10. Aroskar, "Anatomy of an ethical dilemma: The theory," p. 660.

11. Brody, *Ethical Decisions in Medicine*, p. 15. Harron, F., Burnside, J., and Beauchamp, T.L. *Health and Human Values: A Guide to Making Your Own Decisions*. New Haven: Yale University Press, 1983, p. iix.

12. Chriss, N.C. "Doctors down the logorrhea: Debakey sisters cure 'medicalese,'" *Los Angeles Times*, July 17, 1977.

13. Harron et al. *Health and Human Values*, p. 12. President's Commission, *Making Health Care Decisions*. Vol. 1. Washington, DC: US Government Printing Office, 1982, p. 6. Callahan and Bok, *Ethics Teaching in Higher Education*, pp. 72–74.

14. Brody, *Ethical Decisions in Medicine*, p. 6.

15. Stanley, Sr. T. "Ethics as a component of the curriculum." *Nursing and Health Care* 1:63–72, September 1980.

16. Thompson, J.B., and Thompson, H.O. *Ethics in Nursing*. New York: Macmillan, 1981, pp. 49–58.

17. See Smith and Davis for discussion of differentiation of legal and ethical rights, duties, and obligations. Smith, S.J., and Davis, A.J. "Ethical dilemmas: Conflicts among rights, duties and obligations." *AJN* 80(8):1463–1466, 1980.

18. Brody, *Ethical Decisions in Medicine*, p. 100. Raiffa, H. *Decision Analysis: Introductory Lectures on Choices Under Uncertainty*. Reading, MA: Addison-Wesley, 1968, pp. 262–264. Eraker, S., and Politser, P. "How decisions are reached." *Annals of Internal Medicine* 97:262, 1982.

19. Davis, A.J., and Aroskar, M.A. *Ethical Dilemmas and Nursing Practice*, 2nd ed. Norwalk, CT: Appleton-Century-Crofts, 1983, pp. 199–214. Health policy issues include justice in the allocation of limited health resources and the promotion of the general welfare of all people.

20. President's Commission, *Making Health Care Decisions*. Vol. 1, pp. 2–6. Brody, *Ethical Decisions in Medicine*, p. 98.

CHAPTER 7

Step Two: Gather Additional Information

One of the most common concerns in health and illness care is the need to make decisions without knowing all there is to know about the patient's condition. Bioethical decision making often carries the same limitation,[1] that is, patient or professional may need to make an ethical decision and take action based on incomplete information. From the patient's perspective, this incomplete information may be related to the unknown effects of treatment or the prognosis of an illness. From the professional's perspective, the incomplete data may include lack of a specific diagnosis or prognosis for a patient. It may also be not knowing what a comatose patient might want done or not knowing how to allocate staff or other finite resources.

One way of dealing with this need for decision making based on incomplete information is to accept the fact and take the risk. Health professionals are all risk takers when it comes to choosing a treatment for a given condition. There are few guarantees that the treatment will work this time with this person. Likewise, there is risk involved in ethical decision making. Because of the inability to get certain information, we may make an error in ethical judgment. These errors in judgment, like the errors in clinical judgment, may occur when there is still time to try a new approach. However, unlike an error in clinical judgment, ethical misjudgments are less likely to cause death or disability. More often, frustration, anger, and misunderstanding result when, for lack of full information, an error in ethical judgment occurs.

Ethical judgments based on incomplete information are often a reality. However, these should not occur because the decision maker did not take the time to gather needed information. The concern is information that would be helpful, but circumstances prevent access to that information. These circumstances include such things as emergencies when there is little or no time to gather ethical information. Perhaps a key individual in the situation is unavailable or unable to communicate (infant, society, other staff member) so that needed information from them is unavailable.

Step Two in the decision model concerns the identification and gathering of critical information that will help one analyze the ethical components of a health care situation and contribute to the final choice of action. Without determining what information is needed and trying to gather as much as possible, we are neither ethical nor reasoning. The temptation once again may be to respond at the emotional level, ignore the ethical components, and believe we know best. Here again, ethical practice requires resistance to that temptation and the following of Step Two as you move toward moral reasoning and ethical decision making. Even when you think you have all the information needed to make a decision, ask other participants for their input.

WHAT FURTHER INFORMATION IS NEEDED?

Analyzing the ethical components of health care situations moves us beyond the scientific or medical data (laboratory reports, diagnosis, prognosis). This includes critical social, economic, cultural, legal, and psychological information as well.[2] To simplify the presentation in this section, we will concentrate on patient care situations. This decision model can be applied to ethical considerations at the policy or professional staff level, but these will not be included here. Categories of critical information vary somewhat for policy level and professional staff ethical situations.[3] However, the need to determine what further information is needed remains constant.

Once again ethics suggests noting the type of information you and others identify as critical to the situation and noting the value judgments therein. Ask the question, "To what extent does the list of missing or needed information reflect my own values in this situation?" This secondary level of analyzing can strengthen your ability and commitment to understand your own actions in an ethical situation. Listening to others define the missing information critical to making an ethical decision often provides another perspective. This presents an opportunity for dialogue among participants about the important variables for them to consider and why.

What Categories of Information Should Be Included?

A case study may differ from an immediate situation. The categories of information presented or missing from the initial presentation may be determined by the person(s) who is presenting. The purpose of the presentation may also determine the completeness of information presented initially. A case study with health care professionals new to moral reasoning may include a limited number of facts. Thus, participants will have the opportunity to determine what else they would like to know or need to know. In an immediate patient situation, you want all the critical information you can get. However, the completeness of the information presented initially may be determined by the moral reasoning skills of the presenter.

Categories of information may include demographic data, health status and prognosis, patient knowledge, level of understanding, preferences, and competence, family members or significant others involved, the legal perspective on the proposed action, and options already presented to patient and family. Other options will be developed more fully later in the reasoning process. Societal concerns and interests should be considered.[4] Likewise, one must ask about the professionals' investment in the outcome (e.g., research) so that personal biases surface for discussion.[5]

Demographic data are such items as age, ethnicity, sex, and marital status. Socioeconomic considerations might include level of income, family role and dependents, and educational level. The educational level may influence the patient's ability to participate knowledgeably in the decision. Note again the need (court mandated in some cases) to communicate without medical jargon to facilitate patient understanding of the situation.[6] If the patient is comatose or otherwise not competent, the family's knowledge or educational level is significant. One may not choose to use a specific demographic item, such as age, as the only determinant on which action should be taken. How heavily weighted any one of these items becomes in the final decision will once again depend on who makes the final decision and the moral justification for it.

Ability to pay for care (source of payment) is often refuted as having a place in the discussion of what should be done for a patient. However, finite health care resources do not allow the provision of all types of treatment for all patients. Our society's experience with the government subsidy of kidney dialysis teaches a good lesson.[7] There is tremendous expense in providing just one technology for all in need. This expense could reinforce the ongoing need to use good judgment in deciding who should receive treatment. We are back to the earlier ethical question, "Just because we can, should we?" Economists as well as ethicists are questioning whether we can or must provide dialysis to all.

The significant others involved in the situation were identified in Step One. At this point, the importance of their role increases in this analysis. Part of this is their self-interests and their interest in the patient. A preliminary knowledge of what both patient and family would prefer, as well as options already presented, is helpful as a guide to the group discussion. What will actually be decided comes later, however, when these preferences are examined along with those of others in determining the ethical basis of the final choice.

The health status and prognosis of the patient are obvious data needed for determining alternative actions and potential consequences (Step Eight). These data also provide participants with some idea of the time available for moral reasoning. If the patient has a long-range, slow-acting illness, there may be more time for making needed decisions on what treatment, if any, will be offered. In contrast, a severely ill person may need a more immediate decision on treatment if the condition is to be reversed or alleviated.

Other categories of information are patient knowledge and understanding of the patient's condition, preferences for action, and competence to participate in the decision process. Participants in the discussion group without first-hand knowledge of the patient can benefit from learning what the patient knows about his or her health status and proposed treatment plan. The ethical/legal concept of informed consent is one issue here. Certainly, knowing that a patient is in a coma puts a different light on the decision process than knowing the patient is alert and capable of expressing needs and preferences. For many health care professionals, working through a difficult ethical decision with the help and knowledge of the patient is preferable to having no input about what the person might want done. The President's Commission reflected this interest in its suggestion that the major goal in ethical decision making is "shared decision making based on mutual respect."[8] Shared decision making requires knowledge, understanding, and the capacity for making decisions. The patient's ability to participate in the decision is vital information to have early in the moral reasoning process.

Whether or not one needs to seek a legal opinion is in large measure determined by the nature of the problem. For example, law currently dictates how late in pregnancy an abortion can be done, the need to report child abuse and venereal disease, and the protection of handicapped individuals. The current uncertainty of whether anyone can make a decision not to treat a severely ill or defective neonate may cause some health care institutions to be less willing to allow such a discussion without legal opinion even though politics, not law, are intervening in such decisions. Ethics and law often interface in health care. The concept of informed consent is both an ethical and legal one. In large hospitals and government-funded health care settings, legal review of ethical dilemmas is sometimes encouraged. The major use of this review at present is to decide whether one can even consider a proposed action. This is often an unfortunate position for legal counsel, since ethics is not law, and the lawyer may be no better prepared for ethical decision making than the nurse or physician. The reality of our time and culture is that we often turn to the legal system for help in defining our ethics (abortion, Baby Doe).[9] Whether right or wrong, law does influence and, at times, complicates ethical decision making with patients.

The final category of information one may need to gather is consideration of societal and professional interests in the patient situation outcome. Universalizability appears here and in the final decision. "What would happen if all of society decided to do this?" Other questions of societal concerns include, "Will society at large be expected to pay for this decision?" "What are society's rights in this situation?" Brody notes that societal interests must always be kept in mind in bioethical decision making, although conflict between individual and societal interests may occur.[10] During such conflict, the general tendency is to go along with the individual if societal risk is not too great.

The professional investment in the patient situation is a given, although we often need time and thought to clearly state the level of that investment and interest. It is beneficial for all concerned to identify this investment early so that all participants know. We have already discussed knowing patient and family preferences and interests. The same knowledge must be available about the professionals involved. One example of professional interest relates to scientific inquiry (research). Much of medicine and nursing is experimental in the sense that if one thing does not help, we try another. Calling this the "art of nursing or medicine" does not change the experimental nature of patient care. We often hope to learn more about how certain treatments or drugs work. Thus we may push for a given decision so that we can have another experience with that treatment. It is important to be aware of such biases in order to come closer to understanding our own motivations and values in health care.

This discussion of information to be gathered as Step Two in the decision model is meant to illustrate some of the critical facts that one may find helpful in ethical decision making. You may not need all of the items presented, or you may need others not discussed. The intent is to offer suggestions as to what questions might be asked or information sought so that one can proceed towards ethical decision making. The situation will help dictate what else is needed. As you practice moral reasoning, you will find the questions easier to think of and the needed information more clearly defined.

WHAT FURTHER INFORMATION CAN BE OBTAINED?

One of the important corollaries to determining what further information one would like to have is whether it is reasonable and possible to collect such information. The test of reasonableness includes knowing whether there is a source for the needed information, time available to collect the data, and resources to cover the cost of same. There are limits on our ability to get answers to our questions. Sometimes the better option is to recognize and accept these limits. Where and when an individual stops looking for information, however, will also be determined by the personal value placed on the data.

As you compile your list of questions for further information, it may be helpful to also identify the potential source of information and how much time and money, if applicable, would be needed for each. For information you would like to have but for which you do not have a source (patient cannot tell you her preferences, family does not really know what they want done), note the lack of a source and set it aside. For information that is identified as costly and requiring more time than currently available, note these as well and set them aside. Retain the original list for reference during the rest of the decision-making process so that participants can be reminded of the missing data. This reminder can help you determine whether the missing data might have altered the list of alternative actions or the final decision. You cannot obtain the data, but its absence can be noted during the reasoning process. In future situations you may be able to gather some of that data, so you do not want to write it off as always unobtainable.

The action phase of Step Two is searching out the needed information that is both possible and reasonable to obtain. This may require joint efforts, group discussion, or individual time. Just as there are a variety of ways of telling the truth, there are a variety of ways one can collect needed information for ethical analysis. The medical record is a source of demographic information. We are especially concerned here with data needed from patient, family, and other professionals. This requires personal interviews if these persons are not currently involved in the discussion and analysis. One may need to ask who is the most appropriate person to gather this personal information. Sometimes it will be the primary nurse, sometimes the physician, sometimes the patient or family, sometimes the clergy or social worker. All of these possible information seekers imply relationship with one another. A climate of mutual respect and trust is essential, and good communication skills are necessary. Pressures of time, verbal manipulation, ambiguity of language and use of medical jargon, and emotional distance are major obstacles to good communication.[11] It is important to remember that how one communicates with another also derives from one's view of that individual. If children, women, or the elderly are viewed as nonpersons, communication is often one way (talking down to) if attempted at all.

It is at this point of information gathering that the nurses need to articulate their role in taking action. Certainly personal preferences can be shared directly with the decision group. Consideration of how well one knows the patient and the potential influence of the nurse–patient relationship should be kept in mind. The nurse should also consider how much personal information about the patient and family can be shared without consent. Like anyone else, the nurse should strive to protect the confidentiality of the patient.[12] Group discussion of moral reasoning is not the place for hearsay information. Data presented on behalf of another person are best presented as near verbatim as possible without comments that could be interpreted as judgmental. For some, direct involvement of patient and family members in the discussion is preferable. Thus all persons involved have an opportunity to present their views, defend their positions, and learn of alternative positions from others. Whatever the role of the nurse in gathering information, it should be well thought out and presented knowingly and responsibly.

SUMMARY

Step Two of the decision model is to determine what further information is needed. This comes early in moral reasoning, providing data needed in order to appropriately choose what action to take. As with Step One, you may find yourself returning to this step later as you realize that a piece of information was overlooked or not obvious at first glance. We encourage this review of early steps as you proceed in the decision process. It is useful in reinforcing critical inquiry skills, and it is essential for an adequate decision. With the basic situational information gathered in Steps One and Two, you are now ready to move to Step Three and identify the ethical issues involved in the situation. Before doing that, here is a sample of information gathering for "Birth of a Family."

THE CASE

What Further Information Is Needed?

For some, it may be important to know the ages of Sara and Tom. Whether they wanted a child may also be important information. Others may need more information on the pregnancy and the health status of the infant and of Sara. This could be necessary to determine if it was indeed safe for Sara to hold her son. If Sara and Tom were not emotionally or psychologically ready for intimate contact with their son, the timing of this could be counterproductive to the bonding and to the joy intended. This concern would seem to have been addressed, however, by asking them if they wanted to hold their child rather than simply handing or placing the infant on Sara's abdomen.

In the interests of informed consent, it would be important to know if Sara and Tom gave permission to have the nurse–midwifery student assist in the birth. This is a teaching hospital, and all may expect or be expected to have students caring for them, while not overlooking the need for informed consent. One might also ask whether Tom and Sara contracted with the nurse–midwife or gave their consent knowledgeably for midwifery instead of physician care. In other words, what type of contract, if any, did the parents have with the professionals or the institution? How much did they know about such professionals and their philosophy of caregiving? And why did the nurse–midwife not know Sara and Tom's preference for the birth and bonding before delivery?

Clarification of current hospital policies and the reasons for them is additional information needed in this situation. This may include staffing patterns as well as the responsibilities of each professional. It would also be of interest to know why Sara asked whether she could hold her own son. Was it a question about her own capability? Or was it a question of permission? If it was the latter, what events led up to Sara or any mother having to ask permission to hold her own child? This might lead one to ask what type of prenatal care Sara received and whether she received any prenatal or childbirth education before the birth of her son.

We know very little of the nurse–midwifery student's views in this situation. Since she is in a student capacity, what were her responsibilities and views, especially on bonding? What was she thinking about in terms of how to direct the situation in the delivery area? Knowledge of the institution's contract with the nurse–midwifery program and type of physician back-up agreed upon are important details in evaluating the appropriateness of the current delivery scene.

NOTES

1. Veatch, R.M. *Case Studies in Medical Ethics*. Cambridge, MA: Harvard University Press, 1977, p. 39. Brody, H. *Ethical Decisions in Medicine*. Boston: Little, Brown, 1976, p. 93, notes that ethical decisions are made in a state of relative ignorance that can be reduced but never eliminated. Davis, A.J., and Aroskar, M.A. *Ethical Dilemmas and Nursing Practice*. Norwalk, CT: Appleton-Century-Crofts, 1983, p. 217.
2. Shelly, J. *Dilemma: A Nurse's Guide for Making Ethical Decisions*. Downer's Grove, IL: Intervarsity Press, 1980. Veatch, *Case Studies in Medical Ethics*, pp. 38–40. Kreps, G.L., and Thornton, B.C. *Health Communication*. New York: Longman, 1984, pp. 201–202. Curtin, L., and Flaherty, M.J. *Nursing Ethics: Theories and Pragmatics*. Bowie, MD: Brady, 1982, p. 60.
3. Davis and Aroskar, *Ethical Dilemmas and Nursing Practice*, pp. 207–214, note that distributive justice pervades health policy decisions when we do not have resources to provide services for all. Other ethical issues include who pays for health care, who should evaluate quality of care and costs, and is health a right or a privilege. Regarding the allocation of scarce resources, Kenneth Vaux has noted, "We don't live on a lifeboat; we live on a luxury liner. We could fund all the neonatal intensive care units in the country for the cost of one nuclear submarine." Quoted by Lyon, J. "New treatments, new choices." *Nursing Life* 4(2):47–49, March–April 1984.
4. Abram, M.B., and Wolf, S.M. "Public involvement in medical ethics." *New England Journal of Medicine* 310(10):627–632, March 8, 1984. Thompson, J.B., and Thompson, H.O. *Ethics in Nursing*. New York: Macmillan, 1981, pp. 184–185. Veatch, *Case Studies in Medical Ethics*, pp. 61–88. Brody, *Ethical Decisions in Medicine*, pp. 95, 209–211.
5. Brody, *Ethical Decisions in Medicine*, p. 94. Veatch, *Case Studies in Medical Ethics*. Huttman, B. "A crime of compassion." *Newsweek* August 8, 1983:15. Hamilton, A.J. "Who shall live and who shall die." *Newsweek* March 26, 1984:15.
6. Kreps and Thornton, *Health Communication*, pp. 73–76.
7. Davis and Aroskar, *Ethical Dilemmas and Nursing Practice*, p. 207.
8. President's Commission, *Making Health Care Decisions*. Vol. One. *Report*. Washington, DC: US Government Printing Office, October 1982, p. 3.
9. Fenner, K. *Ethics and Law in Nursing*. New York: Van Nostrand Co., 1980. Curran, W.J., and Shapiro, E.D. *Law, Medicine and Forensic Science*, 3rd ed. Boston: Little, Brown, 1982, Chaps. 5–8.
10. Brody, *Ethical Decisions in Medicine*, p. 95.
11. Kreps and Thornton, *Health Communication*, pp. 43–47.
12. *American Nurses' Association. Code for Nurses With Interpretive Statements*. Kansas City, MO: ANA, 1976.

CHAPTER 8
Step Three: Identify the Ethical Issues

The ethical situation has been prepared by clarifying the health problem, the decision(s) needed, the individuals involved, and the need for further information. Now it is time to more clearly identify the ethical issues. Many will already be evident from the preliminary analysis, and others will require more thought and searching before they can be clearly stated. The major value of identifying the ethical issues clearly at this point in the decision process is that it helps participants focus on specific ethical concerns. It is at this point that the ethical decision process distinguishes itself from the problem-solving process normally used by health care professionals. We are now entering the realm of philosophy and theology. It may be helpful to consult experts in those disciplines as we develop our own knowledge in bioethics. Consultations with specialists are now standard practice in health care.[1] Chapters One and Two of this text provide theoretical background for identifying the ethical issues in a health care situation. The reader may wish to review their content at this time.

Ethical issues can be categorized in several different ways.[2] Almost any grouping involves extensive overlapping. Yet some scheme of organization is helpful in getting a grasp on identifying the issues in a health care situation. We find it useful to categorize ethical issues as follows:

Issues of Principle
1. Autonomy self-determination of patients and professionals
2. Do good do no harm (beneficence, nonmaleficence)
3. Justice fairness (allocation of resources)

4. Truth-telling (veracity)
5. Informed consent
6. Quality of life/sanctity of life
7. The Golden Rule

Issues of Ethical Rights

1. Right to privacy (confidentiality)
2. Right to decide what happens to oneself/one's body (self-determination)
3. Right to health care (currently debatable; some say equal access only, others say not a right at all)
4. Right to information (informed consent, access to records)
5. Right to choose whom you care for (frequently limited to physicians in nonemergency situations)
6. Right to live, right to die
7. Rights of children

Issues of Ethical Duties/Obligations

1. Respect persons
2. Be accountable for decisions/actions
3. Maintain competence (professionals)
4. Exercise informed judgment in professional practice
5. Implement and improve standards of profession
6. Participate in activities contributing to profession's knowledge base
7. Safeguard clients from incompetent, unethical, or illegal practice of any person
8. Promote efforts to meet health needs of public
9. Participate in the formulation of public policy

Issues of Ethical Loyalty

1. Professional–patient relationship (covenant fidelity, contract, seller of services)
2. Accountability to whom as employee
3. Professional–professional relationships
4. Professional–patient family relationship
5. Who decides

Issues of Concern in Life Cycle

1. Contraception and sterilization
2. Genetic engineering and embryo transfer
3. Abortion (When does life begin?)
4. Infanticide
5. Adolescent sexuality
6. Allocation of scarce resources
7. Lifestyle
8. Euthanasia

Again, this is a guideline for participants in ethical decision making to identify ethical issues in a health care situation. We acknowledge the overlap with the understanding that different individuals may describe (name) an ethical issue in different ways. This is evident among philosophers and theologians as well. Issues might be added, subtracted, or combined. Additions to the list can be made in any way that will facilitate your completion of Step Three. Once you have completed your list or tentative list in a given case with input from others, consider the historical, philosophical, and theological basis of each issue listed.

WHAT IS THE HISTORICAL BASIS OF THE ETHICAL ISSUE?

Discussion of the historical basis of the ethical issues is helpful from several perspectives. Knowledge of the history of the ethical issue furthers understanding of why it is an issue as well as how individuals over time have viewed it. There is a famous line by the philosopher, George Santayana (1863–1952): "Those who cannot remember the past are condemned to repeat it."[3] A variation of this statement is that those who do not know the mistakes of the past are doomed to repeat them. There is then a negative value in knowing history as it may help avoid mistakes in ethical judgment. The positive side of knowing history is that it helps us to understand how we or others came to value what we value or believe what we believe.

As health care professionals, we need to understand others. One cannot understand others without having some knowledge of their morals, ethics, values, beliefs, and customs.[4] Where did these come from? For example, the strictures against contraception date back nearly to the dawn of history, the beginning of writing. The efforts to prevent childbearing are equally ancient. There would have been no need for laws against contraception if it were not being practiced. As noted throughout this text, one aspect of ethics is to study the reasons, the principles behind the moral codes. As we review the historical basis of the ethical issue we need to ask ourselves, are the reasons behind the ethical issue still valid or are there other (higher?) principles to be applied in the situation today? If so, why? Whether we agree or disagree with the historical reasoning behind the ethical issue, we can understand what it was and how it evolved over time. We can know more about why we may hold a similar position or others hold different ones. We may choose to change our position on the issue or keep the present position, and we can make a reasoned decision on the matter because of our increased understanding of the historical development of the ethical issue over time.

WHAT IS THE PHILOSOPHICAL BASIS OF THE ETHICAL ISSUE?

As we noted in Part One of this text, ethics is commonly seen as a branch of philosophy. Others define moral philosophy as a branch of ethics. Whatever perspective one has, it is difficult to separate ethics and philosophy. When we discuss the philosophical basis of an ethical issue, we are exploring how philosophers viewed or view the ethical concern. Immanuel Kant's view of persons as ends in themselves, for example, is helpful in understanding the ethical concept of respect for persons.[5] Aristotle and Plato are often referred to in discussions of when life begins (ensoulment).[6] The writings of ancient philosophers aid current understanding through history as well as philosophy.

Philosophers and moral theologians have probably spent more time than anyone else in exploring ethical issues, both ancient and modern. They are skilled in moral reasoning and ethical inquiry. Discussion of their work helps us to learn these valuable techniques as well. This discussion also contributes to our understanding of how ethics is defined, how ethical issues are identified, and how one can morally justify a position on the issue.

WHAT IS THE THEOLOGICAL BASIS OF THE ETHICAL ISSUE?

The theological basis of ethical issues is helpful for understanding the religious perspective on ethics. A major portion of our moral prescriptions have been defined by theologians. They have often spent years examining, defining, redefining, and explicating moral codes of behavior and rules.[7] Both theists and nontheists probably follow some of those rules without conscious thought. Taking the time to examine the theological basis of an ethical issue is important in clarifying our own moral positions as well as those of others. Time spent in such discussion also encourages personal reevaluation of what we believe about the issue at hand. We may choose to retain the belief or change it. The hope is that such a decision will be a conscious, reasoned one.

The nature of health care situations often involves basic life issues, such as birth and death and the core emotions of hope, caring, mercy, and love. When we come to the time of making a decision, one may ask, "What is the loving thing to do?" Love is a standard common to many religions. This question is often raised by people who believe in a supreme being. It may also be part of one's culture. Nontheists and theists alike can benefit from understanding the theological perspective on ethical issues. Health care professionals and patients may hold similar religious views, or they may differ. Understanding religious perspectives can encourage ethical decision making.

SUMMARY

Step Three in the decision model continues the analyzing phase of moral reasoning while directing us ever closer to the ethical dimensions of the health care situation. This step is concerned with the identification and understanding of the ethical issues specific to the case at hand. Knowledge of the historical, philosophical, and theological bases of the ethical issues continues our growth in understanding others. It strengthens both our theoretical and practical bases for making ethical decisions. We continue our application of Step Three to "Birth of a Family."

THE CASE

What Are the Ethical Issues in the Situation?

There are several issues in this case. We began with the concept of informed consent involving care by the student and certified nurse–midwife. The self-determination or the autonomy of the parents for choosing the type of care received is part of this concern. Autonomy is also an issue regarding their immediate bonding with their newborn. The Kantian respect for persons, for human dignity, is at the core of the parental autonomy promoted in this situation as well. Allowing the parents to enjoy and bond with their son is an example of doing good, whereas exercising judgment that the infant is healthy before handing it to the parents is an example of avoiding harm.

Parental rights to determine who will care for them as well as where they will receive care are a part of this situation. The ethical issue of the professional responsibilities or duties of the nurse is raised when one questions whether the nurse should insist on moving the infant to the warmer for his safety, while also being concerned about not being fired from her job if she does not perform correctly. The ethical responsibility of the nurse–midwife to exercise informed judgment was noted in Step Two, i.e., giving the parents a chance to hold their son. The midwife may have an ethical responsibility to her professional colleague (new on the job) to either explain that the hospital does not have a policy against parents holding their newborn or an ethical duty to take responsibility for her action to relieve the delivery room nurse of unnecessary anxiety. However, if the nurse had responsibilities to other patients, the midwife may have been interfering with her colleague's professional responsibilities. The nurse may have been concerned with the ethics of the allocation of the scarce resource of her time. If the ethic of nursing is patient-centered care, the center in this case is the parent–infant relationship. We do not know if this is interfering with the nurse's relationship to other patients.

What Are the Historical, Philosophical, and Theological Dimensions?

Historically, one might note the enormous change from home birth (about 95 percent of all births before 1900 AD) to hospital births (about 95 percent today). Part of this change has been a change of attitude. Where birth was once thought to be a natural phenomenon, it has become a sickness or disease to be controlled by hospital care. The whisking of neonates off to the warmer with all the attendant procedures is part of this 20th century perspective. In recent years, there has been a movement back toward home births and intermediate facilities, such as birthing rooms within hospitals and birth centers separate from but near to hospitals. Some want the freedom and lessened expense of out of hospital birth but still want the safety net for those 5 percent (250,000 babies) of births with anomalies or emergency situations. We can note in passing the cultural element of the father's presence at birth. In some cultures and subcultures, this is permissible and even required. In others, it is not required and perhaps forbidden.

As noted earlier, the rubric of do good and, if you cannot do good, at least do no harm is attributed to Hippocrates in the 4th century BC. The Hippocratic Oath in its present form may actually date to a later period, but the concept goes back to a philosophical and theological movement of which Hippocrates was a part. Western ethics draws on the two sources of philosophy and religion, and in this case, the two are one. The concept can be interpreted also from the Judeo–Christian and other religions' tradition of "Love thy neighbor." This thought and the Golden Rule, also found in many religions, may be seen as the source of respect for persons. Philosophically, this can be traced to Immanuel Kant and others. In a way, so can autonomy, self-determination.

In the real world, however, relatively few people have the wealth or power or health for autonomy. It often remains an ideal toward which people aspire. In the face of poverty, ignorance, and disease, one may not have the luxury of autonomy. In recent decades, however, bioethics has been shifting the focus from health care provider to the patient as decision maker. As long ago as 1916, the courts declared a patient's right to refuse treatment, with or without what others consider a good reason. This right, however, is limited to the self. Parents do not have a right to make martyrs of their children. Realistically, one can be aware that a portion of the patients' rights movement (including parents' rights, the pregnant patient's rights) has been an attempt to relieve the threat of malpractice, on the one hand, and, on the other, a relief from decisions that have become too massive and too complex for one or even a few persons. Beyond these pragmatic and utilitarian concerns, there has also been an awakening of conscience in the face of the new complexities brought on by the success of modern health care. In the old days, the patient got well or died pretty much regardless of what the provider did. The advent of antibiotics and new techniques now make very real differences.

Modern health care is not so much in evidence here. The issue of informed consent comes out of a more negative history than the successes of modern health care. As noted earlier, the health care establishment helped Hitler's Nazi regime eliminate the retarded, gypsies, Jews, and others the regime did not like. The war crimes trials after World War II spotlighted this involvement in which so-called experiments were run on the hapless victims without informed consent. The new emphasis on informed consent has become more apparent with the passing years. There are times when researchers and other members of the health care team see informed consent as a threat at worst and a nuisance at best in relation to their work. Some, however, recognize it as an ally in helping patients to receive ethical health care.

The professional duty to exercise informed judgment is a reminder of the earlier note that ethics turns on reason, whereas morals are the shoulds and oughts of life, society, faith, but we would not bother with any of this if we did not feel its importance. Judgment is an example of the feeling element in professional life. It might be seen as a mixture of reasons and sensing or feeling or intuition. It could also, of course, be an example of Jean Piaget's formal operations or abstract intellectual functioning, with the various elements of the judgment coming together at abstract levels. We stop short of mystifying this process, however, for in this case, the nurse–midwife could point to concrete, specific elements that make up the judgment regarding the baby's health and the psychological concept of bonding. Still, there is no denying the feeling of joy experienced by the parents, the student midwife, and the nurse–midwife nor the feeling of distress experienced by the delivery room nurse. The moral–ethical spectrum is not just cold, objective, machine-like rationality, and, of course, neither is it merely a matter of emotionality and feeling. Both mother and baby were doing well and so was the father, by objective, reasonable health care standards.

NOTES

1. Jonsen, A.R., Siegler, M., and Winslade, W. *Clinical Ethics*. New York: Macmillan, 1982, p. ix.
2. Kieffer, G.H. *Bioethics: A Textbook of Issues*. Reading, MA: Addison-Wesley, 1979. Beauchamp, T.L., and Childress, J. *Principles of Biomedical Ethics*. New York: Oxford University Press, 1983, pp. 59–209. Barry, V. *Moral Aspects of Health Care*. Belmont, CA: Wadsworth Publishing Co., 1982, pp. 360–497. Munson, R. *Intervention and Reflection: Basic Issues in Medical Ethics*, 2nd ed. Belmont, CA: Wadsworth, 1983.
3. Santayana, G. *The Life of Reason*, Vol. 1. 1905–1906, off print.
4. Steele, S., and Harmon, V. *Values Clarification in Nursing*, 2nd ed. Norwalk, CT: Appleton-Century-Crofts, 1983, pp. 18–27. President's Commission, *Making Health Care Decisions*, Vol. 1. Washington, DC: US Government Printing Office, October, 1982, pp. 41–51. Kreps, G., and Thornton, B. *Health Communication*. New York: Longmans, 1984, pp. 190–202.
5. Kant, I. *Groundwork of the Metaphysic of Morals*. New York: Harper & Row, 1964.
6. Aristotle, *Politics*. VII. 16, 1335. Plato, *The Republic*. V. 460 ff.
7. Thompson, J.B., and Thompson, H.O. *Ethics in Nursing*. New York: Macmillan, 1981, pp. 24–26, 28–29, 49–56, 74–77, 106–108, 109–111, 163, 185.

When in doubt, tell the truth. It will confound your enemies, and confuse your friends.

—Mark Twain
Pudd'n head Wilson

CHAPTER 9

Step Four: Identify Personal and Professional Values

Personal and professional values influence our daily lives. Some of these values are known and recognized. Others are hidden and unknown. When nurses choose to be involved in moral reasoning, they cannot escape the task of clarifying their own values. Even though one is committed to ethical nursing practice, there is often some anxiety attached to this step of the decision model. Not all of us are ready to examine the very roots of our beliefs. What if I don't like what I find? What if I don't want to change? The decision model does not require that people necessarily change what they value. It does require that you be willing to clearly state what it is you value and why.

We noted in Chapter Four the importance of trust and mutual respect in group discussion of one's values. People may choose to examine their value stand in private on the ethical issues identified in the situation, or one may be ready and willing to participate in a group exploration of individual values. Whichever route is chosen, the process of value clarification is very important as we enter the central core of ethical inquiry.[1] The reader may wish to review Chapter Four at this point in preparation for proceeding with the decision model.

Step Four of the decision model calls for clarification of one's personal and professional values. This is especially relative to the ethical issues identified during Step Three of the process. This type of values clarification helps to focus your value exploration. It provides some security in knowing what it is you will be expected to respond to. The major goal of this step in the decision model, therefore, is to facilitate a personal understanding of why we respond as we do when faced with a particular ethical issue. In the normal activities of the day, we allow our values to govern our actions on a subconscious level. Once values are stated explicitly, they are no longer unconscious.[2] We can function less from a gut-level and more from a reasoned approach to life and our nursing practice. This reasoned approach to professional practice is in your own best interests as well as the best interests of one's patients and colleagues.

WHAT ARE YOUR PERSONAL VALUES ON THE ISSUES?

The process of value clarification is simpler if you begin with one issue at a time. Select one from the list developed during Step Three. Your choice allows you some control over when you will discuss the difficult issues. Focus on the issue as listed, such as quality of life or informed consent. In this way there will be less initial confusion in understanding where you stand on the issue itself. It is taken out of the context of the entire patient situation. This separation also allows you to clarify your general value on the issue before considering any components of the situation. If you find yourself asking about specific details from the situation (age of patient, how ill, what are chances for survival) before taking a stand on the issue, note these for later discussion. These requests for further information often indicate that we sometimes do take certain patient variables (situation ethics) into consideration before deciding how to respond. After noting what further data you asked for, try to return to the ethical issue and state what you believe or value.

A note of caution is appropriate here in our discussion of personal values. It is often difficult to separate our personal values from our professional values. We usually choose a profession for personal reasons, i.e., it supports our values in life. What one values personally may be what is valued professionally, and vice versa. This is neither good nor bad in itself, although a unified ethic can give a sense of wholeness or congruity.[3] Our concern here is to clarify the two—whether they are the same, different, or some of both. One method we have found helpful in determining if one's current values have resulted from personal or professional perspectives or both is to ask such questions as these: "Can you remember a time earlier in your life (before entering nursing) when you thought differently about this ethical issue? To what extent has your nursing (professional) training influenced how you respond to this ethical issue? How do you think your parent(s) would respond to this issue? When you were growing up, what position would your best friend have taken on this issue? Did you agree with your best friend then?" Of course the ever present philosophical question, "Why?" would follow each response.

One of the final approaches to clarifying personal value positions on ethical issues is to ask, "What do I believe about this issue?" If the issue is quality of life, one might ask more specific questions. "Is it more important to be alive than to be conscious or seriously ill?" "Under what circumstances would I be willing to die (or live)?" It may help to think of a family member or friend who is seriously ill or handicapped and ask, "How would I respond if I were in that situation?" You may work out other questions that help you to clarify your value position on a particular ethical issue. The goal is clarity and understanding of personal values.

WHAT ARE YOUR PROFESSIONAL VALUES ON THE ISSUES?

As noted in Chapter Four, professional values are instilled throughout the educational program and practice of the professional role. Nurses learn of the importance of viewing individuals as wholistic individuals who live in relationship with others, influenced by culture, place in society, and state of health.[4] This philosophy of nursing is laden with value statements. It is expected that as people take on this professional role, they will also take on the values ascribed to by the profession.[5] In reality, individuals do value different things, and nurses do not always take the same value position on an ethical issue.

One of the clearest statements of professional values comes in the ANA *Code for Nurses.* One helpful exercise in clarifying the values of the profession of nursing is to ask the discussion group to read the *Code.* Then ask each member to list the moral positions implicitly and explicitly stated therein. This often can be described as the duties and obligations of nurses as defined in the 11 moral statements of the code (see Chapter Eight for the list of ethical duties and obligations taken directly from the *Code for Nurses*). One may also begin with a different question and ask for the character traits of the ethical nurse as defined in the *Code for Nurses.* Any one of these approaches may facilitate the individual's understanding and listing of the value positions of nursing as defined in the ANA *Code.* Results of one of these exercises are given here as an example of how one may approach the clarification of professional values.

The character traits of an ethical nurse as defined in the ANA *Code* include respect, competence, advocacy (protector), responsibility, accountability, and collaborative actions. The AMA *Principles of Medical Ethics* similarly analyzed often produces the character traits of physicians as dedicated, compassionate, competent, respectful, and honest. An interesting exercise that may follow the character trait identification and further clarify how an individual values the profession's values is as follows. Once the participants have made a list of the character traits, ask them to rearrange them in descending order of importance, that is, ask the people to rank those traits that are the most crucial to high quality professional practice. For best results in the use of this exercise, encourage participants to share their ranking as well as the reasons why they gave a certain rank to a given trait.[6] Interdisciplinary groups of health professionals may add an increased understanding of each other's profession during this type of value clarification exercise.

In our experience, relatively few nurses have read and studied either the ANA *Code for Nurses* or the ANA *Standards for Practice.* One is tempted to ask how these standards can be put into practice (both clinical and ethical practice) without a clear understanding of them, whether one agrees or disagrees with any specific point. Perhaps this is part of the reality shock of new nurses as they graduate and begin working with other nurses. This lack of awareness of professional values fits with the general lack of awareness of personal values for a large segment of our society. It does not, however, fit with our concept of the ethical nurse who is able to clearly state both personal and professional value positions on a given ethical issue. Perhaps this is the best justification for including Step Four in this decision model.

WHAT GUIDANCE DOES THE ANA *CODE FOR NURSES* OFFER?

There is considerable agreement that the ANA *Code for Nurses,* 1976, offers general guidance for ethical decision making.[7] It does not, however, offer nurses the specificity needed to know how to act or decide in a given situation. The decision model presented in this text was developed for more specificity in guiding ethical decision making. The model incorporates the ANA *Code* at this point in moral reasoning. It is viewed as the consensus ethic of professional nursing and is therefore of vital importance to ethical decision making for nurses.

The general guidelines for ethical nursing practice are listed in the 11 moral prescriptions or statements of the *Code.* These include such things as providing services with respect for human dignity and without discrimination, safeguarding the client's right to privacy, and assuming responsibility for individual nursing judgments and actions. (See Chapter One for the ANA *Code for Nurses.*) As noted earlier, some of the reasons behind these moral statements can be found in the interpretive statements related to each of the 11 moral statements. These interpretive statements can help one understand why the nurse should practice in accord with the *Code.* These statements also help identify some of the situations where the ANA *Code* might direct the nurse's decision. Let us examine some ethical issues and what the ANA *Code* has to say about them for the nurse.

One of the questions often raised in a patient situation is whether the patient should have any choice in what treatment or drug will be prescribed. This would be the ethical issue of self-determination.[8] The first interpretive statement defines "respect for human dignity" as supporting the client's right to self-determination. Therefore, the nurse could respond that, in general, the profession of nursing states that patient self-determination is to be valued. Whenever possible, the patients should be allowed to decide to what treatment, if any, they will agree. For many, this general statement of self-determination is not sufficient to know how to proceed when the patient and health care professionals disagree or when the patient is under age, in a coma, or otherwise incompetent. It does offer some important guidance, however.

Another example of using the ANA *Code* for guidance in decision making involves the question of whether nurses should participate in research. The seventh and eighth statements of the *Code* suggest that this participation is expected. They do not, however, necessarily help the nurse decide what type of research. What we define as "activities contributing to the development of the profession's body of knowledge" may not be the same ones that you define. What is the guarantee that either of our definitions is ethical? One might have to look further than the *Code* statements themselves to determine what is ethical research activity.[9] The *Code* does, however, establish the importance of research activities in nursing, just as it speaks to many other components of ethical nursing practice.

SUMMARY

Step Four of the decision model has encouraged you to take the time to identify, examine, and clarify your personal and professional values related to the ethical issues in Step Three. We hope this personal examination has been worth the effort as you move toward greater understanding of yourself and what you value as a person and as a nurse. It is now appropriate to take time to examine the value positions of others, Step Five. Before we do that, however, we can apply Step Four to our sample case, "Birth of a Family." The personal values are presented in terms of the certified nurse–midwife (CNM). While these perspectives appear reasonable, they are not presented here as the official position of any individual CNM or any organization. They are presented here only as an example.

THE CASE

What Are Your Personal Values on the Issues?

It would appear that the instructor values respect for all persons—the student, the parents, the baby, the circulating nurse. This is implemented in the way she interacts with them and her concern for everyone's understanding why the infant is safe in the mother's arms. This respect may support her value of the mother's right to determine if the mother wants to hold her child immediately. By virtue of her willingness to offer this option to the mother, one might also surmise she values family development and family-centered maternity care.

What Are Your Professional Values on the Issues?

The professional values evident include support for patient rights to self-determination and informed consent. The caution here is that we do not know what prior agreement she had with the parents for her own care of the labor or for involving her student. The nurse–midwife appears to define "doing good" as promoting bonding with the consent of the parents and avoiding harm by judging the infant stable enough to go directly to the parents. She also appears to value education and learning balanced with safe, satisfying care for the childbearing family.

What Guidance Does the ANA *Code* Offer?

The *Code for Nurses* supports the nurse–midwife's respect for all persons, self-determination and informed choice for the parents, and the exercising of her own informed judgment in her position.

NOTES

1. Steele, S., and Harmon, V. *Values Clarification in Nursing*, 2nd ed. Norwalk, CT: Appleton-Century-Crofts, 1983, pp. 13–18. King, E.C. *Affective Education in Nursing: A Guide to Teaching and Assessment.* Rockville, MD: Aspen Systems Corporation, 1984, pp. 17–19.
2. Brody, H. *Ethical Decisions in Medicine.* Boston: Little, Brown, 1976, p. 12.
3. Steele and Harmon, *Values Clarification in Nursing*, pp. 7–13.
4. Brooks, J.A., and Kleine-Kracht, A.E. "Evolution of a definition of nursing." *Advances in Nursing Science* 5(4):51–85, July 1983. Spicker, S., and Gadow, S. *Nursing: Images and Ideals.* New York: Springer, 1980. Muyskens, J. *Moral Principles in Nursing: A Philosophical Investigation.* Totowa, NJ: Rowman and Littlefield, 1982, pp. 30–40. President's Commission, *Making Health Care Decisions.* Vol. 1. Washington, DC: US Government Printing Office, 1982, p. 145.
5. Steele and Harmon, *Values Clarification in Nursing*, pp. 7, 9–13. Kelly, L.Y. *Dimensions of Professional Nursing*, 13th ed. New York: Macmillan, 1975. Curtin, L., and Flaherty, M.J. *Nursing Ethics: Theories and Pragmatics.* Bowie, MD: Brady, 1982, pp. 67–74, 79–93.
6. Steele and Harmon, *Values Clarification in Nursing*, pp. 96–106.
7. *Perspectives on the Code for Nurses.* Kansas City, MO: ANA, March, 1978. *Guidelines for Implementing the Code for Nurses.* Kansas City, MO: ANA, 1980, pp. v, 19. Payton, R.J. "Pluralistic ethical decision making." *Clinical and Scientific Sessions.* Kansas City, MO: ANA, 1979, p. 11.
8. ANA *Code for Nurses with Interpretive Statements.* Kansas City, MO: ANA, 1976, Interpretive Statement 1.1.
9. *Human Rights Guidelines for Nurses in Clinical and Other Research.* Kansas City, MO: ANA, 1975.

If values are "gut-level" in their normal state, they are no longer "gut-level" once we have transformed them into language by stating them explicitly.

—Howard Brody[1]

CHAPTER 10
Step Five: Identify the Values of Key Individuals

As we come to Step Five in the decision model, we encourage group sharing and discussion even more than before. After spending time identifying and clarifying what you value as an individual and as a health professional, it is time to listen to others and their values. The focus of discussion is the list of ethical issues prepared in Step Three. The key individuals are those identified in Step One and anyone else who may have been identified during the steps of the decision model.

If it is not possible to carry out Step Five with the key individuals involved in the situation (not available, not able, inappropriate, timing), you can proceed alone. The danger in attempting to understand another's value position without the benefit of hearing the person describe and clarify what is meant is one of misinterpretation. We can observe or listen to someone else's view of what the patient or family or physician value, or we might watch their behavior. However, we cannot be certain that our interpretation of the behavior or words is the correct or intended view. Human beings are often inconsistent in their beliefs and values, especially if they have not been consciously examined and freely chosen. This often results in a gap between what we say we value and what we actually put into action. Raths et al. note that this gap may be the distinction between an attitude and a value.[2] An attitude reflects what we say we believe about a given issue. Whether we actually value that issue is determined by how we act when faced with that issue. Therefore, if we have only statements of attitude available for understanding another's value position, we may not be able to interpret what they actually value.

Another possibility for misinterpreting another's values from their actions or words without further clarification involves our own view on the issue at hand. We may, in fact, inadvertently impose our own values during our interpretation of another's behavior or request. The cultural context of one's beliefs and values often attaches meaning to one's behavior. If we are of a different culture, we may not understand that meaning.[3] We may see only what we want to see in the situation, i.e., those actions or words that can be interpreted as supportive of what we think should be done.

Values and beliefs are subject to individual interpretation and therefore are best presented by the person holding them. This personal interpretation allows for time to question "Why?" and a clearer understanding of what is actually valued versus what is an attitude or feeling about the issue. This time for dialogue gives individuals the opportunity to decide for themselves whether a current value remains appropriate for the present time and circumstances. When this is not possible, however, one would do well to remember the notes of caution in trying to interpret what another person values as objectively as possible.

WHY BOTHER WITH THE MORAL POSITIONS OF OTHERS?

Step Five asks us to identify the moral positions of other key persons in the situation at hand. It is quite appropriate to ask "Why?" Of what importance is it to know what others believe and value about the ethical issues in the situation? How will this knowledge facilitate ethical decision making? Any of you who have tried to understand the values of others in ethical dilemmas may be tempted to comment that trying to know the values and beliefs of others (even if only those of the patient) takes time and often contributes to the confusion and difficulty of knowing what to do. It may cloud the path of decision making by suggesting more options. You may already be hassled by having to decide between merely two different actions.

One can acknowledge that spending time and the potential increase in frustration and confusion may be necessary corollaries in understanding others. However, there is value in knowing what others believe and value. First of all, knowing what another person believes and values in the situation contributes to our understanding of that person and the situation. Understanding others is a moral imperative in nursing and other health professions. It is a necessary step in providing care "with respect for human dignity and the uniqueness of the client."[4] Providing the best care possible for all our patients is central to the practice of nursing or any other health profession. The professional must understand patients as fully as possible. That includes their health and prognosis as well as beliefs, values, and culture. It includes anything that contributes to their understanding of their health and their acceptance or willingness to change that health condition. This patient understanding contributes to our knowing of what is the best thing to do in our care of others. It does not, however, clearly tell us what the best thing is. It is one guide toward ethical decision making.

Understanding the moral positions of key individuals involved in an ethical dimension of health care can help to clarify the issues. It can identify the possible areas of moral conflict in the situation (Step Six of this decision model). Knowledge of these areas of moral conflict is helpful in clarifying the situation prior to taking action. The first sign of possible moral/ethical conflict in health care situations often appears as an emotional response of "Something is not quite right here." We may feel uneasy or irritable or uncomfortable in the patient situation. Sometimes these feelings are ignored because we believe that the physician or patient needs to make the decision. They have done so; therefore, it must be right. The nurse's feelings, though strong, really do not matter or would not be listened to, and therefore, they are stifled.[5]

The danger in ignoring early feelings of unease in a patient situation or decision is that one may end up tacitly supporting an unethical decision. Your own feeling of discomfort may have been the moral sensitivity that was needed to initiate moral reasoning and ethical analysis in the situation. The result could have been in the best interests of the patient, even though your own value position may not have been supported on the issue. The least you could have gained was understanding of how and why you differ with the final choice of action. Knowledge of why we are ill at ease with health care decisions contributes to our conscious selection of what type of patients/physicians we can work with most comfortably. We can then choose to avoid these situations ahead of time, rather than be trapped in them. Self-knowledge of gut-level reactions can also help us provide better nursing care by sensitizing us to situations where we might be uncomfortable so that we do not unconsciously avoid that patient or professional colleague.[6] Note that here again we have the interplay between feeling and reason, with reason applied to feelings.

Knowing the moral positions of others contributes to alternatives and the prediction of consequences for those actions (Step Eight of the decision model), including which are acceptable and which are not.[7] We mention Steps Six and Eight here to help you understand more clearly how the model fits together in an orderly manner. They are also a reminder of where we are headed—toward ethical decision making based on critical information and reasoned analysis of the moral variables in the health care situation, which includes information about feelings, as noted earlier.

HOW DOES ONE IDENTIFY VALUE POSITIONS OF OTHERS?

These are a variety of strategies one can use to identify the value positions of other people. These include values clarification exercises, personal discussions within a trusting relationship and environment, and application of moral development theory to the interpretation of behavior and actions.[8] Each of these strategies will be discussed as they apply to identifying the values and moral positions of others involved in health care situations.

Values Clarification Exercises

The use of values clarification exercises can help identify what individuals and groups value in a health care situation. The historical, philosophical, and religious background of the ethical issues helps one understand why individuals may hold different values on the same issue. Some of the exercises we have used to contribute to values clarification are case situations with directed value questions, preference lists, and the use of the Rest Defining the Issues Test (DIT) described in Chapter Three.

Much of our teaching in ethics utilizes case studies for the application of the theoretical bases of ethical decision making. When we have sufficient numbers available for study, we divide them into groups of about 10. The relatively small size of the groups facilitates discussion. There are several ground rules for this discussion. These include listening to others—do not interrupt until the person indicates he or she is finished. Respect the values and beliefs stated by others as being their own and therefore of value. Resist the urge to judge others' beliefs/values as right or wrong. They may be different from one's own but not necessarily better or worse. Be willing to share one's own values with reasons for them. Encourage everyone to go beyond the statement of values to an explanation of why they hold them. The role of the group leader is to assist participants to stay on the track of ethical inquiry, to focus on values and their clarification, and to see the variety of moral positions presented as another important step in understanding other people.[9]

We use actual case situations for ethical analysis while protecting the identity of all persons involved. We have found that real life cases increase the interest of the participants. They can often identify with the type of situation. They have been there. The cases for values clarification are presented with a series of questions directed at personal awareness and moral positions on predetermined ethical issues. For example, when we focus on value positions on the ethical concept of autonomy or self-determination, we may ask the following type of questions at the end of the case study. Following the principle of self-determination, what would you do in this situation as the nurse and why? The more critical part of this question is the "why?" for ethical reasoning. "How should the principle of autonomy guide the final decision in this case? Do you agree with this direction? If you were the patient in this situation, what would you like to have done? Why? What would you like done if the patient were your father (mother)? Why? As you responded to the earlier questions, what common ideas or pieces of information kept repeating themselves? Can you begin to identify your personal value position from your wanting this kind of information? Now state clearly why and to what extent you value the ethical principle of autonomy/self-determination." The group facilitator may think of other questions that will help individuals explore their value position on autonomy or any other ethical issue. The major benefit of these directed questions is the guidance offered participants who may be unfamiliar with values clarification.

Preference lists also help individuals get started on values clarification. Steele and Harmon developed several such lists. The one we have found helpful as an introductory exercise is the preference exercise.[10] One of the great advantages in this and other such exercises is that they can be used alone or within a group. If used alone, one may find a companion to share results. If used in a group, this exercise often promotes a lively discussion of the "Why?" we believe as we do. The preference list in particular sensitizes the taker to sometimes unknown value positions, since the underlying values are not stated in the questions. The questions are stated in language common to everyday use. Later analysis reveals the value positions. These may then be followed by prizing and cherishing exercises so that one begins to understand their hierarchy of values as well.[11]

Personal Discussion of Moral Positions

We have hinted at the nature of personal, one-on-one discussion of values and moral positions. The environment for this sharing implies participation in a trusting relationship. Nurses and patients often are involved in such a relationship. It follows that discussion of what one believes and values may take place within this context. Some views of nursing as a profession include the belief that nurses are not supposed to share any personal information with patients (or become emotionally involved). This may interfere with the nurse's ability to be objective in providing needed patient care.[12] One of the current criticisms of health care professionals is that they have left the humanity out of care, and patients are suffering needlessly from this omission. There are arguments supporting this position. However, there may also be a time and place for the sharing of personal value positions between a health professional and a patient.

Physicians and nurses sometimes disagree on what should be done for a given patient. Time taken for the individual doctor and nurse to discuss why they vary in their view of what is best for the patient may be most beneficial for all concerned. This approach can be seen as preferable to arguments in front of the patient and family or, worse, subversive attempts by professionals to get back at each other, often at the expense of the patient. Needless to say, the trusting environment, respect for others, and listening requirements hold for professional–professional value discussions as much as they do for patient–professional discussions. Just as there are varying value systems among clients, there are varying value systems among nurses and other team members. Respect for persons implies taking the time to understand our colleagues as well as our patients.

Stages of Moral Development

The final strategy for understanding the moral positions of key individuals involved in a health care situation is knowledge of stages of moral development. The ideas presented by Kohlberg, Rest, and Gilligan related to stages of moral development can be reviewed in Chapter Three. Here it is important to learn how these theories may be applied in understanding why individuals value as they do. For example, in a situation involving the ethical issue of informed consent, a person in Kohlberg's Stage Four, concern for law and order, may utilize the legal force of informed consent in determining what action to take. Another individual functioning primarily at level two (you scratch my back and I'll scratch yours) may value informed consent only if they perceive they will benefit from it in the situation.

It is important to emphasize once again that persons in various stages of moral development may end up making the same decision for action, though it is supported by a different rationale. The value in knowing the stage of moral development in addition to understanding the reasons for choosing a specific action is helping one understand the variety of possible actions that might be taken in the situation. The stage of moral development may also be insightful for the individual as one works toward self-understanding and decisions on whether to change one's value positions or reasoning about them.

SUMMARY

Step Five in the decision model calls for time to understand what key individuals in a health care situation value on the ethical issues. We are heading toward the time for deciding who is best able to make the needed decision as well as what options are available for action. Deliberate examination of what individuals in the situation believe and value assists us in determining where or whether there are moral conflicts. It is also a way of exploring the options for action and the consequences of the action for those involved as well as society as a whole. We are nearing our goal of ethical decision making based on moral reasoning. We can apply this step now to our paradigm case, "Birth of a Family," and then go on to identify moral conflicts in the situation that need clarification before deciding who should make the final decision.

THE CASE

The key individuals identified in Step One were Sara, Tom, their newborn son, the circulating nurse, the nurse–midwifery student and the nurse–midwifery instructor. The instructor's values were described for Step Four. Possible others include the nursing supervisor and other patients and nurses on the unit. We will focus on the values of the key individuals. The values are probably represented by the action and words or nonactions described in the initial presentation of the case. As discussed earlier, there are limitations in this interpretation. It may be necessary to note again that the values are not to be taken as the values of all nurses or parents or of any specific institution. We think the interpretations are reasonable inferences, however. In current practice, individuals are encouraged to speak for themselves of course.

What Are Sara's and Tom's Value Positions?

Although we know little of their background (age, religion, education, ethnic group, financial status, views of pregnancy, or if the child was wanted), their working together during labor and delivery is indicative of values in their relationship, the importance of sharing the experience (informed participation), and the right of Tom to be present at the birth of his son. It would also appear that their cultural norms support male participation in childbirth. Their choice of a tertiary level hospital clinic may imply a value of safety with unknown professionals over a do-it-yourself home birth.

Sara and Tom may or may not have had the final decision in nurse–midwifery care with student involvement. Informed consent should, of course, have been a part of that decision. They may have simply trusted that any provider allowed to work there would be competent.

The final parental value considered here is informed choice in holding their son. They both enjoyed doing so but would not have asked. We do not know from the presentation what kept them from immediately reaching for him. It may have been respect for the hospital rules or for authority. This is reflected in their initial questioning. When permission was granted, they responded with eagerness and enthusiasm, so their hesitancy was probably not any sense of incompetency on their own part.

What Are the Circulating Nurse's Values?

One of the issues in this case is informed consent. For the nurse, this appears to be secondary to her perceived duties to care for the infant. She may have simply not thought about parents' rights to hold their own child immediately after birth. She may not believe that physicians or nurse–midwives have the prerogative to decide where the infant would go after birth. She understood the child was to come to her for additional care. She was new to the area. She may have been functioning in an uncertain situation from Kohlberg's fear of punishment Stage One or in respect for what she thought were the rules, as in Stage Four. She was not looking at the whole situation and the good of all, though she did show respect for persons. Sometimes people do lose their jobs for violating the rules, and she appears to value that reality.

What Are G.W.'s Values on the Issues?

The presentation gives very little of the student's values in this case. Her words or thoughts are not recorded. We could conclude that she supports the instructor's value of bonding and parent autonomy because she gave the infant to the parents. She may, however, simply value doing what her instructor says (Stage Three in Kohlberg's outline) rather than having thought through the issues for herself. The observation was made earlier though that people may enter a profession because their own values are the same as the profession's. Nurse midwifery is synonymous with family-centered care based on patients' rights to self-determination. The chances are good that the student also values these concepts even as she is also aware of her student role, which may mean respect for authority figures. These values include the professional obligation to exercise informed judgment in carrying out her duties and making sure that the infant is in good condition so it can be held and that the parents want to hold him.

NOTES

1. Brody, H. *Ethical Decisions in Medicine.* Boston: Little, Brown, 1976, p. 12.
2. Raths, L.E., Harmin, M., and Simon, S.B. *Values and Teaching.* Columbus: Merrill, 1966, pp. 6, 170–171, 197–200.
3. Steele, S.M., and Harmon, V.M. *Values Clarification in Nursing.* Norwalk, CT: Appleton-Century-Crofts, 1983, pp. 24–27. Kreps, G.L., and Thornton, B. *Health Communication.* New York: Longmans, 1984, pp. 191–207.
4. ANA, *Code for Nurses with Interpretive Statements.* Kansas City, MO: ANA, 1976, Statement 1.3, p. 4.
5. The deference to authority can be seen as Kohlberg's Stage 3. The low self-image or lack of self-worth or apathy may be his preconventional level—there is nothing in it for the nurse—neither reward nor punishment. B.P. Hall points out that if nurses do not have a sense of self-worth or a belief in their worth as individuals, they may not be able to value others either. Hall, B.P. *Value Clarification as Learning Process.* New York: Paulist Press, 1973.
6. Thompson, J.B., and Thompson, H.O. *Ethics in Nursing.* New York: Macmillan, 1981, p. 3.
7. Brody, *Ethical Decisions in Medicine,* pp. 12, 16. Aroskar, M. "Anatomy of an ethical dilemma: The theory." *American Journal of Nursing* 80(4):659–660, 1980.
8. Steele and Harmon, *Values Clarification in Nursing,* pp. 13–18.
9. Berkowitz, M. "The role of discussion in ethics training." *Topics in Clinical Nursing* 4(1):39–41, April 1982. Bridston, E.O. "An educational strategy for enhancement of moral-ethical decision-making." *Topics in Clinical Nursing* 4(1):58–61, April 1982. Callahan, D., and Bok, S. (eds). *Ethics Teaching in Higher Education.* New York: Plenum Press,1980, pp. 64–69.
10. Steele and Harmon, *Values Clarification in Nursing,* pp. 212–216.
11. See Raths et al., *Values and Teaching,* for a full discussion of prizing and cherishing one's values.
12. King, E.C. *Affective Education in Nursing: A Guide to Teaching and Assessment.* Rockville, MD: Aspen Systems Corporation, 1984, pp. 11–12.

The test of a first-rate intelligence is the ability to hold two opposed ideas in the mind at the same time, and still retain the ability to function.

—F. Scott Fitzgerald
The Crack-up

CHAPTER 11

Step Six: Identify the Value Conflicts, If Any

Inherent in clarifying values is the discovery of when and why we disagree with others on what is the best thing to do in a health care situation. The previous two steps in the decision model have focused on techniques and reasons for identifying and clearly stating your values as well as those of others. With this understanding of what individuals value relative to ethical issues, you are now ready to clearly identify when and if those values are in conflict. Value conflict often contributes to the confusion and difficulty of making ethical decisions in health care. It, therefore, is important to know when and where that conflict lies. Then the people involved can decide how to resolve such conflicts so that decision making can proceed.

The resolution of value conflicts in a health care situation is predicated on clear identification of conflict. It includes determining the value hierarchy that will be followed in the rest of the situation.[1] Value conflicts do not necessarily result in moral dilemmas, that is, we may differ in our value position on abortion, but unless we need to make a decision on whether to perform the abortion or not, we may not be in a dilemma. Since this text is about making decisions, ethical decisions, we focus on the moral dilemmas. For purposes of discussion here, we will equate a value conflict with a moral dilemma.

The criteria for a moral dilemma were presented in Chapter Five. Briefly, these included (1) an awareness of different options, (2) the ethical or moral nature of the issue at hand, and (3) the existence of two or more possible actions with the freedom to decide between or among them. We are especially concerned with the first criterion at this time, the awareness of differing options. These differing options are often highlighted during individual and group exploration of values. The historical, philosophical, and religious bases for our value positions may also provide different options. As we listen to each other, we begin to realize how different we are as individuals, as well as how similar. When pushed to explore an ethical issue or principle, our differences may come out as conflicts—value conflicts. Let us first explore some of the situations in which value conflicts may appear.

WHAT ARE THE VALUE CONFLICTS?

Conflicts Within the Individual

Value conflict may occur within an individual, between individuals, and among groups. As nurses explore what they believe and value as persons and as professional nurses, sources of potential conflict may appear. One way to help individuals identify such conflicts has been the use of three main questions.[2] The first is, "What are the characteristics of the ideal patient?" We allow time for individual writing or the use of a blackboard to compile the list of characteristics. Once the list is completed, one can ask, "Why did you select that particular characteristic or quality?" After discussion, there is a second question. "What are the characteristics of the ideal nurse?" The individual lists can be shared while also asking why a characteristic was chosen. We ask individuals to keep a copy of their own lists so that they may identify their own values in the exercise, rather than affirming the group consensus of values.

The nurse's individual list of characteristics of the ideal patient and nurse also provides the basis for the third question in this exercise. "What characteristics do you have listed for the ideal nurse that would describe yourself?" Frequently we do not ask for group sharing of this part of the exercise. The individual is encouraged to give it further thought.

The next step is to compare the characteristics of the ideal nurse and patient. This helps identify potential conflict between the way nurses should practice and the type of patient they would prefer to have. For example, gerontological nurses sometimes define the ideal patient as one who can participate in decisions, take responsibility for actions, and be willing to learn how to take better care of themselves. Elderly patients in nursing homes do not always fit this description. The next step may be to explore ways that nurses can care for such patients who do not fit their expectations. Many other examples of conflict in values of professionals as persons and their potential conflict with moral duties or obligations as professionals (care for patient without discrimination) could be given.

The exercise of identifying one's personal view on what constitutes good nursing (the ideal nurse) can be expanded. One can compare the final list of nurse attributes with the ANA *Code for Nurses,* standards for practice, and ANA *A Social Policy Statement.*[3] One can then encourage discussion of which characteristics one can support and practice and which are in conflict with what one personally believes about nursing and, therefore, may not put into practice.

Patients may find they hold conflicting values. One may value self-determination. Yet, when severely ill or in pain, the patient may want someone else to take care of them and make the decisions. Discussion of values and the influence of the situation on what the patient would like to have done also helps to clarify when an individual's values may be in conflict.

Conflict Between Individuals

The majority of value conflicts identified in health care situations arise between or among individuals. These may include patient, family, physician, nurse, clergy, lawyer, hospital administrator, and others in any number of dyadic combinations. The most common value conflicts occur between patient and health care professional(s) and between professional and professional. There are also conflicts between patient and family that sometimes end up with a legal opinion on the competency of the patient.[4]

There are many reasons why patient and health care professional might value different things in health and illness care. Prominent among these is the view that since the professional is highly educated and more knowledgeable about the patient's need for treatment, professional values differ markedly from those of the patient. We note that nurses and physicians are socialized to value health, life, and the pursuit of each. Does this socialization result in our being less understanding of others who may not value these? Not necessarily, though it may create value conflicts with patients who value death more than life full of disease or pain or suffering. Some authors suggest that the cultures of medicine and nursing do place different value on health and illness, treatment and cure.[5] If we are products of our culture in value formation, we may hold different values on life, death, and illness than nonhealth professionals.

Value conflicts between physician and nurse occur. One explanation of such conflict is the emphasis nursing places on caring for the whole person (not just the disease). That care should continue even when we cannot cure. This emphasis on caring, while not absent in medicine, is often replaced in the value hierarchy of physicians with the emphasis on curing.[6] Many physicians face the reality of death, however. They know the inevitability of not being able to keep all persons alive and reasonably healthy. They also value caring. For others who cannot admit to being unable to cure all ills, the decision to keep trying may override an ethical concern for mercy.[7]

Another variable in the practice of nursing that contributes to value conflict is the role of patient advocate. The nature of nursing practice requires more extended time contact with patients than is available to the physician. Because the nurse has developed a relationship with the patient based on extended contact, the physician may, in effect, be caring for a stranger. The nurse thus seems justified in accepting the role of advocate. The ANA *Code for Nurses* dictates that respect for human dignity with support of patient's right to self-determination is an integral part of nursing practice. This value supports patient decision making. It supports what patients would want if they could decide for themselves. In such situations in which the patient lacks the capacity to decide, the nurse tries to speak on behalf of the patient in support of self-determination.[8] This may be in conflict with what the physician thinks is best in the situation, even though personally the nurse may agree with the physician's view. Value hierarchy places the patient's choice above those of the professionals in this situation.

Understanding when and why patient and family disagree on what is best is sometimes difficult. Human beings operate from mixed motives, perhaps most of the time. Even when we take the time to examine our own motives and values, we may be surprised at the outcome and confused about what to do. Health care situations that involve disagreement between patient and family need to be analyzed to determine if the disagreement is a moral or value disagreement or something else. Deciding to let "Aunt Tilly go" may be an act of mercy or an eagerness to lessen the burden of caring for her or even to get the profits from her will. If Aunt Tilly is awake and capable of making her own decision, more and more health care professionals would accept her position before that of the family. A value conflict remains, however, if Aunt Tilly is hanging on to cause problems for the remaining family or is placing unrealistic expectations on her family or society to care for her. Whether or not she has a right to decide that limited resources be used to prolong her life is a difficult moral dilemma.[9]

Family members can also disagree among themselves about what is best for the patient. Sometimes this disagreement is caused by imposing their values on the patient, and sometimes it results from guilt. Extraordinary measures may be pushed by family members out of deep love and care. Then again, they may feel guilty about the patient's condition or about past neglect of the patient. Values clarification is particularly useful here. It helps everyone involved decide what is the best thing to do. It also helps people understand why they have chosen a given action. It may be viewed as a positive force in encouraging individuals to work through their own psychological blocks (with professional counseling) with growth toward self-actualization.

Conflict Among Groups

Value conflicts among groups may have little bearing on an individual patient situation. Some believe that the interests of groups and society at large should have little place in the discussion of what to do for an individual patient. This rugged individualism is especially prominent in Western thought. Others suggest that if we do not keep society's interests in mind, we will have expended our limited health care resources in ways that may not be morally defensible. We are back to the ethical question, "Just because we can, should we?" This question is of particular importance in the use of biomedical technology, just distribution of scarce (limited) resources, and who will pay for these. We are also back to the issue of the adolescent who wants the privileges of adulthood without the responsibility.

Health care providers have a responsibility to society. If you are using this decision model alone, you need to ask such questions as these. "What is society's position on the ethical issues in this situation? What would happen if everyone decided to take the action(s) we are considering? What are the costs and benefits to society of providing care for this patient? Why should society pay for this person's care? To what extent should society's interest be allowed to influence the final decision made for this patient?" These same questions would be helpful in group discussion as well, though often individuals within the group will have presented a similar value position during the earlier steps of the model.

Conflicting Loyalties

A final word on value conflicts is related to the issue of conflicting loyalties for health care professionals. When nurses and physicians are employees of an institution, they must be aware of their duties and obligations to that employer as well as to the patient. Sometimes these duties or loyalties are in conflict. For example, the hospital as a major employer of health care professionals is often managed on a utilitarian concern for the greatest good for the greatest number. This utilitarian ethic may be in conflict with the nurse's principled concern for the autonomy of the individual patient.[10] The patient wants or needs a special touch from home (food, a prized possession, a visit from a child). This need is supported by the physician and nurse. The hospital administrator says "No" to the request, however. The administrator reasons that if we allow it for this one person, we will have many more requests. Besides, animals or outside food will only cause health hazards for other patients in the hospital. The nurse or physician is now faced with the dilemma of deciding to allow the food or pet anyway. They may claim a higher value of what is best for this patient versus what the hospital reasons is best. On the other hand, they may agree with the decision of the hospital administrator and tell the patient they cannot meet his need.

Issues of staff assignments and shortages also create value conflicts with professionals at times. If a hospital makes its decision on how many nurses or physicians to hire based on pure economics without regard for the quality of care, the health care may suffer. Health care professionals need to actively participate in such decisions in order to define the help needed to implement the quality of care demanded from ethical professionals. If you know a given institution cuts corners in personnel in order to save operating costs, you may decide not to work in that setting. We have now moved to a concern for preventing value conflict for an individual, but what about the patients and professionals who are working in that institution where quality is second to productivity? Do we not all have a moral obligation to help to change the pattern of staffing when patient care is diminished or threatened?

Whether you identify a value conflict within yourself, between individuals involved in the situation, or among groups, take time to understand why it has occurred. Note the particular values in conflict for further analysis. The hierarchy of values evolved will form one of the key elements in finally deciding what should be done in this situation.

WHAT IS THE VALUE HIERARCHY?

Rokeach has written that once a value is internalized, it becomes a standard or criterion for guiding one's actions and morally judging the self and others.[11] However, values are also dynamic—they change. Burns takes a strong stand in relation to values and being a professional. He suggests that a professional is willing to state and change personal and social values in order to more effectively use special knowledge and skills to solve the health problems of communities and individuals.[12] In other words, solving health problems is at the top of the hierarchy. The process of choosing, then prizing, values implies a willingness to change value positions or at least rank them so that the predominant value is clear. This predominant value will then guide one in deciding what should be done in a given situation.

Prizing one's values implies a hierarchy.[13] This ordering of values is a rational process that identifies where potential or actual value conflict lies. If we have conflict within ourselves, we cannot proceed to decision making until we determine the rank order of the values in conflict. In other words, which value is most important to me right now? I may not be able to act on two values in conflict at the same time; therefore, I may rank one higher than the other for the moment and take both the risk and responsibility for the outcome. Likewise, in situations of value conflict between two or more individuals, the conflicting values must be clearly stated and then rank ordered or prized. This prizing requires time and discussion in much the same way that values clarification does. It is often done simultaneously with the decision about who can best make the needed decision in the situation. That is, preference may be given to those values of the person who will probably end up making the final decision. We discuss this further in Chapter Twelve.

For discussion purposes, we will assume that team decision making is expected. We are also assuming that value conflicts require an intelligent appraisal of the merit of competing values. One way to rank order values is to list the values in conflict and to whom they originally belonged.

If several values are in conflict on the same ethical issue, group them together for discussion and decision making. If only two values are in conflict, pair them as well. The next step is to ask, "Which of these two (or more) values do I accept as most important in determining action? Why?" Then place the number 1 next to the value ranked highest in the list. Go on in descending order of importance until all values in conflict are ranked. For each decision on ranking, you might ask yourself or group members the following questions. "Can I (we) live with the decision if it is based on this value? Will I (we) be proud to openly state this value to others and acknowledge that the decision was based on this value?" If you are doing this ranking as part of a group, share your ideas on ranking as well as asking for the ideas of others. You will probably need to decide ahead of time whether consensus will rule (unanimity may be very difficult, if not impossible, in questions of value). That is, will a vote be taken and the majority determine the value ranking? And will dissenting voters be expected to support the vote of the majority?

SUMMARY

Value ranking is a difficult and time-consuming process for individuals who have not used this technique before. The more it is used, however, the easier the process. The more it is used, the greater the chances that moral conflict will be resolved in the best interests of all persons involved. Keep your list of value conflicts as we proceed to the next steps of the decision model. Understanding why we had the conflicts and keeping a record of how they were resolved will help us move closer to the final decision that is best for this situation. We still cannot predict the right answer, but we are becoming clearer in our understanding of who should make the decision and from what list of alternative actions. Step Six might have this result for "Birth of a Family."

THE CASE

What Are the Value Conflicts?

The most obvious conflict is between the instructor and the circulating nurse. Both appear to be concerned with the adjustment of the newborn to extra-uterine life. They disagree on where that adjustment should take place in the best interests of the newborn. The nurse appears comfortable with caring for and monitoring the infant if she has him. She is uncomfortable carrying out the procedures with the baby lying on the mother. Perhaps she has never done this, or perhaps she believes it unsafe. Her expressed reason is a fear for her job and the need to follow presumed policies. The nurse may have a personal conflict of values.

The instructor appears to be carrying out her duty to exercise informed judgment. She presumably checked the health of the child and then promoted the values of bonding, parent choice, and safety after seeking parental agreement.

If there were a hospital policy against the midwife's procedure, this would be a conflict. If the procedure spreads to other delivering mothers, it may bring conflicts with the staff, the patients, and the hospital in the use of time and carrying out other procedures.

What Is the Value Hierarchy?

The value hierarchy is established by the instructor. It begins with safety for the infant, which is followed by infant–parent bonding and informed choice by the parents to hold their son, and then an explanation of safety to her nurse colleague. The nurse–midwife is in a position of authority, making decisions and apparently willing to accept responsibility for her actions, although she does not actually say that.

NOTES

1. Steele, S., and Harmon, V. *Values Clarification in Nursing*, 2nd ed. Norwalk, CT: Appleton-Century-Crofts, 1983, pp. 13–15, 20–22. Callahan, D., and Bok, S. *Ethics Teaching in Higher Education*. New York: Plenum Press, 1980, pp. 67–69, 70. Raths, L.E., Harmin, M., and Simon, S.B. *Values and Teaching*. Columbus: Merrill, 1966, pp. 6, 170–171, 197–200. Muyskens, J.L. *Moral Problems in Nursing*. Totowa, NJ: Rowman and Littlefield, 1982, pp. 21–24.
2. Uustal, D. *Values and Ethics: Considerations in Nursing Practice*. South Deerfield, MA: Uustal, 1978, p. 73.
3. ANA, *Nursing—A Social Policy Statement*. Kansas City, MO: ANA, 1980.
4. Curran, W.J., and Shapiro, E.D. *Law, Medicine and Forensic Science*, 3rd ed. Boston: Little, Brown, 1982, pp. 821–845. Veatch, R.J. *Case Studies in Medical Ethics*. Cambridge, MA: Harvard University Press, pp. 43–48.
5. Steele and Harmon, *Values Clarification in Nursing*, 2nd ed, pp. 20–22, 24–27. Kreps, G. L., and Thornton, B.C. *Health Communication*. New York: Longman, 1984, pp. 195–202.
6. Muyskens, *Moral Problems in Nursing*, pp. 30–40. Hull, R. T. "Defining nursing ethics apart from medical ethics." *The Kansas Nurse* 55:5, 8, 20ff, September 1980. Brooke, J.A., and Kleine-Kracht, A.E. "Evolution of a definition of nursing." *Advances in Nursing Science* 5(4):51–85, July 1983.
7. Huttman, B. "A crime of compassion." *Newsweek*, August 8, 1983, p. 15.
8. Curtin, L. "Human advocacy: A philosophical foundation for nursing." *Advances in Nursing Science* 1(3):1–10, 1979. Ashley, J.A. *Hospitals, Paternalism and the Role of the Nurse*. New York: Teacher's College Press, 1976. Beauchamp, T., and Childress, J. *Principles of Biomedical Ethics*, 2nd ed. New York: Oxford University Press, 1983, pp. 136–143.
9. Beauchamp and Childress, *Principles of Biomedical Ethics,* "The principle of justice," pp. 183–217. President's Commission for the Study of Ethical Problems in Medicine and Biomedical and Behavioral Research. *Making Health Care Decisions*. Washington, DC: US Government Printing Office, October 1982, Vol. 1, p. 3, says, "Patients are not entitled to insist that health care practitioners furnish them services when to do so would violate either the bounds of acceptable practice . . . or would draw on a limited resource on which the patient has no binding claim."

10. Thompson, J.E. "Conflicting loyalties of nurses working in bureaucratic settings." *Professionalism and the Empowerment of Nursing.* Kansas City, MO: ANA, December 1982, pp. 27–37. Smith, S., and Davis, A. "Ethical dilemmas: Conflict among rights, duties and obligations." *American Journal of Nursing* 80(8):1463–1466, August 1980. Jameton, A. "The nurse: When roles and rules conflict." *HCR* 7(4):22–23, August 1977. Davis, A., and Aroskar, M. *Ethical Dilemmas and Nursing Practice,* 2nd ed. Norwalk, CT: Appleton-Century-Crofts, 1983, Chap. 5, "Professional ethics and institutional constraints with nursing practice," pp. 49–65.
11. Rokeach, M. *Beliefs, Attitudes, and Values.* San Francisco: Jossey-Bass, 1969.
12. Burns, C.R. "Comparative ethics of the medical profession outside of the United States." *Humanities and Medicine* 32:181, Spring 1974.
13. Steele and Harmon, *Values Clarification in Nursing,* pp. 4–5, 15.

Absolutizing the authority of any one of these—the patient, the physician, the lay and professional, social networks, and the larger society—would be moral disaster.

—Robert J. Veatch[1]

CHAPTER 12

Step Seven: Determine Who Should Decide

We have come to that step in moral reasoning when it is time to identify who will be making the final decision. This decision could wait until alternative actions and their consequences have been identified. However, a preliminary indication of decision maker may help to clarify how much time will be needed (group discussion versus individual). If the decision maker, e.g., a court judge, is not present, it may take time to reach her. Identification of the probable decision maker also allows that person time to review the steps in this decision or the moral reasoning in the case.

Our previous six steps in the decision model have shown that there may be several candidates for the role of decision maker in health care situations.[2] In the past, the physician has often been assumed to be the most appropriate person to make the decisions. This is not so widely accepted today, even among physicians. The nurse's role in this area is increasing, as is that of other health care professionals. Ethicists and philosophers are also providing guidance, though they are not the final word on what should be done either. The patient, of course, is the primary decision maker. There is a new or renewed emphasis on the patient's role. Changing norms in society, an increasing emphasis on the rights of individuals or personal freedom, and a general dissatisfaction with persons in authority have contributed to a new situation.[3]

Yet the patient is not always the best person to make a needed decision, either, even though that health care decision directly affects him or her. The fetus, neonate, and comatose adult cannot speak for themselves at the moment of decision making. Others are left with determining who can best speak on behalf of these patients. Even then a selected individual may not be the best person to make the final choice. The government is vying for a role in some ethical dilemmas in health care (Baby Doe), speaking ostensibly on behalf of society in general.[4] The courts have made ethical decisions, sometimes stepping in unbidden to protect human rights, sometimes when concerned parties in the case could not reach an agreement on such procedures as amputation, abortion, or declaration of incompetency.[5] Family members have been asked to decide in some situations, especially if patients were incapable of deciding. They have been consulted when the health professionals thought the patient was choosing the wrong course of action, though not necessarily left with the final decision. Each of these and other potential decision makers are discussed in this chapter.

There is a major perspective to keep in mind at this point. Who decides may be less important than the basis for the decision making.[6] To put it another way, how one makes a decision in health care ethics (moral reasoning, orderly and critical analysis, and choice from alternatives based on ethical justification) may be more important than who makes that decision. In deciding who decides, consideration of that person's ability and willingness to use moral reasoning is normally crucial. Among the difficulties that may arise is the claim to support client choice when the choice may be mere whim. If key persons are unwilling to reason morally, one might have difficulty supporting their final decision. If the key persons have participated in the steps to this point and are committed to completing the process (Steps Eight, Nine, Ten), it may not make any difference whether the nurse, the physician, the patient or someone else makes the final choice. Let us take a closer look at the list of decision makers and how one might decide who will make the final choice.

WHO OWNS THE PROBLEM?

Sometimes when one is involved in the thick of controversy and uncertainty, it is helpful to focus thoughts by asking, "Who owns the problem I've identified?" Ownership may become a convenient excuse for nonowners to drop out of the controversy and let others decide. It may also be the rationale used to keep others from imposing their view, values, or power on the decision maker.

Asking "Who owns the problem?" in situations involving health care ethics can be a good introduction to thinking about who might be the best decision maker. However, it may become an oversimplified approach to a serious and difficult critical inquiry. You have, no doubt, already realized in the early steps of this decision model that the patient as well as many other key individuals may own the problem in health care ethics. Needless to say, definition of the problem may also vary from participant to participant, just as examination of value positions may highlight new problems not recognized during the initial presentation of the case for analysis. So you might well be thinking, "Why put any effort into identifying who owns the problem at hand?"

There are a variety of reasons one might wish to spend some time on identifying the person(s) most directly connected to the problem(s). First of all, this exercise may help to focus problem identification more clearly. The problem from an ethical perspective may be the initial patient request for a given action (no further treatment, request for relief of pain that might hasten death, abortion for wrong sex fetus). As you have moved through the decision model, you have begun to realize that what might have initially seemed a problem for just one patient and the health care provider goes beyond them. These two individuals are not living in isolation. Other providers might be asked to carry out a patient request that they cannot morally or ethically support. The problem is expanded and becomes theirs as well. While the patient thinks only he or she will be affected by the outcome of the decision, family members may disagree and become part-owners of the problem as well. In the process, they may also redefine the problem, and the final partner in the problem may be society at large.[7] Each of these may help to define the problem more clearly, including its potential effects on themselves. As noted earlier, this type of introspection and sharing is beneficial in defining the issues. It is helpful in identifying areas of value conflict that can then be resolved or integrated into the final list of alternatives and consequences.

The second reason one may wish to explore the ramifications of "Who owns the problem?" is as a check on the moral reasoning process. Step One included the identification of key individuals involved in the ethical dimensions of the health care situation. Another look at this list was noted for Steps Two and Five. Now is the time to ask whether individuals currently involved are really key. Are some of the persons involved in the decision making really involved in the problem? This may be the time to consider society's concerns and the extent to which these influence a decision for an individual patient. The legal representative of the hospital may have asked to participate, but the problem now clarified does not have a significant legal dimension. A nurse from another unit may have participated in early discussions because of personal interest in the outcome, but may not be appropriate in the decision making now. Deciding who owns the problem not only helps to clarify the problem but also helps to clarify who should be involved in the final decision making.

In nonpatient decisions, problem ownership is important in identifying ethical issues and the groups affected by the impending decision. Health policy decisions often take place at the administrative levels (government, hospital). It does not necessarily follow that administrators or politicians are the most appropriate persons to make these decisions.[8] By identifying the individuals and groups potentially affected by the proposed policy, one can involve spokespersons from these groups in the decision analysis. The problem may not be identified as simply a health policy statement. It may involve how this statement will affect the individuals and groups for whom it is intended. Administrators, elected officials, and business executives are not above moral reasoning. They, too, may need help in identifying when they are involved in the ethical dimensions of health care. They need to work through the situation in an orderly fashion, utilizing critical reasoning skills. Asking the question, "Who owns the problem?" may facilitate this identification of ethical dimensions in health policy decisions.

WHO DECIDES WHO DECIDES?

Several people may be available as decision makers. Current health care ethics implies the involvement of patient, physician, nurse, and patient family at a minimum. Social worker, hospital administrator, chaplain, legal affairs officer, and others may also become involved. At some point in the moral reasoning process, a decision needs to be made on who should make the final choice for action. Veatch has stated that absolutizing the authority of any one of these participants in health care situations would be moral disaster.[9] We agree. The elements of a given ethical dilemma change from situation to situation. The person or persons who made a good decision at one time may not be the one(s) to decide the next time.

The person who has invested the time and energy needed to learn and apply moral reasoning may have an advantage in decision making now and the next time around. Veatch warns, however, that repeated exposure to difficult ethical dilemmas in health care may inure an individual and actually decrease one's effectiveness as decision maker through lack of sensitivity to the new situation.[10] How many times can one live through the heart-rending, emotional aspects of severely ill or defective neonates and their parents before wanting out or turning off your hearing because you have seen this before and know what to do? Respect for persons requires listening, caring, understanding, feeling. It also requires ethical decision making. Will you be the one to participate and should you be the decision maker?

The Patient As Decision Maker

The President's Commission for the Study of Ethical Problems in Medicine and Biomedical and Behavioral Research issued a recommendation on making health care decisions in its report of October 1982. The Commission said that patients who have the capacity to make decisions about their care must be permitted to do so voluntarily based on ethically valid informed consent. They added that the decision process is one of shared decision making based on mutual respect and complete information.[11] This supports Veatch's idea that if there is to be individual responsibility and dignity in health care, the individual must retain significant control over decisions that most directly affect one's own welfare.[12]

The Commission noted that patient choice is not absolute, however. The patient cannot insist that health care professionals provide services that violate acceptable practice or the professional's moral beliefs. They also noted that the patient cannot expect services that would draw on a limited resource on which the patient has no binding claim.[13]

This clarification of the limits of patients' personal choice is valid. However, people might interpret these identified limits on patient autonomy as maintaining the power status of health professionals over patients. For example, why should the professionals deeply held moral or religious beliefs carry any more weight in the situation than the patient's? Presumably the patient's request is in keeping with personal, deeply held moral beliefs. Should the professional be able to veto actions that are not in keeping with their own personal values? The ANA *Code for Nurses* suggests that when nurses are caught in the dilemma of personal beliefs in conflict with those of the patient, they may elect not to care for that person only if another person can be found to provide the needed care.[14] We would agree that professionals not be required to do what they have defined as morally wrong for themselves. But they may retain a higher responsibility (moral obligation?) of caring for the patient or at least referring the client to another professional who can care for the patient. If this is not done, the health care professional risks imposing an unethical or immoral action on the patient (from the patient's perspective).

The Professional As Decision Maker

We are living in an age of complex technology, and much of that technology has been applied in health care. Nurses and physicians are already in danger of becoming mere technicians rather than professional care providers. They are tempted to apply technology without trying to understand how it works and why. Technology in health care has created choices for patient care that did not exist a short time ago. These new choices require new approaches in clinical and ethical decision making.[15]

Likewise, the era of the automatic acceptance of physicians or nurses as competent in ethical decision making is coming to a close. People are becoming more aware of the special knowledge and skills needed for this type of decision making, that is, we need to know the how and why of ethical decision making. As stated earlier, technical expertise and clinical skill cannot be generalized to ethics.[16] This does not preclude health care professionals from learning how to make ethical decisions, however. Your reading of this text suggests your interest in expanding your knowledge and skill in ethical decision making. However, because you develop skill in moral reasoning, it does not follow that you should always be the decision maker in ethical dimensions of practice.

There are some patient care situations where it seems most appropriate for the health care professional to make the final choice for action. This may appear obvious when the patient asks the physician to make the decision. A situation like this may seem easy at first glance, but it is probably one of the most difficult for the physician to be in. Patient deference to physician decision making may reflect a deference to authority (the doctor knows best). It may be a reasoned plea for help in a difficult situation or something in between. It is important for the physician to understand why the patient has asked him or her to make the needed decision. Physicians must ask themselves, Are you being set up for a later lawsuit if the patient does not like your decision or the outcome? Are you being asked to take responsibility for an adult who is capable of taking responsibility for personal decisions? Should you take on the responsibility, and why?

We add a note of caution that the patient request that the physician make the needed decision should not be seen as an ego-inflating statement. "The patient has chosen you because you are good and do know best." Physicians and other health professionals do strive to make decisions in the best interests of patients, but we need help in identifying what those best interests are. Physicians and all health professionals would do well to remember the Oracle of Delphi's definition of why Socrates was the wisest of all men. He was wise because he knew how ignorant he was, how little he really knew. Health care professionals are relatively ignorant in making ethical decisions. Knowledge of this fact leads toward wisdom in caring for patients. This is especially true if the patient refuses to take part in any critical analysis of the situation and offers no input on preferences or potential value conflicts. Seeking out significant others in the situation for this information and trying to understand why the patient deferred decision making to the physician indicates that the responsibility for decision making is not taken lightly.

Others As Decision Makers

Another concern raised by the President's Commission is the "capacity for decision making." This concern has a number of value judgments, such as who determines whether the patient or professional or anyone else is capable of participating in decisions about health care? And what basis or definition of "incapacity" should be used? At present, there is general acceptance of the definition of incapacity that includes mental retardation, lack of consciousness, and younger chronological age (infants and young children—the debate continues on when a child is old enough to give informed consent).[17]

However, conscious rational human beings are not always able to make decisions about what to do, even when healthy. The additional strain of being ill may further alter one's ability to decide, yet willingness to participate may be present. One needs to note also that personal investment in the outcome (research, personal moral bias) for the professionals or the family may preclude their capacity for deciding what is best in the situation. Following the steps of the decision model and personal values clarification may offer insight on who can best make the decision in the situation if the patient is incapacitated.

Legal precedent has been set in cases involving comatose individuals, and guidance from this can be helpful. Family members or close friends have often been cited as appropriate spokespersons. In general, if the comatose or incapacitated person has previously expressed preferences or values, the person who knows this should be involved in the final decision. Cases of no prior capacity are more difficult and require spokespersons who try to imagine what that person would want done if they were able to decide.[18]

Team Decision Making

Many people involved in current health care ethics have found it helpful to submit ethical decision making to a team. The advantages of group or team work are clear in the earlier discussion of the steps of the decision process. Sometimes a group of individuals is best for the decision making as well. The group may be those key individuals identified in the earlier stages of ethical inquiry. Involving the total group in selecting the final choice of action may appear to be relatively easy providing there are no major value conflicts. If conflicts do arise, however, the decision making becomes more difficult as the team determines which values should determine the decision and why.

Team decision making may still be the best way to approach ethical decisions in health care, providing the team follows the orderly steps of moral reasoning and the patient is involved. If the group simply meets briefly to take a vote from a list of options, the resultant decision may be neither ethical nor in the best interests of the patient. Ethics committees in health care settings are increasing in number across the United States in response to the need for a forum for ethical discussion and decision making. These committees, however, usually do not function unless requested by a patient or professional. They tend to deal with the more complex and critical (life and death) decisions rather than the day-to-day ethical dimensions of health care practice.[19]

Team decision making requires time and interest from a number of people. Neither of these is always available in health care practice. The patient's need for an immediate decision will certainly obviate lengthy team discussion. A few members trained in ethical reasoning may be consulted by the physician, patient, or family when time is limited. After an emergency, the decision can be submitted for discussion and analysis. We have discussed the value of retrospective analysis of decisions as one prepares for future similar situations. The interests of individuals vary, though health care professionals do value the need for moral reasoning and ethical decision making. Other demands for their time may vote against lengthy ethics meetings. People with interest and background in moral reasoning can be named to the ethics committee. When a need for discussion arises, available people can be selected from the total list.

WHAT IS THE ROLE OF THE NURSE?

The role of the nurse in ethical decision making situations follows the same line of reasoning offered above, that is, the nurse needs to begin by answering the question "Do I own this problem? If so, to what extent, and why? Are my claims to active participation in moral reasoning justified in this particular situation? On what basis? Am I willing to examine and share my personal and professional values on the ethical issues just as I expect others to share? Am I willing to commit time and effort to values conflict resolution and other aspects of moral reasoning? (We noted earlier that to be professional is to be ethical.) Do I have a personal or professional stake in the outcome of the decision that qualifies or disqualifies me as a decision maker? Is there a need for anyone other than the patient to decide on the final course of action?"

The ANA *Code for Nurses* claims that the nurse protects or safeguards the patient against the unethical, illegal, or incompetent practice of anyone else.[20] This may be interpreted as the role of ethical watchdog, though many would shudder at the thought. In fact, there are instances of nurses who were so busy watching each other, they forgot to take care of the patients. It is doubtful that the squeal sheet offers much, if any, ethical guarantee to the patient, and yet, the public expects and deserves no less from educated and licensed professionals than ethical, competent, and legal practice. Practical application of this advocate role includes responsibility (albeit shared with other professionals) for ensuring that the ethical dimensions of practice have been identified and moral reasoning has preceded ethical decision making. This does not mean that the nurse is always the final decision maker. She assures the client that an ethical approach to decision making has been or will be followed.

One final note on the role of the nurse involves sharing one's personal belief of what should be done. A patient may offer much more information and concern about a pending decision in care to a nurse than to the physician. You will need to determine whether this information needs to be included in the discussions of what should be done and, if so, encourage the patient to do so. If this is not possible, you may decide to offer the information on behalf of the patient, being careful to maintain needed confidentiality.

At times, the patient may also have asked, "What would you do if you were me?" These questions raise the issue of when, if ever, it is appropriate to share one's personal ideas on what should be decided with the patient. We know from many studies in clinical practice that patients can be easily influenced by nurses and physicians because of their "authority and knowledge" status.[21] We therefore need to be careful when asked to share what action we would take in the situation. First of all, we may not have complete information. The response would be unexamined in the light of the decision model. If your response is clearly a personal one, it may not fit the patient's situation without question. Just as it is unethical to unconsciously impose one's values and moral stands on patients, it may be inappropriate to consciously share these as well. We cannot ever completely know what another person is thinking or what factors they use to make decisions. We may, therefore, wish to share this with the patient and explore why they asked the initial question rather than volunteering our personal stand on the issue.

SUMMARY

Recent articles have appeared in professional journals that call the President's Commission reports the consensus ethic in health care.[22] Time will tell if that becomes a reality. We accept these reports as the results of reasoned analysis and critical inquiry by an interdisciplinary group of professionals (including one nurse), and therefore worthy of consideration by anyone involved in health care ethics. However, following their recommendations without personal thought and moral reasoning could lead to unethical decisions in health care. One cannot escape the effort needed to learn moral reasoning if one truly wishes to make ethical decisions in professional practice. One can recognize the value of the ideas. One can try to understand the reasoning behind the ideas. One can ask if any particular recommendation fits your own situation. To blindly follow the Commission's report without further thought, however, is to substitute authority for reason, as in Kohlberg's Stage 3.

At the completion of Step Seven, it may be apparent that more than one individual may qualify as the decision maker in the situation. It may be the patient or a health care professional or a combination of people. Realistically, health care has not moved completely beyond the old days when decisions were made by those with power and status. However, the current emphasis on patient rights reinforces the patient as decision maker. But those who are to carry out the decision and other interested parties (family, hospital, society) also have rights to participate in the decision-making process.

Determination of the decision maker should include the following as the person(s) proposed is reviewed. "Are these persons involved in and significantly aware of the critical elements of the situation? Are they willing to use moral reasoning to reach a final decision? Do they know themselves well enough to identify the personal values and potential biases they bring to the decision? Are they willing to make the final choice from a list of alternatives with moral justification?" Potentially anyone who can respond positively to these questions could also decide what is best for the patient in the situation. This may be the patient, the family, the health care provider, or others.

Before proceeding to Step Eight to clearly identify the alternatives for action and their consequences, Step Seven can be used to further analyze "Birth of a Family."

THE CASE

Who Owns the Problem?

In this case, the health problems of neonatal stability and the need for bonding were identified. Secondary concern for the allocation of nurse time was also raised. A successful transition to extrauterine life is of direct benefit not only to the newborn but to his parents and the professional staff who have accepted responsibility for overseeing that transition. The allocation of professional time involves the professionals immediately included and the supervisory personnel who determine staffing patterns and assignments. The patients are, of course, the primary concern, both those immediately included and others who are present elsewhere in the facility and future patients who will be involved in this facility and in the practices of the professionals.

Who Decides Who Decides?

In this situation, the nurse–midwifery instructor appears in control of the entire situation. She is responsible not only for her student but also for the care of Sara, Tom, and their son. She made a decision to allow Sara and Tom to hold their baby over the objections of her nurse colleague. She helped the nurse to understand why she made this choice but without reassuring her that she, the instructor, would take responsibility for the choice. Before actually handing the boy to his parents, she asked them if they would like to hold him, giving them the right to refuse, i.e., a choice. In this, she was in a position of power, but she also shared that power with the parents by asking their preference first. She appeared to be aware of the infant's health status and thus exercised informed judgment in sharing of that decision making. It is, however, not clear what happened in terms of additional procedures in the birth process. Presumably, these were carried out while the parents were holding their son.

What Is the Role of the Nurse?

The circulating nurse thought she was correct in asking for the infant to take to the warmer for observation. She would appear to have the infant's best interest in mind, at least initially. However, was she wrong in insisting on taking the infant when it seemed alright in the mother's arms? Or was she not keeping her duty to protect the infant and physically taking it from the mother? When the instructor pointed out that the infant was doing well, she then admitted that her concern was more with policy and fear of losing her job than the infant's safety. Are these appropriate rationale for ethical decision making in this situation? What would you have done?

NOTES

1. Veatch, R.J. *Case Studies in Medical Ethics.* Cambridge, MA: Harvard University Press, 1977, p. 36.
2. Veatch, *Case Studies in Medical Ethics,* Chap. 2, "Responsibility for the decision," pp. 35–56. Harron, F., Burnside, J., and Beauchamp, T. *Health and Human Values: A Guide to Making Your Own Decisions.* New Haven: Yale University Press, 1983, pp. xi–xiii. Brody, H. *Ethical Decisions in Medicine.* Boston: Little, Brown, 1976, pp. 95–110. Aroskar, M. "Anatomy of an ethical dilemma: The practice." *American Journal of Nursing* 80(4):661, April 1980. Thompson, J.B., and Thompson, H.O. *Ethics in Nursing.* New York: Macmillan, 1981, pp. 4–5. President's Commission for the Study of Ethical Problems in Medicine and Biomedical and Behavioral Research. *Making Health Care Decisions.* Washington DC: US Government Printing Office, October 1982, Vol. 1, pp. 2–6.
3. President's Commission, *Making Health Care Decisions,* pp. 2–8. President's Commission. *Deciding to Forego Life-sustaining Treatment.* Washington DC: US Government Printing Office, March 1983, pp. 3–9.
4. Abrams, M.B., and Wolf, S.M. "Public involvement in medical ethics." *New England Journal of Medicine* 310 (10):627–632. March 8, 1984.
5. Curran, W.J., and Shapiro, E.D. *Law, Medicine and Forensic Science,* 3rd ed. Boston: Little, Brown, 1982, pp. 785–845. Shapiro, M.H., and Speece, R.G., Jr. *Bioethics and Law: Cases, Materials and Problems.* St. Paul, MN: West Publishing Co., 1981, pp. 690–723.
6. Jonsen, A.R., and Garland, M.J. *The Ethics of Newborn Intensive Care.* San Francisco: Health Policy Program and Institute of Government Studies, University of California, 1976, "Introduction," p. 7. Robinson, D.L., Shaffer, J.A., and Bowker, J.W. "Pain and suffering." *EB* 3:1177–1189, 1978.
7. Veatch, *Case Studies in Medical Ethics,* pp. 59–88. Brody, *Ethical Decisions in Medicine,* p. 95.
8. Abrams and Wolf, "Public involvement in medical ethics," p. 310. Davis, A.J., and Aroskar, M.A. *Ethical Dilemmas and Nursing Practice,* 2nd ed. Norwalk, CT: Appleton-Century-Crofts, 1983, Chap. 12, "Public policy and health care delivery," pp. 199–214. Harron, Burnside and Beauchamp, *Health and Human Values: A Guide to Making Your Own Decisions,* Chap. 6, "Health and the 'right' to health," pp. 111–139; Chap. 7, "Health care . . . for whom?" pp. 140–164.
9. Veatch, *Case Studies in Medical Ethics,* p. 35.
10. Veatch, *Case Studies in Medical Ethics,* p. 40.
11. President's Commission, *Making Health Care Decisions,* pp. 2–3.
12. Veatch, *Case Studies in Medical Ethics,* p. 36.
13. President's Commission, *Making Health Care Decisions,* p. 3.
14. ANA, *Code for Nurses with Interpretive Statements.* Kansas City, MO: ANA, 1976, Statement 1.4, p. 5.
15. President's Commission, *Deciding to Forego Life-sustaining Treatment,* pp. 1–2. Veatch, *Case Studies in Medical Ethics,* p. 3. President's Commission, *Making Health Care Decisions,* p. 15. Childress, J. "Who shall live when not all can live?" In Munson, R. (ed) *Intervention and Reflection: Basic Issues in Medical Ethics,* 2nd ed. Belmont, CA: Wadsworth, 1983, pp. 497–498. Kelly, L.S. "High

tech/high touch—now more than ever." *Nursing Outlook* 32(1):15, January–February 1984. Veatch, R.M. "The technical criteria fallacy." *HCR* 7(4):15–16, August 1977.

16. Aroskar, M.A."Anatomy of an ethical dilemma: The practice." *American Journal of Nursing* 80(4):661, April 1980.

17. Beauchamp, T., and Childress, J. *Principles of Biomedical Ethics*, 2nd ed. New York: Oxford University Press, 1983, pp. 70–74, 136–143.

18. President's Commission, *Deciding to Forgo Life-sustaining Treatment*, pp. 5–9. Curran and Shapiro, *Law, Medicine and Forensic Science*, 3rd ed, pp. 785–845.

19. Abrams and Wolf, "Public involvement in medical ethics," pp. 630–632. Veatch, R.M. "Hospital ethics committees: Is there a role?" *HCR* 7(3):22–25, June 1977. Francouer, R.T. *Biomedical Ethics: A Guide to Decision Making*. New York: Wiley, 1983, Chap. 15, "Consensus decisions for public policies," pp. 173–179.

20. ANA, *Code for Nurses with Interpretive Statements*, Statement 3, pp. 8–9.

21. Payton, R. *Information Control and Autonomy*. Philadelphia: Saunders, 1979.

22. Jonsen, A.R. "A concord in medical ethics." *Annals of Internal Medicine* 99(2):264, August 1983.

CHAPTER 13

Step Eight: Identify the Range of Actions and Anticipated Outcomes

In Steps One to Seven, we talked about the identification of possible actions or decisions. The early identification of the decision needed in Step One usually raise the question, "Should I (patient/others) do X or not do X?" Listing the ethical issues (Step Three) may suggest other possible actions or decisions. Further discussion with key individuals may identify even more options.

As noted earlier (Chapter Five, Criteria for an Ethical Dilemma), two or more choices with equal value or importance may raise an ethical conflict. Absence of conflict, however, does not mean the absence of ethical dimensions in a health care situation. The very nature of nursing implies an ethical dimension to all care situations that warrants critical inquiry and moral reasoning.[1] Each situation raises at least two choices—action or no action. The "no action" option is often forgotten in the intensity of the moment, especially when it is apparent that the patient will become worse or die without some intervention. It is important, however, to always consider the "no action" option in ethical reasoning. This helps to clarify one's values about the patient and profession and will facilitate overt decision making.[2]

Clear identification of options helps one see the possible consequences. This in turn helps the decision maker make a reasoned choice of which action to choose (Step Nine). The task of Step Eight is to list the range of actions with their anticipated outcomes.

WHAT IS THE RANGE OF ACTIONS?

The range of possible actions may be simple at first glance. Step One began with the early decision requested. A series of questions may help to clarify alternatives and consequences. These questions include, "What does the patient want done? What does the physician want done? What does the family want done? What do you (the nurse) want done?" All key individuals need to identify what they want or think should be done in the situation. Do not be concerned with the issues of paternalism or maternalism (I know best) or self-determination (patient knows best) at this point. Simply record the actions suggested or requested. Begin your list of options with the answers to these questions. Include the option of "no action" as well.

The next source of possible actions comes from an individual or group mental exercise to think of other actions not mentioned in the situation. These come from past exposure to similar situations, clinical experience in general, and personal experience grappling with the ethical issues. Try to free your thoughts from the specifics of this situation and focus on the ethical issues for a few moments of discussion. This is the creative side of moral reasoning when anything goes in discussion. You will not be taking action yet, and it is better to err on the side of ridiculous options rather than omit a viable alternative. Later, you can eliminate those that, on second thought, are inappropriate or unavailable as choices in this particular situation. Some of these options will also be eliminated once you begin to list the potential consequences for each.

Another source of alternatives comes from the literature on the ethical issues identified in the situation. Texts on bioethics often take an issues approach. Personal study may highlight actions appropriate to the situation. Professional codes may be helpful. "What action(s) would be dictated by the ANA *Code for Nurses*, the AMA *Principles of Medical Ethics*, or the *Hospital Patient's Bill of Rights*?" This provides another check on the completeness of your listing of possible actions. Aroskar[3] suggests that one take into account the setting or context of each proposed action as well as the intention of purpose of the action.

A final suggestion on completing your list is to ask for a review by an outside consultant, such as an ethicist or an ethics committee. Even if they have no further suggestions, they can offer review and reassurance that you have carried out the steps of critical inquiry and determined the range of actions.

WHAT ARE THE ANTICIPATED OUTCOMES OF EACH ALTERNATIVE?

The comprehensive list of possible actions or decisions must now be explored for potential consequences. The list can be narrowed to only those actions possible in the current situation. As you begin this step of critical inquiry, it is simpler to consider one alternative at a time. Listing the action on the left of the paper or blackboard and anticipated consequences on the right can be helpful in organizing your (the group's) thoughts. Visual stimulation can also facilitate the process of comparing alternatives when one is ready to make the final choice.

In asking, "What would happen if we did this?", consider physical, emotional or psychological, social, economic, and cultural effects on each person. You may also ask, "What are the legal ramifications of this action, if any?" (The ethical ramifications will be considered in Step Nine as we search for the moral justification of a given action.) When working within an institution, it may be helpful to ask, "What would the hospital administrator say about this action?"

A larger concern is found in Immanual Kant's concept of universalizability.[4] "What would happen if everyone did this?" This brings in the interests of society and the ethical concept of justice (Chapter Fourteen).

SUMMARY

You have now come to the end of Step Eight with a completed list of the range of actions and their anticipated outcomes. You have applied the test of reality and eliminated those options that were unavailable or unrealistic. You may not wish to eliminate an option prohibited by hospital policy, law, codes of ethics, or bills of rights, or personal preference of any key individual at this time. Part of the moral justification of each option that follows in Step Nine will include the exploration of what is ethical even though it be illegal or against hospital policy or personal preferences. We know there are actions in health care that are both ethical and legal, some which are legal but unethical, and some which are ethical but illegal. Which of the latter two risks you are willing to take in health care decisions is an important consideration. It is part of moral reasoning as well. We return to "Birth of a Family" to apply Step Eight before proceeding to Step Nine and the choice of action.

THE CASE

The decisions made were presented in the case. There are other choices that might have been made, and these would have had consequences. The choices presented are based on the infant's healthy and stable condition.

What Was or Is the Range of Actions?

The possible actions include (1) present the newly delivered infant to the parents without asking (simply place him on the mother's abdomen), dry, and suction, (2) give the boy to the waiting nurse for quick evaluation and then ask her to return him to his parents once he is dried off and suctioned, (3) give the child to the nurse and not offer the parents the option of holding him until he is weighed and identified, (4) have the student hold the baby, dry and suction him, and then give him to the parents if they so desire for a short time (the cord might or might not be cut immediately), (5) allow the parents to hold their son for an unlimited time period as long as he is alright, (6) request a different circulating nurse who is supportive of parent bonding, (7) call the supervisor to clarify hospital policy.

What Are the Anticipated Outcomes of Each Alternative?

1. The parents could be frightened, angry, or pleased to find their son forced on them without warning or consent. This action could have broken their trust with the health care provider or evoked gratitude at her thoughtfulness. If their reaction was negative, it would of course destroy bonding rather than aiding it. Information gleaned in Step Two would facilitate our prediction of the consequences of this alternative.

2. Both nurse and parents may have accepted this option without question. The nurse expected it and the parents did not seem to expect or know what the procedure would be. The mother's question suggests she expected not to be able to hold him. We are not sure how the student would have responded or what she was expecting.

3. This option places the nurse in control of the infant and allows her time to carry out her duties. The parents may have been too shy to ask for anything different. The instructor would have had negative feelings for not offering or encouraging immediate bonding.

4. This option was carried out with positive outcomes for all but the nurse.

5. If the parents were allowed to hold their son for an unlimited time, official weighing and identification would be delayed. This would mean the nurse would also be delayed in returning to other patients and duties. This would probably not be a profitable use of her time. Parents can be offered the option of holding their baby again after these procedures. However, if this nurse also becomes the postpartum recovery nurse, the time problem would be diminished.

6 and 7. Requesting another nurse or clarification from the supervisor could result in confusion and unnecessary use of their time. Such a request could also create bad feelings among the health care providers.

NOTES

1. Thompson, J.B., and Thompson, H.O. *Ethics in Nursing.* New York: Macmillan, 1981, p. 2. Muyskens, J. *Moral Problems in Nursing: A Philosophical Inves-*

tigation. Totowa, NJ: Rowman and Littlefield, 1982, pp. 15–16. Curtin says "Nursing is a moral art." Curtin, L., and Flaherty, M.J. *Nursing Ethics: Theories and Pragmatics.* Bowie, MD: Brady, 1982, pp. 86–87. Brody, H. *Ethical Decisions in Medicine.* Boston: Little, Brown, 1976, pp. 1–3.

2. Compare slow code, no code, or the delayed (slowed) response to a physician's request for assistance that may represent covert decisions for "no action." Thompson and Thompson, *Ethics In Nursing,* pp. 3–4.

3. Aroskar, M. "Anatomy of an ethical dilemma: The theory." *American Journal of Nursing* 80(4):660, April 1980, and "Anatomy of an ethical dilemma: The practice," *American Journal of Nursing* 80(4):662, April 1980.

4. Kant, E. *The Metaphysical Elements of Justice: The Metaphysics of Morals,* Part I. Indianapolis: Bobbs-Merrill, 1965, p. 22.

All that is necessary for the triumph of evil is for good people to do nothing.

—*Edmund Burke*[1]

CHAPTER 14

Step Nine: Decide on a Course of Action and Carry It Out

Step Nine is the final choice for action in the health care situation plus carrying it out. Nurses and other health professionals make decisions daily in their practice. Many of these decisions have an ethical component that may not always be recognized. Many ethical or moral decisions are made on the basis of what the health care professional feels is best in the situation. This concept is intuitionism and ethical egoism.

The heart or feelings do not always make right or ethical choices. We have also discussed the merits and pitfalls of the mental exercise of moral argumentation using ethical principles and theories. Pure reasoning in a philosophical mode can rationalize almost any action in health care, especially when applied to justify an action already taken. Thus, the mind may also lead to choices or actions that are wrong or unethical. The ethical question "Why?" might be seen as a reasoning check on both the heart and the mind.[2]

The ten-step approach to ethical choices is an attempt to clarify the process by distinguishing the kinds of decisions to be made, the ethical issues involved, and the combination of values held by the various parties concerned. This and other models for ethical decision making may be used after the fact. A decision has been made, and you want to check to see if it was the correct or best one. This is valuable, but health care providers must do their primary reasoning prior to making decisions. The danger in always looking backward is that you end up rationalizing your morals rather than reasoning morally in order to determine what action to take.

In preparation for choosing one action from the list of alternatives listed during Step Eight of the decision model, we offer a brief review of Beauchamp's four levels of moral justification. (See Chapter Two for discussion of these levels.) These levels or action guides begin with (1) a particular judgment about what ought to be done in the situation that is justified by (2) moral rules. The moral rules are justified by (3) principles that are ultimately justified by (4) ethical theories.[3] The four suggest different levels of justification. Under ordinary conditions, we often function at the lower levels in health care. The final choice, however, may require the use of various levels.

The process of moral justification, once again, is appropriately done prior to choosing the action to be taken. Moral justification helps to narrow the choices. Instead of rationalizing a choice already made, it should help one to understand the basis for the choice in the face of conflicting moral claims. Moral reasoning, including moral justification for choices, is vital in all health care situations, not just the ones where obvious conflict or disagreement is present.

While all participants may agree on the choice of action during the initial presentation of the situation, that action may be neither appropriate nor ethical.[4] Following the ten-step decision model or any other form of moral reasoning may highlight previously unknown differences in opinion, value conflicts, or the need to include others (patient/family/society) in the process. Moral justification of alternatives may demonstrate that the initial action desired was, indeed, unethical and not in the best interests of the patient or others involved in the situation. In the best of circumstances, you may realize that the initial action was both best and ethical. Now you understand why and may be able to reinforce your correct pattern of moral reasoning for future use.

Other health care situations have known or identified conflicts or disagreement on what should be done. The decision model will assist you to sort out the nature of the disagreement (values, personal beliefs, power struggle) so that ethical issues are clearly identified and grappled with. When the disagreement is found to be on other than ethical grounds, these can be considered accordingly.

One final note of caution is that justification and ethical choice may be difficult and frustrating. Putting your feelings (heart) into words so that they may be considered as well as engaging the mind's reasoning is hard to do, even for those skilled in expressing feelings. The temptation is to give up and return to former patterns of making decisions for and about patients. Yet patients are complaining more and more that their care lacks human warmth, emotion, feeling, genuine concern. Both heart and mind are important in ethical decisions.[5]

We encourage you to persevere. Though ethical decisions may not get easier because of the increasing complexity of health and illness care, the process for arriving at these decisions can become easier to use. Humanistic, ethical health care can be the result.

APPLICATION OF ETHICAL THEORY TO EACH ACTION

With Steps Five, Six, and Seven, you have already completed levels one and two of moral justification according to Beauchamp's outline. You also began to highlight the ethical principles involved in Step Three with the definition of ethical issues. You can finalize the analysis of moral principles by asking what principle supports the moral rule identified in the discussion of value positions.

Now you are ready to consider the fourth level of moral justification, ethical theory, in relation to each alternative or action on the list generated during Step Eight of this decision model. You may wish to refer back to Chapter Two and the discussion of the major ethical theories. These include utilitarianism, deontology, and natural law. Some, perhaps most people, function with some combination of the various approaches to morality or ethics. In natural law, people are usually concerned with both means and ends, both the consequences and the rules or principles. With this in mind, Payton developed a pluralistic decision-making model. She combined the earlier work of Brody, who designed separate deontological and utilitarian models for ethical decision making.[6] These three models have been included in Appendix C for your information. Whether you stand more fully in one tradition than another, knowledge of all ethical systems aids your understanding of your own ethical decisions as well as those of others who may make different choices.

We end our preparatory notes with the reminder that we are often called upon to make decisions based on incomplete information. You have done your best to gather all pertinent data about the health care situation up to this point. You still may not have complete information. You assigned weights to each action in your list. Sometimes in this process, one will stand out more clearly than the others, but this may not happen. You may be left with making a choice between two apparently equal alternatives. In the end, you will make that choice based on what you think is best. The difference between this final choice of what is the best of the alternatives and the first gut-level idea of what you thought should be done is clear. Your choice is now made from a list of actions that survived the previous eight steps of this model. The selection is based on reasoned choice rather than on the basis of personal unexamined bias or values.

Utilitarian Approach

The application of utilitarian ethical theory to the health care situation at hand would subject each action on the list to this critical analysis. Those that clearly do not conform to the utilitarian perspective would be noted and eliminated as utilitarian choices. For purposes of discussion and to be comprehensive in the review of the most appropriate alternative, note the actions not appropriate to the utilitarian perspective but do not discard them yet. They may be appropriate in the deontological perspective or in natural law.

As you compare our decision model with the act utilitarian ethical method of Brody, you will note that problem perception, alternatives listing, and prediction of consequences of each alternative have already been done. The remaining task is to assign the value of satisfaction or utility produced by each consequence or action. When this is completed, providing you have accurately predicted consequences and estimated utility value, you select the alternative with the highest utility.

This approach may be appealing at first glance. It may seem relatively easy. However, experience suggests that it may be quite difficult for the average person. We noted earlier the problem of defining happiness (or the greatest good) and for whom and the problem of assigning a weight to that happiness. We do not presume to have the final answers on what is happiness or the greatest satisfaction or for whom. Once again, we offer questions to stimulate your own thinking on these issues. You might begin by asking, "Which action will produce the greatest amount of pleasure or good for the greatest number of individuals?" If several actions qualify at first glance, there may be a need to assign a weight of utility to each and then ask the question again.

How one assigns the weight of happiness or good to a given action is a difficult concept. Utilitarians note that the standard of value for judging happiness must be both impartial and universal. Impartiality means every person is counted as having equal value. Universality is the assumption that every person in similar circumstances would select the same action.[7] Therefore, a simplified application of these concepts might include asking, "Does this action treat all persons equally? Would this action be selected by all persons exposed to a similar situation?" The final assignment of weight to the actions and consequences that meet the affirmative test of these questions is less clear. It can be set by the individual with the best perspective of utility theory or group consensus.

Deontological Approach

The deontological model for ethical choice as proposed by Brody consists of a comparison of proposed actions (alternatives) with the list of ethical principles (moral rules). The immediate problem with this model is agreement on the list of principles to be used for comparison. Once again the reader is referred to Chapters One and Two for a fuller discussion. Beauchamp and Childress gave priority to autonomy or self-determination, beneficence (do good), nonmaleficence (do no harm), and justice or fairness. The ANA *Code for Nurses* and others also include the principles of informed consent, truthtelling, confidentiality, accountability.[8]

Once you have agreement on the ethical principles to be applied in the situation, you can compare the list of actions to them. The basic question will be, "[To what extent] does this action conform to the principle of Y?" Those that conform to one principle may not conform to another, as noted earlier. Aroskar[9] suggests that one also ask which ethical principles are negated by the proposed action. For example, upholding the principle of non-maleficence (do no harm) may be in conflict with truth-telling in situations where knowing the truth (disease state, prognosis) may potentially cause harm to the individual at the moment. Your task, then, is to apply the list of principles to each action and note which conform, which do not, and which are in conflict.

Once the comparison of principles and actions is completed, you are ready to decide which action is best. If you have only one action consistent with the principles, the decision is obvious. If you have several alternatives consistent with the principles, the final choice may be made on other bases. If you have an action that is consistent with one principle and conflicts with another, you will need to appeal to a higher level principle or rule. This implies a hierarchy in ethical principles. It is best to recognize this hierarchy prior to this Step Nine. If not done before, you will need to define the hierarchy at this time. If the appeal to a higher moral principle is successful, you will have the choice that stands above other actions. If there is no higher level principle to resolve a conflict of principles, other help may be needed, or the decision may be made on other grounds.

Natural Law

A pure model of the Brody type has not been developed for the natural law approach to ethical decision. One method is the use of several questions. As you review each action proposed, you might ask, "Does (to what extent) this action reflect the original intent of nature or the will of God?" This question may be followed by, "Is this action the natural thing to do? What is or was the original purpose or intent of the body system to be affected by the decision? Will the action suggested promote that original intent?"

Lawrence Kohlberg's natural law approach was discussed in Chapter Three. A proposed action might be considered in terms of Kohlberg's six stages or three levels of moral development. Is the purpose preconventional, conventional, or postconventional? Does the choice protect the choosers from harm or reward them in some way (Stage One)? Is it a political solution, as in the aphorism that sums up Stage Two, "You scratch my back and I'll scratch yours"? Are we following a personal authority or the authority of law and order, for Stages Three and Four? Is the concern for the whole of society or for justice, as in Stages Five and Six? One strong tendency in the health care system is for providers to cover themselves (Stage One) or to conform to the law (Stage Four). This may not be wrong in itself. The question is one of reaching for the highest stage possible in the situation. Kohlberg's ideal of course is Stage Six, "What is the just thing to do?" The patient's welfare is considered within the context of society and the whole of humanity.

We discussed in Chapter Two and elsewhere the naturalistic fallacy highlighted by the question, "Does is mean ought?" Just because something exists, does that mean that it is right? We have also extrapolated to the more frequent concern today in our complex health care system, "Just because we can, should we?" Natural law followers may respond affirmatively to the first question but either way to the second. If one cannot determine what is the natural thing to do in the situation, one may appeal to other ethical systems for assistance in the final decision. Intuitively, we are supposed to know what is right and wrong. This is not always the case in complex ethical decision making in health care. What is good and right for me may not be so for you, and vice versa. This leads toward pluralistic ethical decision making in our society today.

Pluralistic Approach

As noted earlier, human beings are capable of rationalizing almost anything one chooses, but not all reasons are good reasons. Some reasons do not conform to moral justification. Payton notes that very few, if any, professional nurses make decisions according to pure utilitarian or deontological ethical reasoning.[10] For one thing, we are subject to a variety of conflicting claims and loyalties because of our status within the health care hierarchy. For another thing, reality dictates that we be concerned with both the means and ends of our actions, often simultaneously. This simultaneous concern for means and ends can be called "bioethical pluralism." It implies that the morality of an action is determined by consideration of both.[11]

The decision model described in this text is based on bioethical pluralism, as you have probably already realized. We do not promote one pure ethical system over another, nor do we suggest that you must use all of them. The model is designed to promote freedom of inquiry, understanding of how different individuals make difficult moral and ethical decisions, and encouragement to take the time needed to learn how you can best make ethical decisions in your own practice.

You may use a combination of deontological, utilitarian, and natural law questioning as you evaluate each action option. You will then need to determine which principles or moral justification you will use in order to make your final choice. Those actions that conform to none of the ethical systems can be avoided. Those actions that conform to some but not others will be discussed further, and those lists that result in only one action that is morally justifiable will lead you to the ethical choice. Many ethical decisions fall into the middle category of two or more correct actions that affirm both caring and reasoned analysis of what is right. How to finally decide in these situations is a delicate balance of reason, emotion, art, science, and respect for all persons involved.

WEIGHING THE GOODS AND HARMS

Another technique for making a choice can be summarized by the weighing of goods and harms. This technique involves many different methods of weighing consequences and weighting actions. They include consideration of cost–benefit ratios, decision tree and decision matrix analysis using mathematical probabilities, and ethical principles translated into decision models. A brief description of these is offered to broaden our discussion of bioethical decision making.[12]

Cost–benefit discussions often raise the questions of "defined by whom and for whom?" Costs are not only financial but emotional and physical as well. The costs are not only to the patient but to society, the family, the health care professional, and others. Consideration of benefits follows the same line of questioning. The ratio of cost to benefit is not only a major principle in a deontological approach to decision making. It is a practical reality that is being considered more and more as the costs of health care increase.

Decision tree and decision matrix techniques are both based on the list of alternative actions. The decision tree requires that you assign probability estimates to the events associated with each action. The final step is calculation of the payoff or consequences for each combination of actions. In order to do this, assign a value for each outcome and a probability estimate for each event.[13] Each of these steps requires your personal, albeit reasoned, interpretation of mathematical probability. For some, the model may be less than optimal for ethical decision making. It is sometimes difficult to quantify human responses to illness.

The final weighing method to be discussed here is the application of weight to specific ethical principles. McCollough has developed two such models, the autonomy model and the beneficence model. He calls these models of "moral responsibility in medicine." Their common goal is acting on or promoting the best interests of the patient.[14] The models are used to discuss physician responsibility in decision making. They may be applied to other health professionals also. Each model is based on a moral principle that provides a basis for understanding the patient's best interests, duties, or obligations that are generated for the health professional by this principle. They also define the virtues requisite to the fulfillment of those duties or obligations.

The beneficence model requires the health professional to behave in such a way that the important and legitimate goods of the patient are pursued while avoiding harms. The goods and harms in this model are defined (understood) from the perspective of medicine (health professional). This model is often equated with the paternalistic approach to decision making in health care. The goods in this model include health, prevention, elimination or control of disease, relief from pain and suffering, ameliorating handicapping conditions, and prolonging life. The harms include illness, disease, pain and suffering, handicaps, and premature death.

The autonomy model likewise requires professional behavior that pursues goods and avoids harms for the patient. However, the patient defines the goods and harms (individual values and beliefs). Therefore there is no independent, common list of goods and harms. The health professional has both a duty and an obligation to pursue the patient's goods and avoid self-interest.

McCollough notes that neither of these models should be taken as absolute guides for decision making. He admits to a complicating factor of third-party interests and perspectives (other than patients and physicians). Rarely are patients and physicians the only individuals involved in health care or in an ethical decision. People do not exist in isolation. Ethical decisions should not be made in isolation. However, this type of decision model based on ethical principles could help one organize and evaluate the range of actions.

The final point to be made on weighing and weighting actions prior to choosing one involves the universal dimension. This concept is raised in the question, "What would happen if everyone did this?" Brody suggests that the principle of universality distinguishes ethical statements from commands.[15] It also provides an important measure of the validity of ethical positions, according to the deontological position of Kant. It is helpful to consider this principle throughout the moral reasoning process as a way to maintain sensitivity to the broader concerns of humanity.

CHOOSE ONE ACTION

Throughout this chapter we have been referring to the generic you, the reader, in discussing the selection of a moral justification for action in a health care situation. The role of decision maker changes hands quite frequently in today's health and illness care so that you, the reader, may not be you, the decision maker, at all times. Historically, nurses have had a limited role in selecting the final option for action. This is based partially on the nurse's place in the health care hierarchy as well as the patient's interest. The physician is more likely to decide if the decision is made by a professional. However, increasingly patients are willing to decide for themselves when possible and appropriate. Whoever makes the final choice, it should be made on a morally justifiable basis. You are preparing to do that, whether for practice in case discussion or in current practice. While practice does not make perfect in ethical decision making, it can go a long way to ensure more ethical practice and more ethical care.

As one prepares to carry out the final choice for action, we add an ongoing concern. Ethical choices are often difficult and rarely engender complete agreement among interested parties. You consider how and under what circumstances you can support (and carry out, if necessary) a final action when you do not agree with it. As health care professionals with moral responsibilities, duties, and obligations for patient care, as well as persons who value the autonomy and dignity of our patients, nurses may not simply refuse to participate in the care of an individual because the patient decided differently than we would have decided. Nurses are more often in this bind than physicians, who can refer the patient elsewhere for care. It is vital that nurses especially understand their own values and the situations that they cannot tolerate. Thus they can avoid working in settings where such decisions may be made or learn to genuinely accept the choices of others so that alternate choices do not interfere with care.

Another approach to the acceptance of other decisions is to become aware of the great variety of value systems, moral positions and ethical actions. You have been learning these throughout the nine steps of this decision model. Through understanding, you may find it easier to practice the ethical mandate of respect for persons even when you disagree with their choices.

SUMMARY

You have learned of moral justification techniques and selected one action for implementation. The decision will be ethical if the steps of the model have been followed with understanding, reason, and caring (respect for others and the self). The final choice will be implemented and the results noted for evaluation according to Step Ten. Before moving on to evaluation, however, we pause to consider "Birth of a Family."

THE CASE

The range of options from Step Eight might be analyzed as follows.

The Options

1. *Place the infant on the mother's abdomen without question.* From a deontological perspective, the principles of informed consent, parent self-determination, and respect for parents would be violated by this action. The instructor could be seen as maternalistic in her solo determination that the baby should be placed on the mother and that immediate bonding is good for everyone. Her definition of "doing good" could be viewed as harmful if the parents were not ready for this close contact with their newborn. This action may also be viewed as less than respectful of the student's plans for immediate care of the mother and child and potentially detrimental to her learning to take responsibility for her own actions. It is also important to note that not all newborns can physically tolerate this position, including those with a need for immediate pediatric examination and those with short cords that will not reach to the mother's abdomen or chest. This action also does not take into consideration the circulating nurse's concern for hospital policy and her apparent inability to assess the physical condition of the infant when on the mother's abdomen.

2. *Give the infant to the nurse and ask her to return him to the parents.* This action supports the nurse's concern for stabilizing the infant in the warmer. It does not appear to go against parental expectations of what might happen in the delivery room. It promotes bonding, though with some delay. The instructor's concern with immediate bonding would not be accomplished. It is difficult to know if the 5 or 10 minute delay would interfere (cause harm) with the parent–infant bonding process and the development of the family. The nurse would have to be willing to return the baby to the parents, however, since once the infant is taken to the warmer, she is the only one free to bring it to the parents until the placenta is delivered and the midwives break scrub. Once again, giving the infant to the parents should be based on their informed consent.

3. *Give the newborn to the nurse and do not discuss bonding.* This supports the nurse's view of the appropriate thing to do. It is procedure oriented with no apparent concern for the psychoemotional needs of either the parents or the child. The procedures themselves (suctioning, heat, silver nitrate in the eyes, weighing, and identification) are correct, though their timing is open to discussion and variance. This action might also be viewed as placing the physical needs of the mother and child at the top of the hierarchy of values. It ignores or delays any other needs. This may be viewed as a technical approach to care. Some would view this as less than professional. It follows the rules (Kohlberg Stage Four). It does not fulfill the ANA *Code for Nurses*, with its concern for patients. It violates natural law in the sense that a newborn infant would normally go to its mother. It could fulfill the utilitarian concern of the greatest good for the greatest number if these procedures do in fact fulfill that end or purpose. If one considers utilitarianism in terms of the principle of the greatest good, the principle of utility or satisfaction, we would need further discussion here on what is the good.

This option might raise some anxiety for the parents if they are not sure what is happening to their son. It might also raise anxiety if they perceive that no one is paying attention to their desire to see and hold their baby. Whether the parents would get to the point of asking to see and hold their child is unknown. The instructor may view this action as negating parents' rights, the good of bonding, and a caring concern or respect for all persons involved. It violates midwifery standards of care.

4. *Have the student hold the baby, dry and suction him, and then give him to the parents if they so desire for a short time.* The decision made, the action actually chosen, was made by the instructor. By asking the parents if they would like to hold their son, she brought them into the decision-making process so that it was, in the end, a joint decision. From a utilitarian perspective, this may not have been the best decision if other new parents would not be offered the same option or if the time commitment of the nurses would increase in the delivery area to the detriment of other patients. On the other hand, facilitation of immediate parent–infant bonding with healthy newborns and willing parents may be seen as a universal good for society as a

whole. Joseph Fletcher's situation ethics, a form of utilitarianism, asks what is the most loving thing to do in a situation. The parental response to holding their son appears to fulfill this ethic.

The deontological approach includes, in descending order of importance, the principles of do good and do no harm (mother and child), autonomy and informed consent for the parents, and the allocation of resources. The routine procedure responsibilities of the nurse are secondary in this option to the bonding. The student's perspective here is unknown. She accedes to the instructor's plan with the parents.

A natural law approach would support this concern for parent–child bonding and family development over hospital routines. Theological ethics has supported the family in most religious traditions, so that support would be here. The Golden Rule would apply positively to the family for many people, though not necessarily all. The Golden Rule as applied to the delivery room nurse might ask for additional consideration.

5. *Parents hold their son as long as they want.* This action, predicated on the health of the infant and parental consent, would appear to be supportive of the value of immediate bonding. Questions of justice and the allocation of resources (professional time) might be raised, since this holding could delay such nursing activities as weighing and putting silver nitrate in the newborn's eyes. Identification of the infant could take place with the baby on the mother or in the father's arms. The nurse might see this method as inefficient and awkward and not a good use of her time. Similarly, if the baby is being held by his mother, the instructor may not wish to carry out potentially uncomfortable tasks (placenta delivery, episiotomy repairs) for fear the child might be dropped. If the father were holding the boy, this would obviate this problem, however. The nurse–midwives could then complete their delivery tasks in good time. Another question of justice that might be raised concerns other parents and whether they can be offered this option, i.e., is it practical and feasible to support such a policy in a busy obstetrics unit? Will the care for others be compromised by such a policy for all?

6 and 7. *Request a different circulating nurse who is supportive of parent bonding or call the supervisor to clarify hospital policy.* These actions might result in final agreement on bonding actions in the delivery area, but they would probably be very disruptive to all involved, including the parents. Changing charge nurses in midstream could also present some potential danger to mother and child if there was a period of time without a nurse present at the delivery. This action would not be in keeping with respect for all persons, especially the circulating nurse. It could result in a turf war between nurse and nurse–midwife, during which patient care could be seriously compromised.

Requesting the supervisor to clarify policy and diminish the nurse's concern for practicing safely according to protocols would require time to find the supervisor. This action could result in a needless demand on the supervisor's time, take her away from more essential duties, and contribute to poor professional–professional relationships. It is doubtful whether better care for patients would result from such an action, and it is hard to imagine that Sara and Tom would benefit from it either.

The Choice

Option 4, the decision made, the action taken in the case as presented, is the option of choice based on the reasons stated. However, it is not as clear-cut a decision or action as one might like. The concern with bonding and parental love as the highest good is a utilitarian concern, including situation ethics. It is supported by the deontological, natural law, and religious perspectives. It is supported by the ANA *Code for Nurses* with its concern for patients over procedure. However, the second option might also fulfill these concerns, except for the unknown factor of how much a 5 to 10 minute delay might interfere with the bonding and the joy. Option 2 would have the additional value of allowing the nurse to carry out her responsibilities, with the overtones of professional–professional respect. The resultant hierarchy of the final choice then is patient (family) concerns, professional concerns, hospital routines.

NOTES

1. Burke, E. *Letter to William Smith.* 1795.
2. Midgley, M. *Heart and Mind: The Varieties of Moral Experience.* New York: St. Martin's Press, 1981, pp. 4–14. Brody, H. *Ethical Decisions in Medicine.* Boston: Little, Brown, 1976, p. 16, says that a statement for action derived from an ethical reasoning process will prove to be a better guide to action in important matters "than either one's initial gut reaction or blind adherence to pre-existing rules."
3. Beauchamp, T., and Childress, J. *Principles of Biomedical Ethics,* 2nd ed. New York: Oxford University Press, 1983, pp. 4–8.
4. Brody, *Ethical Decisions in Medicine,* p. 9, points out there is nothing wrong with identifying a course of action initially. He agrees that this is how humans actually function, i.e., we have some early idea of what we want to do. However, he also agrees that the initial reaction must then be analyzed by some rational process. It should be rejected if it fails the test.
5. Kelly, L. "High tech/high touch—Now more than ever." *Nursing Outlook* 32(1):15, January–February 1984. Carper, B. "The ethics of caring." *Advances in Nursing Science* 1(3):11–19, April 1979. Huttman, B. "A crime of compassion." *Newsweek* August 8, 1983, p. 15.
6. Payton, R.J. "Pluralistic ethical decision making." *Clinical and Scientific Sessions.* Kansas City, MO: ANA, 1979, p. 11. Brody, *Ethical Decisions in Medicine,* pp. A-2a, A-2b.
7. Brody, *Ethical Decisions in Medicine,* p. 7.
8. Beauchamp and Childress, *Principles of Biomedical Ethics,* 2nd ed.
9. Aroskar, M. "Anatomy of an ethical dilemma: the theory," *American Journal of Nursing* 80(4):660, April 1980.
10. Payton, "Pluralistic ethical decision making."

11. Childress, J.F. *Priorities in Biomedical Ethics.* Philadelphia: Westminster Press, 1981, p. 13, distinguishes single ethical systems, such as the utilitarian concern for utility or the concept of justice or the single concept of love from what he calls a "bioethical pluralism" that takes into account more than one principle.

12. For a detailed description of weighing and weighting actions consequences using cost–benefit, decision tree, and decision matrix techniques, see Francoeur, R. *Biomedical Ethics: A Guide to Decision Making.* New York: Wiley, 1983.

13. Francoeur, *Biomedical Ethics: A Guide to Decision Making,* pp. 119–137.

14. McCollough, L. "Two models of moral responsibility in medicine." ICS: Bioethics Course Outline, Georgetown University, March 18, 1983.

15. Brody, *Ethical Decisions in Medicine,* p. 7.

CHAPTER 15

Step Ten: Evaluate the Results

We have arrived at the final step in the bioethical decision model. It is now time to review and evaluate the results of the final choice for action. Did the action or decision produce the results intended? Is another decision or action needed? What information about this situation is transferable to similar situations?

DID THE DECISION OR ACTION PRODUCE THE INTENDED RESULTS?

One part of evaluation is determining whether the action chosen was the best in the situation, now that the actual consequences are known. Step Eight of this decision model is concerned with identifying the alternatives for action and possible consequences. One test of our reasoning ability is whether the projected result was indeed the consequence of the chosen action. If the result was not what was anticipated, you may ask, "Why?" "Is the unintended result acceptable, in need of a new decision to reverse it, if possible, or an additional decision to overcome the unacceptable result?" This may be the time to ask if the missing information of Step Two was important or not.

One of the pitfalls of moral reasoning is thinking that once the decision or choice for action is made, there is nothing more to do. Too often this misinformation has left patients dissatisfied (and even harmed) and health care professionals falsely believing they have carried out their moral duties and obligations. Even when patients have determined the final course of action based on thoughtful consideration of all options, they may not be satisfied with the results. These results may have been correctly predicted, but before they were theoretical, and now they are reality and may be difficult to deal with. Consider the theoretical discussion of life without a leg and the reality of having only one leg, or the theoretical prolongation of life with chemotherapy and the reality of severe, depressing side effects of those drugs.

Likewise, when health professionals stop short of evaluating the results of moral reasoning, they may think the process too cumbersome and reject it. They may think the end result has been accomplished without need for further discussion. The patient or professional may feel the need for discussion of the results, especially if the results may not have been intended. If the professional refuses to carry out the evaluation step, however, neither of these situations will be identified. Parenthetically, one may miss the satisfaction of knowing that the time and effort were well spent (correct anticipation of results and satisfaction with same) and the ten steps worth repeating in new situations. Even more important, if one does not review the nine steps, a false sense of security in moral reasoning could result. Current patients may not suffer from this lack of understanding, but future patients might.

IS ANOTHER ACTION NEEDED?

Decisions in health care often lead to the need for more decisions. Ethical decision making is no exception. Once a choice for action is made and implemented, it is time to evaluate whether other decisions are now needed as well. We mentioned above the potential need for a different decision, also, if the selected action did not produce the desired results or is now inappropriate. Whatever the circumstance, review and evaluation of the decision taken will help you identify whether and when another action is needed.

When the key individuals involved are dissatisfied with the results of the chosen action, one may be able to return to the alternatives list and select a different one. This may be done providing the results of the first action did not markedly alter the circumstances of the health care situation. If the circumstances or situation are markedly changed, then the ten-step model should be followed once again. If key individuals have not changed, values identification may take little effort once ethical issues are reviewed. Likewise, each of the steps will probably take less time because the individuals have used them before.

When the chosen action produced different results than anticipated, it is important to understand why that happened. "Did you miss a step in the process or fail to clearly identify the scientific or value dimensions of the situation? Did a key individual not get included in the exploration of alternatives and outcomes? Did something in the situation change during the moral reasoning process that was not identified? Did the patient not reveal complete information about the illness so that the results of therapy could not be correctly predicted? Do you need help to evaluate why the error in judgment occurred?" Whatever the response to these questions, it is important to ask them as one searches for understanding of what happened. This understanding can rebuild one's confidence in continuing to strive for ethical practice.

WHAT INFORMATION IS TRANSFERABLE TO OTHER SITUATIONS?

The final step in the review and evaluation of the decision process and outcome involves the transfer of learning to new situations. The ten steps of the decision model take time and effort. One way to internalize the learning and strengthen your grasp of moral reasoning is to identify what you learned in this situation that may be helpful to you in similar situations in the future. Certainly the exploration of your personal and professional values is valuable information to retain until it is time once again to see if those values remain appropriate for you. The process of value clarification can also be transferred to new situations. Knowledge of other people's value positions is important to remember when facing new patient situations. You may begin to note familiarity with a variety of values as you work with new clients.

Understanding different ethical issues and methods of moral justification can be transferred to other situations. This is especially helpful when a similar ethical issue presents itself, even when the key individuals are different. Be cautious in the application of previous moral work in new situations lest you mistakenly think you know the answers and thereby decide to forego exploration with a new set of individuals, who may have a new set of issues and values. We are suggesting that prior use of the ten-step decision model can help you in new situations. However, experience does not automatically provide the answers to new questions. The ten-step model must be used in its entirety again if you wish to continue making ethical decisions in health care practice.

SUMMARY

We have come to the end of the ten-step decision model based on moral reasoning. Appendix A of this text presents actual cases for the application of the decision model. You may choose to use these cases or apply the model to case studies of your own. Return to each step as needed for review. Evaluation of "Birth of the Family" applies Step Ten to our ongoing case study example.

THE CASE

Did the Decision or Action Produce the Desired Results?

When the instructor decided to ask the parents if they wanted to hold their healthy newborn son, the response was an initial questioning if it was alright. Then they responded with an eager "Yes." If the desired result included informed parental choice, shared decision making, and immediate parent–infant bonding, all appear to have been achieved. The circulating nurse remained uneasy with this choice of action, however, and concerned about her job. We do not know if the student was supportive of the action, though the apparently positive result could offer reinforcement for her to consider this type of action in future situations. Her future patients might also be positively affected by her participation in this case.

Is Another Action Needed?

One might consider the allocation of professional time and decide after 10 to 15 minutes that the nurse needs to carry out her assigned duties with the newborn. This action may accord respect to the nurse and her responsibilities. It would free her to complete the tasks to which she is assigned. Another option would be for the instructor to help the nurse carry out these procedures while the student cares for the mother. Maintaining positive professional–professional relationships has the value of ensuring good care not only for Sara, Tom, and their son but for future patients in this setting. The attention to the nurse's concerns as well as the family's needs may support further action by the instructor such as those cited.

The nurse and the instructor might check the institutional policies to see what they actually say. If the nurse is wrong, this could change her future actions in relation to newborns and parents. This would reinforce the instructor in her actions. If the nurse is right, she might want to share that clearly with the instructor and other colleagues. If the instructor disagrees with the policy, she might want to work with the administration and other hospital authorities to change the rules. She might also want to reconsider what is involved in the violation of the rules in relation to her own covenant, contract, or commitment to the institution that has granted her hospital privileges.

What Information Is Transferable to Other Situations?

Several things have come out of the ten-step process. Sara and Tom may have learned the value of shared decision making in health care as well as participation in the bonding process. Hopefully, the positive regard for them as persons by the health care personnel will encourage their willingness to use other health services knowledgeably and responsibly.

The nurse may have learned more about herself and her motives for working. She may be questioning whether nursing is a job or a professional commitment for her. She may also explore options in carrying out assigned tasks in a less structured manner while maintaining safety and responsibility for these actions. She may have negatively realized the limits of her own autonomy in delivery situations and how those limits cause her to respond to patients and other professionals.

The student may have learned the value of parent choice, immediate bonding, and the importance of using one's control during delivery situations in a responsible fashion. She may have also realized that she needs to discuss her learning needs and plans for managing delivery with her instructor so that she can function autonomously in future situations rather than simply following the direction of others. She also can use this positive parenting experience as an option for action with future clients who may be interested in it.

The instructor learned about the differing values some nurses place on their job and following policies. She may decide to check out a nurse's views of these policies prior to working with new nurses in the future. She may check on the accuracy of the nurse's perception of those policies both to protect her own privileges in the setting and out of respect for the hospital. The parents positive response to immediate bonding will probably reinforce her offering this option to parents in the future.

APPENDIX A
Case Studies in Nursing

Appendix A of this text consists of a variety of case studies. These are for discussion and application of the ten-step decision model presented in Part Two. The cases have been selected to reflect the variety of roles and responsibilities of nurses, the different work settings and relationships with patients, families, peers, and other health team members. These cases do not attempt to present all of the ethical issues and dilemmas facing nurses. We have, however, tried to illustrate some of the more common ethical situations in nursing practice. You no doubt have cases of your own that reflect the ethical concerns of nurses in addition to those presented in this text.

The case studies are presented within the framework of the life cycle that is commonly used in nursing curricula. One can encounter the same type of ethical concern with a different age population, of course.

The case studies are selected for your recognition of the ethical dimensions of nursing practice. The first case has been analyzed according to the decision model. Other cases are included for self-study and use of the model individually or within a group setting. You will want to develop your own case studies of reasoned analysis as well.

All cases are based on actual nursing situations, with names and other identifying data changed to protect the confidentiality of the participants.

PREGNANCY DECISIONS

The three cases presented in this section represent the nurse's interaction with people. One involves a couple who have decided not to conceive and have children. Another involves making a decision about the level of health desired for their child. The third case explores one couple's wish to have significant input into decisions about their care during labor and birth. The nursing roles range from independent clinician (primary care provider) to staff nurse (provider of direct nursing and physician-determined care) in a hospital setting. The first of these cases is analyzed according to the ten-step decision model in Part Two of this book.

Case No. 1: Refusal to Bear Children

Sara has received health care from S.W., RN, a Women's Health Care Specialist, over the last 3 years. Sara is 28 years old and has recently married. Her husband, Bill, has accompanied her on this visit. During her annual checkup, Sara asks what needs to be done to have her tubes tied. Upon further questioning, both Sara and Bill are adamant that they do not ever want any children. All nonpermanent forms of contraception are unacceptable. When pushed for reasons for the tubal ligation, Sara admits that she could never accept the idea of an abortion—morally, physically, or emotionally. She is not willing to take the chance of having intercourse which might result in pregnancy.

A review of Sara's past medical history and current health status reveals no contraindication to any method of contraception or pregnancy. She is very healthy and has no family history of birth defects. She has no unusual fear of pregnancy or children. S.W. is convinced that both Sara and Bill have put a lot of thought into their decision not to have children. They express the view that it is their responsibility to take action to avoid having children they do not ever want. They ask S.W. to help them find the physician who will be willing to perform the tubal ligation.

THE ANALYSIS

Step One: Review the Situation

First of all, Sara appears to be in good physical health, with no apparent medical or physical contraindication to any form of contraception. She is sexually active and wishes to continue this activity. She also is not willing to get pregnant. The health problem can be defined as the need to prevent an unwanted pregnancy. In the fullest sense, health for Sara and Bill can be defined as freedom from the threat or potential for bearing children. From the professional's view, the health problem may be defined as a request for sterilization from a relatively young woman or this couple's refusal to bear children. Another perspective on the health problem could be the potential discrimination implied in the woman seeking tubal ligation versus the man seeking a vasectomy.

Sara and Bill appear to have jointly made a firm decision not to have children. The primary decision for them now is how and who will provide the requested tubal ligation. The nurse might raise the question of whether the tubal ligation should be done at all as well as to whom the referral for surgery should be made. The physician will have to decide whether to perform the procedure on Sara. The nurse may also have to decide whether referral to a trained counselor (psychologist, social worker) is indicated. Have Bill and Sara considered all the critical factors as they decided not to have children? S.W. may decide to take the time to explore their decision process herself if time and expertise allow.

The major ethical component of the situation is whether a relatively young couple have the right to decide not to have children. If so, should they be offered some form of permanent contraception at this time? A physician must perform the surgery and, therefore, will have to decide to agree or refuse. Another ethical dimension of the situation is what responsibility does S.W. have to support Sara's decision and refer her to the appropriate physician?

The scientific component of the decision is whether tubal ligation is biologically safe for Sara. Most physicians would agree that it is.

The key individuals involved in this situation include Sara, Bill, S.W., physician, and potentially other professionals, such as social worker. Society may be affected in the long run if every young couple decided not to have children, but its interest at this time seems minimal. Sara and Bill are adults and presumably competent to make their own decisions. However, other family members might hold a different view.

Step Two: Gather Additional Information

The nurse will probably want more information from Sara and Bill on why they do not want children. Why are they choosing permanent contraception? Why are they choosing the ligation rather than a vasectomy? S.W. has had a long-term relationship with Sara and may choose to ask her these questions in private and the same with Bill. The nurse also recognizes that a value judgment on these issues may be made as Sara talks about her reasons. S.W. may also review all methods of contraception and ascertain Sara's and Bill's knowledge of them. Explanation of risks and benefits of each method, including male and female sterilization, are important components of the informed decision process. Here it is important to identify the level of knowledge and understanding that Bill and Sara have. Knowledge of Bill's health status is important in this situation as well.

S.W. may need more information on what qualities the couple are seeking in a physician referral and their understanding of the costs and other factors. The physician receiving the referral will probably want the same information collected by S.W., though the physician may choose to obtain it personally.

Step Three: Identify the Ethical Issues

The ethical issues in this case include Sara and Bill's right to decide not to have children (quality of life, self-determination) and their right to permanent contraception (autonomy). Other issues include informed decision making (consent), the physician's right to refuse to perform the surgery, and the nurse's responsibility to ensure informed decision making (advocacy) as well as referral to a competent physician (accountability). Contraception has been considered immoral in the past, and some groups and individuals still consider it wrong. The purpose of sexual intercourse was to produce children. This does not appear to be the value system of the individuals here but may influence the choice of a physician. In times past, mutilation of the body has been considered wrong unless it was for a justified reason, such as saving one's life. This does not appear to be a problem for this couple. The choice of tubal ligation over vasectomy raises several questions about the value of male and female virility. In some cultures, tne macho male has tended to identify vasectomy with castration. The ethics of submitting the female to surgery rather than the male appear to be in the background here if the decision has already been made by the couple. However, the reasons may influence the relationship both now and later. The simpler, less invasive vasectomy performed in the office might be considered preferable on the ethical grounds of the allocation of scarce resources or the lesser risk of the two procedures.

Step Four: Identify Personal and Professional Values

S.W. would need to examine how she feels about women (couples) who decide not to have children (value of parenting), about unwanted children (value of wantedness), about women having the responsibility of contraception rather than males, and about clients' right to decide for themselves what their health care and lifestyle will be (autonomy). She may wish to list her personal values on these issues (what she would do) as well as note what the ANA *Code* states is her professional responsibility. The *Code* statements that apply here include respect for persons, accountability and competence, informed decisions, and maintaining confidentiality.

Step Five: Identify Values of Key Individuals

Sara and Bill's values related to lifestyle and children seem clear and obvious. Where these values came from remains unclear, as is their choice of ligation rather than a vasectomy. They appear to accept responsibility for their decision not to bear children by seeking sterilization. They support marriage and sexual intercourse without accepting pregnancy and children. They expect the health professionals to accept their decision and provide the needed surgical procedure. They trust S.W. and respect her judgment on referral to a competent physician. We do not know who will pay for the services (insurance, Medicaid, Sara and Bill themselves). Some would suggest that ability to pay should not influence health providers' willingness to provide services.

The physician or other health professionals are not yet involved in the situation. Presumably if a physician accepts the referral, she would be supportive of permanent contraception for this couple.

Step Six: Identify Value Conflicts, if Any

No value conflicts are evident yet. It is possible, however, that S.W. may not know of a physician willing to perform tubal ligation on a woman of this age for Sara's reasons. It is also possible that S.W. will not be able to support this couple's request once further information on their reasons are explored. S.W. may find it possible to support a vasectomy but not the proposed tubal ligation.

Step Seven: Determine Who Should Decide

The most logical decision makers in this situation appear to be Sara and Bill regarding permanent contraception. Their decision not to bear and raise children affects them directly. The physician, however, must agree to tubal ligation, since it is not something they can do for themselves. S.W. may support and become the advocate for Sara's right to decide if she is satisfied with the information provided on reasons and informed decision making.

Step Eight: Identify Range of Actions with Anticipated Outcomes

The range of actions in this situation include (1) referral to a physician who agrees to perform tubal ligation, (2) referral to a counselor to help Bill and Sara review their decision, (3) the offer of other forms of contraception while Bill and Sara spend more time thinking about tubal ligation, (4) refusal to refer for tubal ligation or offer a nonpermanent form of contraception, and (5) Bill and Sara can decide to use another form of contraception and accept a minimal risk of pregnancy. The anticipated outcomes of (2) and (3) actions may be a loss of trust in S.W. as a health care provider, anger and resentment toward health care professionals, and a review of the decision. The last could strengthen the couple's initial request for tubal ligation or result in a new decision, e.g., for a vasectomy or for nonpermanent contraception. It seems unlikely that the couple would change their minds and have a child. If S.W. refuses to refer the couple to a physician, Bill and Sara can seek a physician on their own. If they agree to another method of contraception and retain the fear of unwanted pregnancy, their sexual activity and emotional relationships may become troublesome.

Step Nine: Decide on Course of Action and Carry Out

If Sara and Bill's decision for tubal sterilization is supported and a physician is willing to perform the surgery, that action can now be taken. It would appear to be most in keeping with informed decision making, self-determination and autonomy of adults, and responsible nonparenting. Contraception and choice are values supported by many people in our society. The refusal to bear children has rarely been discussed openly. Governments tend to oppose it (loss of manpower), as do some individuals and some religious groups.

Step Ten: Evaluate Results of Decision/Action

Evaluation will depend on what decision was made and whether the expected outcomes occurred. At this point, one would review each step of the model and analysis to see if anything was left out or overlooked.

Case No. 2: Amniocentesis—Quality or Sanctity of Life?

T.J. is a nurse–midwife caring for Mrs. R., a 25-year-old woman pregnant for the first time. Mrs. R. is currently 16 weeks (4 months) pregnant, and the pregnancy has progressed normally. As the nurse–midwife begins today's visit, she notes that Mrs. R. seems very upset and nearly in tears. With gentle support, Mrs. R. tells of her concern. It seems that her husband just found out that his brother's infant son died of Tay-Sachs disease. He wants to know if this pregnancy is affected. If so, he wants the pregnancy terminated.

Mrs. R. goes on to say that she can understand her husband's concern, but she does not wish to terminate this pregnancy, "no matter what!" She explains that it took them 3 years for her to become pregnant. She may not have another chance to have a baby. She adds that she believes God will protect their baby from this disease. She then turns to the nurse–midwife and says, "What would you do if you were me?"

Case No. 3: Birth Options—Choice or Coercion?

Jane Jones and her husband, Tom, believe in the Lamaze method of childbirth. They both want Tom present during the labor and birth of their child. The Joneses have a very low income. They arranged with Dr. Goode for prenatal care and delivery at Fine Hospital, the only one in the area where medically indigent people can be attended for childbirth. The closest other hospital is over an hour's drive. Dr. Goode informed the Joneses at the outset that Fine's general policy is not to admit fathers to the delivery room. He added that the chief resident has discretion to alter the policy in individual cases. Finally, he informed them that in the event that he was away or otherwise unable to participate in the birth, the chief resident would take his place.

The Joneses arrived at Fine Hospital with Jane in active labor. J.E. is the nurse in charge of the labor area. She informed Mrs. Jones that the internal electronic fetal monitor (EFM) would be attached to the scalp of their fetus. Tom would have to wait downstairs in the father's waiting area. She also told Mrs. Jones that Dr. Goode had been in a car accident on his way to the hospital. The chief resident, Dr. Smith, was on vacation. Another resident, Dr. Wilson, would be taking care of her. Mrs. Jones questioned the use of the EFM. She shared her birth plans with J.E., emphasizing that she needed her husband to be with her. J.E. explained that the EFM was used to identify any distress in the baby. The hospital required its use on all women in labor.

J.E. was familiar with the Lamaze method and supported Mrs. Jones' need to have her husband present. Just as she was about to say something, the resident came in to examine Mrs. Jones. Dr. Wilson confirmed that Mr. Jones would not be allowed to stay in the labor area. He added that he did not think the Lamaze method was particularly wise. "Most women who deliver at this hospital have some kind of problem." He would permit natural labor unless there were problems. Mrs. Jones, frustrated, alone, and now fearful, looked to J.E. for help. J.E. shrugged her shoulders as if saying, "What can I do?" She walked out of the room.

NEONATES AND ADVOCATES

The ethical dimensions of caring for neonates are often complicated by the fact that someone other than the neonate is required to speak on behalf of the neonate. This factor is also present in caring for comatose adults and other persons who cannot speak for themselves. The major ethical issues that arise for nurses caring for neonates include advocacy, quality versus sanctity of life, beneficence and nonmaleficence, and just allocation of health care resources. Once again, the cases presented here offer time to reflect on these and other ethical dimensions of caring for neonates. They involve nurses in hospital settings, both in the labor room and in neonatal intensive care units.

Case No. 4: Refusal of a Cesarean Section

A 23-year-old woman (gravida 1, para 0) from Nigeria was admitted to the hospital at 0500 hours in active labor. She had been followed in the outpatient department on a regular basis. Her prenatal course was uneventful. She was at 39 weeks gestation. Admitting examination revealed vital signs, including the blood pressure and the general physical examination, to be within normal limits. The uterine fundus was enlarged to 38 centimeters above the symphysis, which was compatible with dates. Estimated fetal weight was 3000 grams (6.6 pounds). Uterine contractions were every 5 minutes and, upon palpation, were felt to be of good quality. Vaginal examination revealed the cervix to be 3 cm dilated and 80 percent effaced. The presenting part was vertex at a −1 station. An external electronic fetal monitoring device was applied to the abdomen, and the fetal heart rate (FHR) tracing was normal. The contractions increased in frequency to every 3 minutes and were of good quality.

At 1000 hours the patient was examined and shown to have made slow progress. The membranes ruptured spontaneously, and the amniotic fluid was clear. On examination, the cervix was 4 cm dilated and 80 percent effaced, and the vertex was at zero station. A scalp electrode was applied to the fetal head for internal heart rate monitoring, and an intrauterine pressure catheter was placed in the uterus to ascertain the frequency and quality of the uterine contractions. At 1100 hours, the contractions were noted to be of good quality and every 3 minutes. Labor continued, but at 1300 hours, the internal FHR tracing demonstrated decreased variability. The uterine contractions continued of excellent quality, and vaginal examination revealed the cervix to be 4 cm dilated and about 80 percent effaced, and the vertex was at zero station.

The attending physician discussed with the patient the possibility of cesarean birth. She was not progressing in her labor in spite of the excellent quality contractions. The patient declined to accept the possibility. In anticipation, however, the primary care nurse and resident in charge had frequent conversations with her describing the possible need. They thought she could understand the consequences of, or lack of, cesarean birth, but because of her religious beliefs, she remained certain she would not have a section. She continued to read her Bible during all this time.

At 1400 hours, the amniotic fluid was meconium stained, indicating possible fetal distress. The FHR tracing now showed persistent decreased variability. Assessment of the patient indicated that she again failed to make progress, and cesarean birth was discussed again. She again refused to accept it.

Case No. 5: Technology—At What Cost?

The headline on an ad for a large Health Maintenance Organization (HMO) read, "37 DAYS OLD. $25,791.82 IN DEBT." At birth, this neonate weighed 3 pounds. The diagnosis was severe respiratory distress. Within minutes he was transferred to a regional neonatal intensive care unit under the care of neonatologists. His breathing was aided by a specialized machine, and his care monitored by the most advanced technology available. His hospital bill was tremendous by 36 days of age, but the reader is told that the parents are not to worry because the HMO paid the entire bill. The reader is not told, however, whether this infant lived.

Case No. 6: Mercy or Research?

A nurse ethicist was asked to visit the university hospital's neonatal intensive care unit (NNICU) and talk with the nurses about the newest arrival there. Amy was born at 26 weeks gestation by elective cesarean section for severe Rh incompatibility. She weighed 360 grams (10 ounces) at birth and was now being cared for in the NNICU. She appeared perfectly formed and fit into the palm of the attending obstetrician. Her parents requested that nothing be done to save her and began their grieving. This was the sixth pregnancy that resulted in an infant with Rh disease. The previous five infants had died, and they knew this one would too. The professional staff, however, seemed determined to keep her alive as long as possible. She had received six exchange transfusions within the first 24 hours of life. Since they did not know what to feed her, they insisted that the mother pump her breasts to give the milk to Amy. When asked what would be done in the event of a cardiac or respiratory arrest, the primary nurse responded, "No one has brought that up yet." She confirmed that the parents did not want the infant resuscitated, but the staff was committed to keeping her alive. The supervisor added, "Just think! We'll be written up in all the papers." Amy died after 14 days of expert technology.

CHILDREN, CONSENT, AND RESEARCH

The major ethical issues that arise in caring for children include the age of consent for all therapeutic procedures, involvement of children in research, and the concerns surrounding child abuse. Nurses provide health care for children in schools or play centers and outpatient facilities and illness care in hospital and homes.

Case No. 7: Informed Consent

Sally is a 10-year-old member of a fourth grade class. The school nurse noted that her immunization record was incomplete and called her mother to inquire about this. The mother responded that she was unable to afford taking Sally to the pediatrician and authorized the school nurse to give the needed injection. Sally was called into the nurse's office. She was told about the need for the immunization and that her mother said it was okay to give it to her. Sally thought for a moment and then said, "No. I don't want a needle. You can't make me have it." How should the nurse proceed?

Case No. 8: The Age of Consent

Jimmy is a 5-year-old with leukemia. He has had multiple hospitalizations since this diagnosis was made 2 years ago. He returned to the hospital 2 days ago in crisis, and there is some doubt about whether he will survive. Donna is the primary nurse assigned to care for Jimmy this time. She is sitting with him when the physician stops by to tell Jimmy that she is going to try some new drugs to make him feel better. In order to know how much of the new drugs to use, she needs to have some

blood samples. With that she approaches Jimmy with needle and syringe. Jimmy cries, "No. I don't want any more needles! Just leave me
be." With that he grabbed Donna's arm and tried to hide under the
covers. The doctor said she was sorry she had to do this and then asked
Donna to hold Jimmy while she drew the blood samples. Donna knew
about the research project that the physician was involved in and won-
dered if the new drugs were part of that project. How should she
respond?

Case No. 9: Child Abuse

Mike is the pediatric nurse practitioner (PNP) working in a well-baby
clinic. This morning W.W. brings her 6-week-old infant, Becky, to the
clinic for a checkup. As Mike begins the physical examination he notes a
rather large (4 centimeter) bruise on the left side of Becky's head and
another bruise across her right buttock. He turns to W.W. and asks her if
she knows when and how the bruises happened. She responds with, "I
think she fell off the bed. It happened while my husband was watching
her a couple of days ago." Mike suspects abuse or neglect. How should
he proceed?

ADOLESCENT CARE

Some of the major ethical concerns in providing health and illness care for
adolescents include provision of contraceptive agents and counseling, ex-
tramarital sexual activity, and whether parental consent is needed for any
type of treatment. Pediatric nurse practitioners, clinical specialists in adolescent care, and staff nurses in hospitals provide services for this age group in a
variety of settings. The cases involve contraceptive and abortion care, venereal
disease and prostitution, and consent for organ donation.

Case No. 10 (A and B): Responsible Parenting at 14?

A. A concerned mother brings her 14-year-old daughter, K.M., to see you
in a family planning clinic. The mother asks to speak with you
alone. She tells you that in the past few months she has been having
many problems with her daughter. K.M. has been cutting classes at
school, staying out late at night, and lying about where she has been.
The mother read a description of sexual intercourse in K.M.'s diary that
suggested "she must of had it. I can't follow her everywhere. She's too
young to be a parent. I'm a single parent myself. I can't raise another
child." The mother asks you to put K.M. on the pill. You talk to K.M.
alone. She is elusive. She denies being sexually active, but there is some-

thing about her manner that leaves you wondering. Then she says she is willing to take the pill even as she continues to deny sexual activity. Do you give her the pill?

B. A 14-year-old female, O.W., presents to the emergency room with the chief complaint of vomiting for 5 days. She is accompanied by her mother. The history reveals that she is one month late for her menstrual period. The nurse practitioner does a pregnancy test, which is positive. As she talks with O.W. alone about this finding, O.W. asks her not to tell her mother that she is pregnant. She fears that "my mother will make me have an abortion." O.W. expresses the belief that "abortion is killing." As the nurse leaves the examining room, the mother approaches her and asks, "What is the problem with my daughter?" How should she respond?

Case No. 11: The Sexual Epidemic—Fact or Fantasy?

D.V. is a 15-year-old male who comes to the emergency room complaining of abdominal pain. He is accompanied by his mother. On physical examination performed with his mother out of the room, Joe, the nurse practitioner, notes a urethral discharge. Gram stain of the discharge reveals gonorrhea. Joe gives him a prescription for antibiotics. When Joe discusses the need for his partner to be treated, he tells him it was an older male. D.V. was paid $10. How should Joe respond?

Case No. 12: Kidney Donor

Thomas is a 17-year-old white male with known hyperoxalosis since age 4. Hyperoxalosis (generalized deposition of calcium ocalate throughout the body) is a rare inborn error of metabolism (autosomal recessive trait). It usually leads to chronic renal failure. Now he needed dialysis. Dialysis therapy relieves the condition, but it removes insufficient amounts of the oxalic acid. Thus, it does not prevent progressive deposition of the calcium oxalate. Theoretically, a kidney transplant could remove sufficient oxalate, the preferred therapy is a transplant. The best transplant is a matched, live, related donor, but even then the success rate is limited. Any temporary decrease in renal function, e.g., acute tubular necrosis (common in transplants) leads to rapid accumulation of oxalate and to permanent and often progressive loss of function.

Thomas is being considered for a transplant. He has two siblings. His brother is in his early 20s and has hyperoxaluria. His 16-year-old sister is a perfect genetic match. Should she be asked to donate one of her kidneys?

HEALTH CARE FOR ADULTS

One of the common ethical issues raised in health care for adults is distributive justice or the allocation of scarce resources. These resources may include illness care for those who deliberately abuse their bodies through poor health habits, drug abuse, or smoking or the allocation of home or community care services. Adults in their middle years are frequently healthy, though communicable diseases and job-related accidents or illnesses occur. Community health nurses, occupational nurses, and primary care nurse practitioners provide much of the health care for adults.

Case No. 13: Primary Care Nurse

C.W. is a family nurse clinician in joint practice with an internist in a large urban community. He has been caring for Ann, a 52-year-old woman, over the past 4 years. Ann has chronic hypertension of 10 years' duration and a long history of cigarette smoking. She does not always remember to take her blood pressure medications and refuses to watch her dietary intake of salt. At her last visit a month ago, Ann contracted with C.W. to quit smoking. When she arrives for her appointment today, she smells of cigarette smoke and admits that she just cannot give up this one pleasure in her life. C.W. reminds her of their contract, but Ann shrugs and says, "Oh well. You know I can't keep a promise like that. I guess I'll just have to accept it. It's a good thing you keep me healthy, right?" C.W. is seriously considering refusing to care for Ann anymore since his time appears wasted.

Case No. 14: Spouse Abuse

Mr. Smith, 61 years old, has cancer of the colon with multiple metastases. Surgical removal of the tumor left him with a colostomy that he is unable to manage by himself. A palliative course of radiation therapy decreased his pain, but he is constantly tired and basically immobile.

Hospital personnel—social worker, nurses, and physicians—talked with the Smiths about several things they could do. The Smiths decided on a hospice-type care at home. He would stay at home, with his wife providing direct care with the help of a community health nurse (CHN). Other support services would be available as needed. The goal was comfort and support rather than aggressive intervention. Both the Smiths agreed to this. Mrs. Smith was willing to take care of him.

The first home visit by the CHN was quite productive. Mrs. Smith was eager to learn as much as possible about her husband's care. She often asked if her actions could hurt her husband. The nurse interpreted these questions as real concern for the husband. By the fourth home visit, it was obvious that the initial impressions were a facade. Mr. Smith had a lot of pain. He had not been given his pain medication for 24 hours. His colostomy was surrounded by ulcerated areas. His back had areas of skin breakdown showing little or no care. He admitted his wife had been neglecting him but added that he did not mind.

The nurse talked with Mrs. Smith. She had remained in the kitchen during the visit. She did not deny the neglect. In fact, she said she did it on purpose, intending to make him suffer. He had abused her for 15 years. Now she could get back at him. She intended to inflict as much pain as possible in his last weeks of life.

Case No. 15: Communicable Disease in a Research Unit

M.D. is employed as a nurse in a research unit of an area hospital. S.W. is a 21-year-old female recently admitted from a local nursing home with a central nervous system degenerative disease of unknown viral origin. There is speculation that the virus may be transmittable via cerebrospinal fluid (CSF). S.W.'s symptoms have been getting worse, and she currently cannot walk or talk.

The unit physicians have prepared a research protocol to isolate the virus. The protocol calls for placing an external shunt for the removal of CSF three times a week for the next 3 months. The nurses are concerned about contamination via CSF, but the physicians think all staff should be supportive of the research since they are working on a unit dedicated to research.

Case No. 16: Denial of Death

W.B. was a 24-year-old single mother of a baby daughter. She was admitted to our unit at the end of the summer. Her admission diagnosis was metastatic cancer of the cervix. Throughout her 2 month stay, W.B. deteriorated despite aggressive therapy. Bone metastasis prevailed throughout her body. At one point, she twisted her leg attempting to use the commode chair and fractured her hip, necessitating internal fixation.

W.B. was a cheerful person. She had a deep religious faith and often asked for someone to read the Bible for her. She knew she had cancer but did not believe the disease was terminal. Nurses would frequently discuss what was physically happening to her, but she selectively listened to what was being said. Toward the end of the first 2 months, W.B. was told that nothing more could be done. Again, W.B. listened and said she understood, but went on talking unrealistically. The future with her baby was now W.B.'s lifeline.

Her support system included her 23-year-old sister, who was taking care of the baby, and their alcoholic mother. After 2 months, W.B. wanted to go home. She wanted to be with her baby. Her sister wanted to take her home. However, W.B.'s calcium level climbed daily. As hypercalcemia advances, it causes increasing confusion, lethargy, and eventually coma and death. The only therapy was injections of mithramycin.

The injections were needed frequently. The drug was expensive (about $100 a shot) and was covered by insurance only for inpatients. The family could not afford paying for it out of pocket. If W.B. went home, her life would end much sooner. Staying in the hospital would extend her life. She did not believe she was dying and would not listen when the subject was raised. Thus the decision was left to others.

The health care team was asked to make the decision. In the discussion, the primary nurse was asked for her ethical judgment, including her reasons.

ILLNESS AND OLD AGE

Among the major ethical issues in the health care of the elderly is the allocation of resources for the elderly. Likewise, ethical concerns for autonomy and self-determination of the aged are pervasive in a society that does not always value those who are old or of little productivity. Preparing for death—the good death, if you will—occupies much of the aged's thoughts as illness strikes and one wonders if this will be the end of living. A newer ethical concern has surfaced recently, that of abuse of the elderly. Health care providers face all of these ethical issues in their care of the aged who are both ill and well.

Case No. 17: Is There Dignity in Dying?

S.B. is a senior nursing student in a BSN program who has been assigned to care for Mr. Ed today. He is 59 and was admitted to the medical service 2 weeks ago for severe myocardial infarction. He has a 10 year history of heart disease. He has had two cardiac arrests in the last week. As she starts his morning care, Mr. Ed asks S.B. to sit awhile and talk with him. During the conversation, he says he wants to "let nature take its course." He pleads for no more resuscitation if his heart stops again. He says he has put his life in order and he is ready to die.

She goes out to the head nurse to ask how his request for a "No Code" might be conveyed to the rest of the staff. The head nurse tells her it is hospital policy that all patients on the unit are coded. S.B. is confused about Mr. Ed's request and the policy. She cannot find her instructor. She slowly wanders back to his room. She senses a calm stillness in the room and realizes he may have had another cardiac arrest. She listens for heart and breath sounds, and there are none.

She leaves the room and calls the resident on the phone. He asks, "Is the body still warm?" S.B. answers that it is pretty cool. The resident responds that he will be there shortly to pronounce Mr. Ed dead. S.B. returns to the room, still uncertain about her decision not to call a code.

Case No. 18: Autonomy and Aging

Mr. B. is a 72-year-old man with the medical diagnoses of nephrotic syndrome, delirium state, herpes simplex of the mouth, and a *Candida* infection of the groin and lower extremities. He is a retired hairdresser who never married and lives alone in a senior citizen apartment building. He has two brothers who are supportive and visit regularly.

Mr. B. is currently hospitalized for a worsened uremic state requiring dialysis. There is a history of poor compliance with the prescribed medical regimen. At the outset of this hospitalization, Mr. B. was treated with peritoneal dialysis. He progressed to hemodialysis. At this point Mr. B.'s mild occasional confusion exacerbated to a delirium state in which he often was disoriented, shouting for nurses, consistently ringing the call bell with multiple inappropriate requests, e.g., "Get me out of bed," when he was sitting in a chair. Mr. B. participated little in his care.

Antidepressant and tranquilizing medications were not helpful, and the psychiatry consultant felt that Mr. B.'s uremic state produced his altered mental status. The attending physician, family, and patient had agreed at the beginning of his hospitalization that he would not be resuscitated in the event of a cardiac arrest. Mr. B. remained confused, though with periods of lucidity. He could recognize faces, remember names, knew he was in a hospital, and generally knew the time of day but not the date. He continuously repeated questions and remarks. His judgment and insight into his situation were poor. He agreed that he wanted hemodialysis but often refused the procedure as it was being started.

The nursing staff were extremely frustrated with Mr. B. They felt he was manipulative and demanding purposefully. No consistent plan of care was developed or implemented. The primary nurse had a difficult team of patients and felt overwhelmed by Mr. B.'s behavior. The nursing staff would leave his call light unanswered, shut his door, or pull the curtain around the bed. All staff members called the patient by his first name, and, nursing staff often spoke in an abrupt, hostile manner.

The attending physician and house staff questioned the patient's comprehension of his situation but considered that his refusal to have hemodialysis indicated that he did not wish the lifesaving procedure. When approached with an explanation, Mr. B. said he would go through with the hemodialysis, but he would then refuse as the procedure was begun. The physicians concluded that the patient did not want dialysis, and hemodialysis was discontinued. This was discussed with the family and agreed to. Mr. B. died 1 week later.

Case No. 19: Nursing Home or Prison?

Mr. D. was a 70-year-old patient in X Nursing Home. In contrast to many of the residents, Mr. D. was ambulatory. In fact, he not only walked, he danced. Sometimes he danced alone and sometimes with others when he could get someone to dance with him. In contrast to the noncommunicative types so prevalent in the home population, Mr. D. talked. In fact, he talked virtually nonstop, yes, even when he was dancing, and occasionally in his sleep. He even talked when he wrote letters, which was frequent. He would ask for paper, borrow paper, and sometimes take paper and write letters. Some of these letters ran to 10 and even 20 pages. Sometimes the talk turned to singing, mostly off key! Whenever he could get a nurse to listen to him, he would tell her that he was not helpless. He was not crazy. He was in the home because his wife wanted to get rid of him. She did not believe in divorce so she had him committed to the home. "Will you help me get out of here? I want to go home." Several times he tried on his own. When the staff found him missing, they called the police, who usually found him walking down the road within a few miles. Once though, he made it home, but his wife had him sent back. He insisted that he liked the nurses. He liked the food. He was not sick, he insisted. He repeatedly asked the nurses, "Why are you keeping me here? I want to go home."

HEALTH CARE PROFESSIONAL RELATIONSHIPS

Many ethical concerns are raised in the day-to-day practice of nursing. The previous cases illustrate some of the ethical issues in the professional to client relationships. Other ethical issues relate to our relationships with other professional colleagues. Once again we speak of respect for human dignity, self-determination, and advocacy—but this time directed at our peers and colleagues. The desire to maintain an ethical perspective in all areas of practice includes examination of our duties, obligations, or responsibilities to other health care professionals and staff. The following are a few cases illustrating some of the common ethical concerns in professional to professional relationships.

Case No. 20: Nurse to Nurse

The charge nurse for the surgical ward of a local hospital has assigned a new staff nurse, D.D., to one of the most complicated cases on the ward. A woman with a total pelvic exonteration has just returned from the recovery room. D.D. protests that she has never cared for such a patient before and would like a different assignment. The charge nurse yells at her that everyone has to learn, and it is now her turn to do so. The young nurse walks away from the report session and goes in to visit the patient, still wondering how she will ever manage to provide safe care. As she approaches the foot of the bed, she notes that the woman is shaking all over. D.D. calls out to her. The patient does not respond, so D.D. comes closer to the bed. She sees a large stain of blood forming on the sheet over the woman's abdomen, and she lifts the sheet. When she sees the open wounds, D.D. gasps and runs out of the room into the bathroom and vomits. Another staff nurse decided to stop by to see how the new nurse was getting along and found the patient in shock. She began treatment that saved the patient's life.

Case No. 21: Unethical Nursing Behavior

J.N. is a nurse assigned to a surgical ward. He is waiting to care for Mr. L., who is about come back from the recovery room after an appendectomy. J.N. sees a nurse colleague drawing up 50 milligrams of Demerol. He notes that the medication card has Mr. L.'s name on it. The nurse has charted his name in the narcotic record. The nurse colleague returns to the medicine room 10 minutes later with an empty syringe. J.N. casually asks who needed the Demerol. "Oh, Mr. L. He just returned from surgery and was in pain." Confused, J.N. checks Mr. L.'s room and finds that he has not yet returned from the recovery room.

Case No. 22: Administrative Responsibilities

W.A. is a nursing supervisor in a church-affiliated rehabilitation hospital. The powerful administrator is paternalistic and conservative in practice. He has also covered up for several incidences of poor medical and nursing practice in the center. The nursing director is viewed by the staff as an ineffective leader, though she often battles with the administrator about nursing's low image, the strict dress code, and the need for changes to improve patient care.

W.A. is scheduled to work days this weekend. She is called Friday evening and told that the administrator just fired the director of nursing. The evening supervisor warns W.A. that the rest of the nursing staff is considering a walkout for Saturday at 8 AM. There is no union involved.

Case No. 23: Accountability and Allocation of Resources

G.W., a 37-year-old man, has arrived in the hospital emergency room in severe cardiac failure after collapsing in his office. The physician–nurse team takes over the resusitation efforts from the emergency squad and works quickly to try to stabilize his cardiac status long enough to transfer him to the medical intensive care unit (MICU). As the medical resident attends to G.W., she asks the charge nurse to call MICU and prepare for G.W.'s transfer. The charge nurse returns shortly and announces that the MICU is full. There is no bed or monitoring equipment available, unless another patient is moved out. The physician knows that transfer of G.W. at this time could mean his death. She decides to call the MICU herself.

Once again, the response from the MICU resident is that transfer is impossible. He does not want to decide who would be moved because there is a nursing shortage on the stepdown unit. Any patient moved could easily die from lack of continuous monitoring. In addition, the nurses in the stepdown unit have refused to accept responsibility for any more patients assigned. They have the support of the hospital administration in this.

APPENDIX B
Codes of Ethics

The codes of ethics of the American Medical Association and the International Council of Nurses are included here for easy reference during the reading of this text. The code of ethics of the American Nurses' Association can be found in Chapter One. All health care professionals can benefit from periodically reviewing the code of ethics for their professional group. These codes offer guidance for professional behavior in relationships with patients, peers, and society.

INTERNATIONAL COUNCIL OF NURSES CODE FOR NURSES (1973): ETHICAL CONCEPTS APPLIED TO NURSING*

The fundamental responsibility of the nurse is fourfold: to promote health, to prevent illness, to restore health, and to alleviate suffering.

The need for nursing is universal. Inherent in nursing is respect for life, dignity, and rights of man. It is unrestricted by considerations of nationality, race, creed, color, age, sex, politics, or social status.

Nurses render health services to the individual, the family, and community and coordinate their services with those of related groups.

Nurses and People

The nurse's primary responsibility is to those people who require nursing care. The nurse, in providing care, promotes an environment in which the values, customs, and spiritual beliefs of the individual are respected.

*Reprinted with permission of the International Council of Nurses.

The nurse holds in confidence personal information and uses judgment in sharing this information.

Nurses and Practice

The nurse carries personal responsibility for nursing practice and for maintaining competence by continual learning.

The nurse maintains the highest standards of nursing care possible within the reality of a specific situation.

The nurse uses judgment in relation to individual competence when accepting and delegating responsibilities.

The nurse when acting in a professional capacity should at all times maintain standards of personal conduct that reflect credit upon the profession.

Nurses and Society

The nurse shares with other citizens the responsibility for initiating and supporting action to meet the health and social needs of the public.

Nurses and Co-Workers

The nurse sustains a cooperative relationship with co-workers in nursing and other fields.

The nurse takes appropriate action to safeguard the individual when his care is endangered by a co-worker or any other person.

Nurses and the Profession

The nurse plays the major role in determining and implementing desirable standards of nursing practice and nursing education.

The nurse is active in developing a core of professional knowledge.

The nurse, acting through the professional organization, participates in establishing and maintaining equitable social and economic working conditions in nursing.

AMERICAN MEDICAL ASSOCIATION PRINCIPLES OF MEDICAL ETHICS (1980)*

Preamble

The medical profession has long subscribed to a body of ethical statements developed primarily for the benefit of the patient. As a member of this profession, a physician must recognize responsibility not only to patients, but also to society, to other health professionals, and to self. The following Principles

*Reprinted with permission of the American Medical Association.

adopted by the American Medical Association are not laws, but standards of conduct which define the essentials of honorable behavior for the physician.

(I)

A physician shall be dedicated to providing competent medical service with compassion and respect for human dignity.

(II)

A physician shall deal honestly with patients and colleagues, and strive to expose those physicians deficient in character or competence, or who engage in fraud or deception.

(III)

A physician shall respect the law and also recognize a responsibility to seek changes in those requirements which are contrary to the best interests of the patient.

(IV)

A physician shall respect the rights of patients, of colleagues, and of other health professionals, and shall safeguard the patient confidences within the constraints of law.

(V)

A physician shall continue to study, apply and advance scientific knowledge, make relevant information available to patients, colleagues, and the public, obtain consultation, and use the talents of other health professionals when indicated.

(VI)

A physician shall, in the provision of appropriate patient care, except in emergencies, be free to choose whom to serve, with whom to associate, and the environment in which to provide medical services.

(VII)

A physician shall recognize a responsibility to participate in activities contributing to an improved community.

APPENDIX C
Models of Ethical Decision Making

Howard Brody developed the act–utilitarian and deontological models for ethical decision making in the early 1970s. These models are helpful in analyzing the ethical dimensions of a health care situation from either theoretical perspective. Rita Payton developed the pluralistic model of ethical decision making based on the work of Brody, and in recognition of the pluralistic nature of many health care situations. These models are reproduced with permission of the authors for easy reference during the reading of this text. You may also wish to apply them during Step Nine of the ten-step model described in this text.

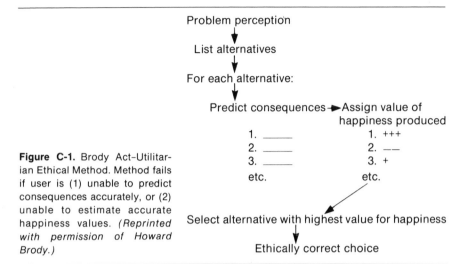

Figure C-1. Brody Act–Utilitarian Ethical Method. Method fails if user is (1) unable to predict consequences accurately, or (2) unable to estimate accurate happiness values. *(Reprinted with permission of Howard Brody.)*

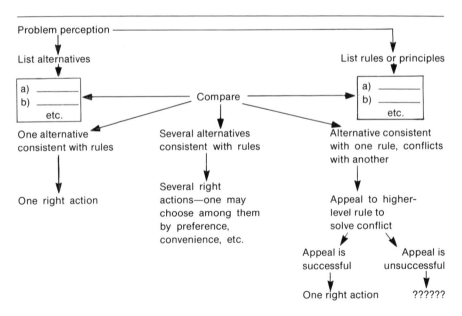

Figure C-2. Brody Deontological Ethical Method. *(Reprinted with permission of Howard Brody.)*

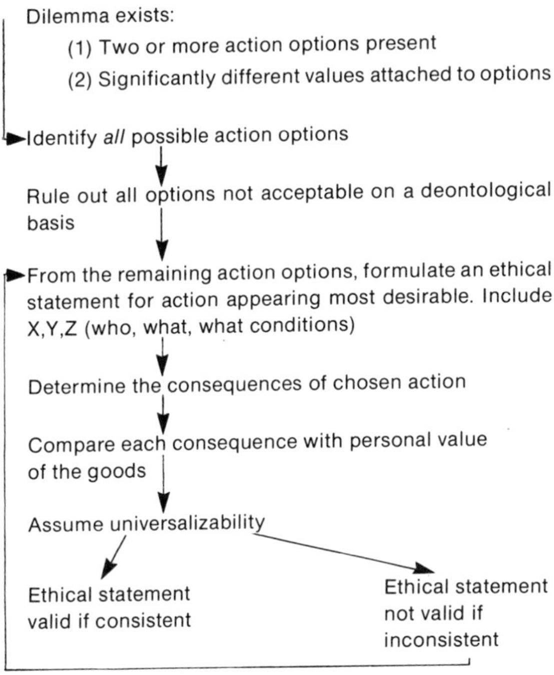

Dilemma exists:

(1) Two or more action options present

(2) Significantly different values attached to options

Identify *all* possible action options

Rule out all options not acceptable on a deontological basis

From the remaining action options, formulate an ethical statement for action appearing most desirable. Include X,Y,Z (who, what, what conditions)

Determine the consequences of chosen action

Compare each consequence with personal value of the goods

Assume universalizability

Ethical statement valid if consistent

Ethical statement not valid if inconsistent

Figure C-3. Payton Pluralistic Ethical Decision-Making Model. For cycle return in case of invalid result: (1) Ethical statement may be reformulated modifying the conditions, or (2) Alternate action option (still available after rule in) may be explored going through all remaining steps. Remember—the decision to take no action is in itself action. *(Reprinted with permission of Rita J. Payton.)*

Glossary

Absolute Duty. A duty is an obligation or responsibility owed to another or an obligation to follow a code of conduct, e.g., the ANA code of ethics. Duty ethics are sometimes equated with deontology, and especially the deontology of Kant. Kant's ethics were absolute, unconditional, i.e., the duty is to be followed at all times regardless of circumstances, consequences, or persons, whether one feels like it or not. In ethical dilemmas, prima facie (Latin, "at first sight") duties may give way to an absolute duty. In Jewish Law, all 613 commandments in the Scriptures may be suspended in order to save a life. This is a common standard in health care, one now being questioned in relation to the quality of life (QOL) potential.

Accountability. This is both a legal and an ethical concept. It is sometimes equated with responsibility. In the vernacular, one could say "The buck stops here!" The temptation in many walks of life is to let someone else take responsibility. One of the issues in the trial of Adolph Eichmann for war crimes was accountability. He claimed he was only following orders and could not be held accountable. The Israeli court disagreed and ordered him executed for murder. Health care workers not uncommonly refer responsibility to others in the hierarchy or to hospital policy, and so on. As recently as 1973, a judge said that nurses could not be sued for malpractice, for they are only carrying out orders. Others note that if nursing is going to be a profession, nurses must be accountable. Nursing will not be a profession until nurses accept responsibility, even if it means going against orders or policy when these are inaccurate or wrong.

Act Deontology. The ethical theory of deontology means rules. In act deontology, the rule is that the individual knows in each situation what ought to be done. See *Intuitionism*.

Act Utilitarianism. Each situation is judged individually according to its utility. There is no reliance on general rules of mortality or ethical principles. Act utilitarianism, however, could be seen as itself a rule. It is a subset of the ethical theory of utilitarianism.

Allocation of Scarce Resources. Allocation refers to distribution. In this case, it is a question of who gets the resources. The latter may be money for health care, a hospital bed, a scarce item of equipment, or the time and energy of health care providers. The just distribution of resources is a major element in the ethical principle of justice in health care.

Applied Ethics. This is sometimes called "normative ethics." There are theories about ethics, such as the systems of utilitarianism or deontology. The application of the theory to real life cases moves health care providers from abstraction to reality. Normative ethics carries the implication of prescription. One can describe ethics as observed in the health care setting. One can prescribe, saying this is what ought to be done. The shoulds and oughts are sometimes equated with morals. Thus applied ethics may be equated with morality or even moralizing, whereas the ethical "Why?" is the philosophical reasoning behind the applied ethic.

Autonomy. The original Greek means independence. The "auto" part of the word comes from the Greek *autos*, meaning "self." The "nomy" comes from the Greek *nemein*, meaning "to hold sway." Thus the word means self-governing. It is used interchangeably with self-determination. A profession is supposedly autonomous—self-governing—though that may be within the limits of the law or society. Individual autonomy may be limited by illness, economics, politics, and any number of other factors. Legally, at least in the United States, the individual can refuse health care for any reason whatever, including a mere whim. If a person is judged incompetent, however, as in suicides, the mentally ill, senility, or some other condition, autonomy is limited or even denied. Whether the autonomous individual can demand or has a right to health care is a heavily debated issue.

Belief. A belief may be a doctrine, such as nurses believing in caring for the whole person, or an attitude, such as patients believing in their nurse or physician. The former is a matter of truth, whereas the latter is a trust. For some, a belief is something that cannot be proven, as in religion where an atheist cannot prove there is no God. A belief is thus like the axioms of science. Some people do not have proof but do have reasons for their beliefs. Aiken's four levels of moral discourse are noted in the text. Belief is sometimes related to his expressive level. A nurse might believe in caring for people. At Aiken's moral rules level, one would say, "Nurses should care for people."

Beneficence. The Hippocratic Oath says to do good or at least do no harm (maleficence). The Latin *bene* means "well," and *facere* means "to do." The concept stands as an ethical principle in itself or in relation to harm, as in the cost-benefit ratio where the issue is the amount of cost (money, suffering) in relation to the good that is accomplished. We inflict pain, e.g., surgery, but for the greater good of health, freedom from the disease, or relief of the greater pain caused by the illness. For some, the cost of maintaining life may not be worth it if the quality of the life saved or maintained is unacceptable. It has been suggested that health care providers have a duty to do no harm, whereas beneficence is supererogation—work beyond the call of duty.

Bioethics. The ethics of life may refer to all of life, including such aspects of living as the environment. In practice, bioethics have come to refer to health care ethics. Thus, technically, instead of talking about ethics in nursing, one should talk about bioethics in nursing. The terms are often used interchangeably, however, although ethics is a larger concern and may refer to many other areas, such as business, politics, law.

Biomedical Technology. Technology comes from the Greek for the study of art or artifice, the study of the practical, or the applied arts. In this context, the reference is to the broad range of procedures, machinery, devices, medications, or other applications of medical science. It may be a new type of hospital bed or the application of an electric current to stimulate bone growth in the nonunion of a broken bone. Many of these developments have come in the past few decades. The enormous number and complexity of modern technologies have been a major stimulus to the rise of bioethics. It is the success of modern health care that has raised so many questions, such as when does a person die if machinery can keep the heart and lungs functioning after they would have normally stopped if left to themselves (natural law)? While one can appreciate the new options available in health care, the questions are getting tougher. In nursing, these developments have given rise to such phenomenon as the physician who acknowledged that modern nurses know more than his physician father knew a few decades ago.

Categorical Imperative. Immanuel Kant (1724–1804) suggested that our actions must be tested by the question, "What would happen if everyone did this or did not do this?" Another version is that human beings are an end in themselves. People are never a means to some other end or purpose. To use people for research or to use them for anything is to violate this essential human dignity. The concept grows out of Kant's belief in human rationality, which is the same at all times and in all places. As noted earlier (*Absolute duty*), this is a universal law, which is part of the deontological system of ethics. The imperative is a part of human nature, which makes Kant a nativist rather than an environmentalist in the old nature vs nurture debate begun in ancient times. Socrates (469–399 BC) was asked if people are good by nature or if they become so by education or training. His intellectual grandson, Aristotle, said the latter. Socrates himself asks, "What is good?" In one sense, Kant's categorical imperative answers that we know (intuitionism) what is good. Some relate this to the idea of conscience, but others consider the comparison simplistic.

Code of Ethics. Professional codes of ethics contain the rules by which a profession governs itself. Some of these are professional etiquette relating to advertising, fees, relationships with other professionals, or the refusal to relate to those who are unacceptable. Other rules are moral or ethical standards, such as do good or, at least, do no harm, or, "The nurse provides services with respect for human dignity . . ." The rules set the standard and in this sense are moral standards. The ethical "Why?" may not appear in the code itself. Codes have been criticized for being too general. They do not always give guidance in specific situations. That is perhaps necessary, since the situations have an infinite variety of details.

No code could possibly cover all situations. It is up to the ethical individual to apply the code to the situation. It is sometimes thought that to be a profession, a group must have a code of ethics. The proliferation of professions has brought a proliferation of codes. But these are often modelled after earlier or related codes, and they are not necessarily all that different. Some have suggested that the purpose of a code is to avoid government regulation. Some have even suggested that codes are window dressing to fool the public. What professionals do in practice may be quite different from the professional code of ethics. Codes remain, however, one guide to what a profession considers its moral or ethical principles.

Cognitive Disequilibrium. "All is right with the world" might be called equilibrium. "There's something wrong with the world" might be called disequilibrium. The one is satisfaction, acceptance, quiet, peace. The other is disturbed or disturbing, disruptive, a sense of something out of place. People may feel or sense the disequilibrium—an emotional or intuitive perception. A rational, intellectual, or mental understanding would be the cognitive counterpart. Disequilibrium may result from or be a clue to the presence of a moral dilemma. In the theories of Jean Piaget (1896–1980) and Lawrence Kohlberg, moral development comes through disequilibrium as the person tries through understanding to overcome the moral discrepancy.

Confidentiality. This ethical principle is related to privacy and to secret knowledge or knowledge known only to a few. Confidential communication refers to personal and private matters shared with a health care provider, clergy, lawyer, or other professional who cannot be compelled by law to repeat that information or be a witness against the client. The concept is more widespread than this, of course, since it may refer to personal friends or professional colleagues. The major exception now widely accepted is when there is the threat of harm to another person, i.e., a threat to murder someone. The violation or potential violation of confidentiality is a source of ethical dilemmas in health care. It may be in conflict, for example, with the responsibility to tell the truth, i.e., a patient has cancer. The family does not want him to know it, but he asks point blank, "Do I have cancer?"

Consensus Ethics. The consensus is the general opinion. The ethics of society in general might be considered as the consensus. The agreement might also be within a subunit of society, such as among nurses or in the intensive care unit. Kohlberg's conventional level of ethics with Stages 3 and 4 (personal authority and law and order) might be considered a consensus ethics. In relative morality theories, it is the ethics of the society, such as the Trobriand Islanders, Islamic society, Western society, or Chinese society.

Consequentialism. In general, this refers to the consequences, the results, what happens. A consequentialist ethic is a teleological ethic—one concerned with the end, the purpose, the consequences, or, in the vernacular, the bottom line. Utilitarianism is a consequentialist ethic. "The end justifies the means" is a consequentialist statement. This ethic is sometimes considered a one-principle ethic in contrast to a pluralistic ethic of two or more principles (see *Deontology*). In health care, one is justified in inflicting the pain of an injection or an operation because of the greater good (the end) that one intends. This is the cost-benefit ratio approach to ethics.

Contract Theory. Thomas Hobbes (1588–1697), John Locke (1631–1704), and Jean Jacques Rousseau (1712–1778) thought that society was based on individuals who banded together for mutual protection. In American Revolutionary history, this meant that people cannot be governed without the consent of the governed, and when the people want to do so, they can change their government. In the Hegel to Marx tradition, human beings are social animals. There is no such thing as the individual apart from society. People are interdependent. John Rawls represents a modern revival of classical contract theory. Rawlsian ethics has been seen as a fourth category of deontological ethics. The revival is not with political obligations but with ethical principles that obligate people to each other. The highest principle is that of justice, considered Stage 6 in Kohlberg's moral development concept. Instead of being inherited from one's ancestors, these obligations are accepted when the individual accepts the benefits of society. The principles relate back to Kant's universalism—freedom, autonomy, dignity, human rights, self-respect, and above all, the just allocation of resources. In health care, contract theory relates to the relationship of provider and patient. Is it just an individual contract—"You pay your money and take your choice"—or is health care a social right, i.e., everyone has a right to health care?

Cost–Benefit Ratio. The cost may be financial or a matter of time or suffering. The benefit is the good that comes from the expenditure. Some ethicists think that one can assign values to various aspects of life and calculate the cost in relation to the benefit—a utilitarian calculus. While money has a kind of value, others think that the value of suffering or of the good may be difficult if not impossible to determine. Some people can tolerate more pain than others. For some, the pain of life is well worth it compared to the alternative! Some see the pain as intolerable. This becomes a special moral dilemma when the expected length of life is very short and the quality of that life is very low. The skyrocketing costs of health care have brought the cost-benefit ratio into particular prominence in the area of public health policy. The costs of many procedures are beyond the resources of the average person. Should society bear these costs? Should society bear the costs when the benefits are great? What about when the benefits are few or limited either in numbers of people served or in the little good that it does the individual?

Cultural Transmission. Society passes on its values and other aspects of its heritage to successive generations. Parents pass on their values and other beliefs to their children. Kohlberg sees this as the conventional level of morality, but cultures and people can obviously pass on their lower and higher stages as well. The American Constitution, for example, is Kohlberg's Stage 5. It has obviously been passed on to subsequent generations. What is at issue here is whether the younger generation merely accepts the morality of previous generations or whether this heritage is thought through and evaluated anew in each generation. Nursing ethics can be passed on through the Nightingale Pledge but each generation might consider the ethical "Why?" for the standards. The same is true for the ANA *Code for Nurses*. Merely repeating the *Code* without thought does not make a nurse ethical. It is of interest that Kohlberg has retrenched his educational effort from trying to help people develop to the postconventional level of Stages 5 and 6 to helping them develop to the conventional level of Stages 3 and 4.

Defining the Issues Test (DIT). This questionnaire was developed by James R. Rest. He worked with Lawrence Kohlberg who depended on oral interviews, with over 120 variables. Rest used six stories with specific questions to create an objective pencil and paper test than can be taken in less than an hour and scored by anyone with the ability to understand the scoring instructions. The DIT has been standardized and used on tens of thousands of people. It supports Kohlberg's thesis about education influencing moral development. It gives no evidence of differences between men and women or between cultural, ethnic, or racial groups beyond that of education. The DIT does, however, result in higher ratios for liberals as compared to conservatives. It generally gives a higher stage rating than Kohlberg's interview process. The latter involves generating a response, whereas the DIT involves recognizing a response, thus tapping a different quality of memory and development. The DIT also differs from Kohlberg's stage theory in being a continuum on a spectrum of development without the sharp distinction between stages presented by Kohlberg's theory. In practice, however, the latter is not a sharp distinct development either but a gradual move over time so a person actually thinks and decides in or across several stages at any given time. The stage assigned in Kohlberg's research is the one where most of the reasoning is.

Deontology. The Greek *deon* means binding, to bind, and hence, rule or principle. The study of these principles is one major system of ethics. There is no set number of ethical principles, but the principles used in health care can generally be grouped under such headings as autonomy, beneficence (do good), nonmaleficence (do no harm), and justice. Confidentiality, professional competence, loyalty, respect for persons, the Golden Rule, truth-telling can usually be considered a part of one or more of these umbrella terms. Deontology is usually contrasted with utilitarian ethics, which is concerned with the consequences rather than the means. However, utility itself may be considered a principle.

Descriptive Ethics. An observer, such as an anthropologist, looks to see what people actually do in terms of ethics. Their actions may be congruent with the spoken principles, the combination called "praxis" in some traditions. Sometimes there are distinct differences. In the vernacular, people do not always practice what they preach. It has been suggested that the real ethics of western society are greed, materialism, money, security, jobs, status, and power, rather than the Golden Rule or some other expression of the ideal. Descriptive ethics may relate to normative ethics or to morals as compared to the ethical "Why?" which asks for the reasons behind the ethics as described.

Distributive Justice. The allocation of resources, especially the scarce resources of money, time, energy, trained personnel, and equipment, has been a concern throughout the ages. Traditionally the rich get first choice, and the poor may get nothing at all. The just distribution of resources usually calls for some type of equity in the distribution. One standard is that all human beings are created equal. In Kantian ethics, human beings are an end in themselves, without regard to wealth, race, sex, ethnic group, nationality, or any other distinction. This standard appears in the ANA *Code for Nurses*. In reality, those with the power or the money usually get the best health care. Some suggest that health care should be available to everyone. Some claim that every person has a right to health care. Distribution, of course, is uneven, even for the powerful and wealthy, so there are a number of problems with the ethical principle of just distribution but the ideal remains.

Duty. See *Absolute duty.*

Egoism. Egoism focuses on the self. Ethical egoism sees self-interest as the standard of morality. It is sometimes considered a separate ethical perspective. Kurt Baier notes it as part of the teleological tradition. The good is what is good for the self. This selfishness is contrasted to altruism, with its concern for others. Kohlberg's preconventional level of moral development is narcissistic. Ethical egoism is Stage 2. It is an ad hominem, "according to the person," perspective—there is no objective, independent truth or principle. It is all a matter of self-interest.

Elitism. The elite are the choice or chosen few, presumably the best of the group. Ethical elitism sees the right or the good as that which is good for the elite. The latter may be the wealthy, the educated, the professionals, or simply those in power. In health care, the ethical issue may be one of who gets the care or who has the power in the health care system. This approach stands in contrast to equality of care. The ANA *Code for Nurses* says the nurse gives care without regard to social or economic status. The *Interpretive Statement* expands this to say irrespective of background or other status. Elitism is similar to but distinct from ethical parochialism.

Ethical Parochialism. This focuses on "my group." "What's good for my company (race, sex, church, class, political party, country) is what is right." The elite may be an objective group, whereas parochialism is again an ad hominem perspective, as in egoism, but the ego identifies with the group. Middle class ethics or WASP (White Anglo-Saxon Protestant) ethics might be elitist as an objective category. It would be parochialism if the moral agent belongs to the group and proposes his group as the standard of what is right. A health care provider might see his professional group as the standard of what is right, as the ones who know what is right or who have the ethical right to decide what should or should not be done.

Ethical Pluralism. Pluralism refers to a concern with or an acceptance of more than one. A one-principle ethic, such as utility or justice, may be called "monism." Deontology as an ethical system usually considers valid two or more principles, such as truth-telling, doing good, autonomy. Another pluralistic approach is the mixture or combination of systems. Some or perhaps many or even most people are sometimes utilitarian and sometimes deontological. Natural law may be understood as a combination of these two systems, for it is concerned with both consequences and principles.

Ethical Theory. Originally a theory was a mental looking at something, an intellectual exercise or speculation as compared to doing something practical. It may in reverse be an attempt to understand the actual, i.e., why does a patient or health care provider behave this way? In time, a theory became an attempt to systematically spell out an idea or relate various ideas in a system. An ethical theory may be an intellectual attempt to understand ethics as contrasted to applied ethics. An ethical theory may be an ethical system that develops an idea of ethics or relates various principles of ethics. Utilitarianism and deontology are two main philosophical ethical theories.

Ethical Universalism. The good is what is good for all humanity. Kant's categorical imperative judged goodness by what would happen if everyone did or did not do the action proposed. He derived his theory from the idea that all human rationality is the same. Universalism stands in contrast to egoism, elitism, and parochialism. It is sometimes related to utilitarianism, but this system does not always relate to all people. The aphorism, "The greatest good for the greatest number," so common in health care policy, implies a lesser number who get left out. "The end justifies the means" says nothing about all humanity, and the concept of utility may or may not relate to all. In theological ethics, this concept may support the principle of equality, as in the idea that God is the creator of all people so all are equal and should be treated as such, e.g., in health care. Theological ethics, however, have also been parochial. The theological concept of universalism says that all people will be saved, in contrast to the belief that one's own group will be saved. This contrast may influence health care, but not necessarily.

Ethics. The English word comes from the Greek *ethos*, meaning "character" or "custom." The term is often used interchangeably with morals from the Latin *moralis*, meaning "manners." Both words are thus concerned with distinguishing right from wrong in attitude or behavior. Some distinguish ethics as the theoretical concern, whereas morals are the applied or practical concern. Ethics are the reasoning aspect of the moral–ethical continuum. Philosophically, ethics asks for the reason behind the moral rule or standard. There are various ways to consider ethics, such as applied ethics or normative ethics (what to do), Biblical ethics, philosophical ethics, social ethics, theological ethics, theoretical ethics, descriptive ethics (this is what people do), prescriptive ethics (this is what people should do). In addition to health care ethics or bioethics, there are business ethics, legal ethics, political ethics, and so on.

Euthanasia. A good or painless death has been a major human concern throughout history. The word has taken on additional meanings in terms of health care and relationships. Passive euthanasia means letting a person die. Under some circumstances—terminal and especially a painful illness—some suggest that this is acceptable. "Let nature take its course" might be a natural law perspective. Active euthanasia, the actual hastening of death, is generally condemned as murder. However, a number of legal cases involving the killing of terminally ill patients in great pain or permanent paralysis have resulted in acquittals or suspended sentences. One of the gray areas is giving analgesics. A dose high enough to deaden the pain may also hasten death. In some cases, this may be acceptable under the law of double effect. Others consider it active euthanasia. "Pulling the plug" has become a euphemism for turning off the machinery, such as a ventilator, and letting nature take its course. A related concept is extraordinary vs ordinary care or treatment.

Extraordinary Treatment. Pope Pius XII said that we are required to use ordinary means to save life. We may use extraordinary means, but we are not required to do so. The distinction has been heavily debated. In the famous case of Karen Ann Quinlan, the use of the ventilator was extraordinary to the family and their priest. However, it was ordinary to the physicians who used such equipment as part of their normal routine. An even more difficult distinction has become public in recent years. Food is generally seen as ordinary. It was continued after Ms. Quinlan was taken off the ventilator. In other cases, people have argued that when life becomes totally empty, i.e., a comatose person without hope of recovery, food may even be considered extraordinary.

Fraternal Charity. Brotherly love may be another term for the Golden Rule, "Do unto others as you would have others do unto you." In its Silver form, it reads, "Do not do unto others that which is hurtful to thyself." This ethical principle is common to many of the religions of the world. It is a norm cited by theists and nontheists, religious and nonreligious. An earlier form of brotherly love is found in the Biblical story of Cain and Abel. After Cain had killed Abel, God found Cain and asked, "Where is thy brother?" Cain responded with a question, "Am I my brother's keeper?" The appropriate answer is usually interpreted as being "Yes." This concept has been cited in health care, i.e., health care providers are their brother's keeper. In paternalistic societies, the concept of brotherly remains common. Other traditions are concerned with all people—sisterly love as well as brotherly love. The religious tradition to "love thy neighbor" is thus extended to all. See *Ethical universalism.*

Informed Consent. This principle relates to Kant's concern for the dignity of all people, the principles of self-determination and autonomy, and the legal concept of the inviolability of the human person. It is thus both an ethical and a legal principle. Consent gives permission to the health care provider to touch the person. This consent is often understood, i.e., when someone enters an emergency room and asks for treatment. The question of "informed" is vague and debatable. One standard is that one is informed when one has had a procedure explained in ordinary language and acknowledges that it is understood. How much patients need to know is part of the debate. One standard is the "reasonable person," which some people call a legal fiction. The concept of informed consent has ancient roots, but its modern significance dates from the Nazi era and the so-called experiments performed by physicians on Nazi prisoners. These experiments were done without the consent of the victims. The war crimes trials after World War II focused public attention on this unethical research. The *Nuremberg Code* (1946) called for the voluntary consent of the human subject in research or human experimentation. The concept has been repeated in subsequent codes and is now widely accepted as a principle in health care. Some, however, call it a farce. They claim that by manipulating the data, they can get anyone to sign an informed consent agreement. When persons are really ill, the doctrine may be meaningless—all they want is to get well.

Intuitionism. Intuition is knowing something without rational thought. It is sometimes compared to instinct or knowing naturally without being taught. In ethics, intuitionism suggests that we know what is right or wrong without being taught. Some relate this to natural law. Nature, or God as the creator of nature, has endowed us with this understanding. Some relate the concept to conscience. Intuitionism may be seen as part of the deontological system of ethics or as a separate approach. It has been suggested that many people, including health care providers, are intuitionists. Some even see it as the bottom line in otherwise carefully reasoned rational philosophical ethics.

Justice. Legal justice is in accordance with the law. Ethical justice may refer to fairness or impartiality. The just distribution of goods is one example. John Rawls has focused attention on justice. Kurt Baier considers Rawls's justice a deontological perspective in the tradition of the social contract.

Law of Double Effect. When the effect, the result, the aim, or the purpose is good, an action may be ethically acceptable even though a secondary effect is wrong. The classic illustration is a pregnant woman with cancer of the uterus. It is acceptable according to this doctrine to remove the cancerous uterus if it is necessary to save the woman's life, even though the secondary or double effect is an abortion, which may be wrong on other grounds. The doctrine is notable as a part of Roman Catholic ethics but is not limited to this tradition. It is in essence a part of health care ethics as part of utilitarianism, e.g., it is ethically acceptable to cause pain, as with surgery, when the intent is the health of the person. As noted under *Euthanasia,* it may be acceptable in terminal illness to give a large dose of analgesic to relieve pain even though the large dose hastens death.

Medical Ethics. Medical ethics are the moral obligations of the practice of medicine. These are sometimes called the "standards of practice." Medical ethics are often or usually identified with physician ethics. Health care ethics, the ethics of health care professionals, are thus the larger concept. There are many areas of overlap, but the professionals do not always agree on everything. In recent decades, medical ethics have sometimes been identified with biomedical ethics and, hence, bioethics. The history of medical ethics is ancient and present in all cultures. Though differing somewhat from group to group, there are commonalities, such as concern for the patient and colleague or professional courtesy. In the Western world, the Hippocratic Oath has been an important source of medical ethics, though it did not catch on until the middle ages. The oath to the Greek gods is usually ignored, as are some other aspects of it.

Metaethics. The Greek *meta* means "beyond." For some, "beyond ethics" means being "above the law." More commonly, it refers to a higher law or to an ultimate ethic, such as the will of God or the law of nature. We can ask for the reason behind a moral standard and then ask for the reason behind the reason, and so on, until we reach a stopping point, an ultimate, or an axiom that is accepted as the final appeal. Another view of metaethics is the study of ethics itself. This study deals with a number of questions, such as "What is ethics?"

Moral Agent. The agent is the person who is acting, i.e., the one who has the power to act. A moral agent is the one making the moral decision. This is "where the buck stops" or "the bottom line." It is sometimes assumed that the moral agent is the one making the final decision. Thus it has been suggested that nurses are not normally moral agents because they are usually part of the hierarchy rather than the final decision makers. To be a moral agent, one must be free, i.e., have the power to decide. A broader view is that the very action of deferring to another is a moral decision. Adolf Eichmann claimed he was not responsible for the murder of Jews by the Nazis. He was only carrying out orders. Others considered him morally and legally responsible, and he was executed accordingly. Nurses are more and more becoming legally responsible and hence, directly or indirectly, are moral agents. Some claim that to be professional, one must accept responsibility. Hence, to be professional is to be a moral agent. Others claim that we are morally responsible whether we accept the label of professional or not. Thus nurses are moral agents regardless of the issue of professionalism. All normal human beings may be considered moral agents. The exceptions are the comatose, the retarded, the mentally ill, children under age. In some cases, older children and the mentally incapacitated are seen as having some degree of moral responsibility.

Moral Relativism. There is a saying that all things are relative. Moral relativism usually refers to the different ethical standards of different groups or cultures. Consensus ethics is that of the group at hand. Ethical egoism, elitism, or parochialism may also be considered relative. In contrast, some claim that ethics is in some sense universal. Ethical universalism would be an example of this. Kant's categorical imperative would be another example. The moral development theories of Piaget and Kohlberg are also nonrelativist.

Moral Theology. Theology is technically the study of God. In more common usage, it is the study of religion or religious doctrines. It is sometimes limited to Christian theology but, more broadly conceived, applies to all religion. Moral theology studies the ethics or moral standards of religious or theological traditions. These might be broken down with a tradition, e.g., Roman Catholic ethics, Brahmin ethics, Rabbinic ethics. Moral theology is sometimes contrasted to moral philosophy. While the distinction can be made in the Christian West, it is not applicable to many religious traditions, such as Buddhism, where there is no distinction between theology and philosophy.

Morals. As noted under *Ethics*, the term or concept of morals is frequently equated with ethics. This might even be seen as the common understanding. Others see morals as applied ethics, or the shoulds and should nots of moral rules whereas ethics is the "Why?" or the reasons behind the morals. The study of morality is concerned with what is right and wrong in conduct, character, or attitudes. In Western culture, moral and immoral often refer specifically to sexual attitudes and behavior, but traditionally the concern is with all aspects of life.

Natural Law. In theistic traditions, this is the law of God who created nature. In nontheistic thought, it is the law of nature without further referent. It is usually thought of as being discoverable by human reason without revelation. See *Naturalistic fallacy*. In the West, Natural Law derives from both Greek philosophy and the Bible. The Apostle Paul may mean natural law in Romans 2:14 when he says non-Jews know the law of God, i.e., without special revelation. Paul distinguishes this law from the concept of conscience, though others relate the two. Thus natural law may be related to intuitionism—we naturally know right from wrong without external instruction. Others suggest that conscience is formed by the environment. In contrast to the naturalistic fallacy, nature as a referent has sometimes been suggested as the source of ethics. For some time, it was argued that such actions as contraception and homosexuality were wrong because they are unnatural, i.e., the lower animals do not practice contraception or homosexuality. Nonprocreative sexual activity has now been observed in animals, and this argument is being dropped. This may be another example of the way in which ethics and scientific data interact. It should be noted that opponents of the two examples still argue against contraception and homosexuality but on other grounds. Natural law has been considered a third system of ethics along with deontology and utilitarianism. Others suggest it is simply a combination of both means and ends, both principles and purposes, and not a third system.

Naturalistic Fallacy. The concept is usually related to the work of David Hume (1711–1776). It is generally thought that nature provides what is. The fallacy is the effort to derive ethics from what is. Hume held that what is does not tell us what ought to be. Science provides data but not values. The concept is sometimes used against Natural Law, where the natural may be the values of the one(s) deciding what is or is not natural. It has been said that much health care passes as scientific clinical judgment when it really reflects the values of the health care provider. On the other hand, it has also been claimed that ethicists and people making ethical decisions need to know the facts or their ethics will be out of touch with reality. While the naturalistic fallacy is widely accepted, it has been questioned in recent years. The debate centers on professionals who think they are the ones who ought to make the ethical decisions, though they have no special understanding of morals or ethics. In a different direction, new developments have brought new choices and a renewal of the old question, "Because we can, should we?" It is claimed by some that the should is a moral standard that must come from ethical considerations rather that scientific ones. A major feature of the renewed debate is the now widespread recognition that there is no value-free science, including health care science. Science itself is a value. Participation in any phase of science or health care science is a part of human values. All health care has an ethical dimension. While it can be separated for analysis and decision making, the separate science or health care is not thereby value free. The mere existence of something, an is, does not provide an ethic. But the is and the ought are closely interwoven and are not separate in real life.

Nonmaleficence. Literally, this means "do no harm," from *male*, which means "evil." It is a major ethical principle usually paired with beneficence, "do good." Both are presented in the Hippocratic Oath, which urges health care providers to do good or at least do not harm. The principle might be seen as a major source of the resurgence of bioethics in modern times. The new technologies and procedures might be seen as the intention of the health care providers to do good. Sometimes, however, technologies do harm. The debate here can be exampled by the extension of life, a presumed good, which turns out to be prolonging dying, which some see as harmful when the QOL is low or the patient suffers a great deal for a very short extension of life. This type of experience led one physician to suggest that neonatal intensive care units are the new horror chambers of the 20th century. The undesirable side effects of chemotherapy have been considered in this light along with numerous other examples

Normative Ethics. See *Applied Ethics.*

Nursing Ethics. Some claim there is only one ethics—human ethics. All other ethics are ethics applied somewhere. Thus bioethics is ethics applied to health care. The narrower category of medical ethics may be seen as physician ethics. In this sense, nursing ethics is ethics applied to nursing or the ethics of nurses. The theory is that the ethics of health care are the same for all 268 health care professions. Nursing ethics, however, uses case studies in nursing or refers to the activities or the ethical decision making of nurses rather than other health care providers. There are some suggestions, however, that nursing ethics is a different ethic in a more thoroughgoing way. Nursing ethics, for example, has been called an ethic of caring rather than an ethic of cure. Proponents of other views see this as overdrawn, for nurses also cure and physicians and other health care providers also care. Since 95 percent of nurses in the United States are women, the development of a women's ethics has some bearing on nursing ethics. The work of Carol Gilligan and others is noted in the text. Women's ethics has been epitomized as an ethic of caring, though here again, not all women are caring, and there are men who care. So too, women's ethics has been described in terms of relationships, though there are also men in relationships. People are sometimes called dependent or independent, although others note that all human beings are interdependent, i.e., in relationship.

Obligation. The word means to bind, and hence an obligation is a duty. The words are often used interchangeably. An obligation may be legal, as in a contract, or ethical, as in a promise. Health care providers have a legal and ethical obligation not to abandon a patient. There is a positive obligation to care, at least in the view of some. Professional obligation requires one to care, though in nonemergency situations the professional may refer care to another.

Paternalism. The Latin *pater* means "father." Health care providers tend to treat patients as though they are children. In time of illness, people tend to psychologically regress to degrees of childlike helplessness. Paternalism may keep them there, partly because they are easier to control, which is helpful to hospital routine. It also discourages questions, and patients are more apt to do what they are told without time to ask for reasons or to argue. In emergencies, paternalism and its female equivalent, maternalism, are more acceptable and even required. Under more normal conditions, this parental attitude may violate informed consent and the autonomy of the patient. In this case, it is unethical though some interpreters insist that some mild form of paternalism is normal and necessary for health care. One perspective is to see the health care providers as having a responsibility to help the patient in a child state to return to adult functioning.

Prima Facie. Literally, this means "first face," which becomes at first glance or what appears on the surface. Prima facie duties were noted under *Absolute duty.*

Principle. The English comes from the Latin for "beginning." It is the origin or cause or basic truth or doctrine. Ethical principles are basic reasons, perhaps equivalent to the axioms or unquestioned laws of geometry. Some ethical principles, however, are intermediate reasons—expressions of more basic or ultimate reasons. There is no particular number of principles, but some, such as autonomy, justice, beneficence, and nonmaleficence, are more prominent than others.

Quality of Life. A good QOL has been a human desideratum for all of history and probably for all of human existence. If one has no choice on the QOL, it may not be a question. In health care, it has become a major issue in recent decades. QOL is often contrasted to quantity or sanctity of life (SOL). The SOL has ancient roots. Jewish law was noted earlier as having 613 commandments, all of which can be set aside to preserve life. Preserving life became part of health care several centuries ago. Prior to the rise of modern health care and even prior to 1950, health care providers did not have much choice in the matter. People recovered or they died. Antibiotics and other new procedures have changed much of that. "Pneumonia is the old man's friend" no longer applies, for it can be cured. If life is preserved for something like normative existence or a meaningful existence, there is little argument with SOL. When it is the extension of comatose life or a life filled with pain and suffering, the QOL takes on greater significance. Some insist that QOL should never be a consideration in bioethics. Others say it is the primary consideration. QOL is not limited to physical life but includes socioeconomic and other considerations. It is a significant element in the abortion debates. One of the major difficulties with QOL is its vagueness. What is tolerable pain or suffering to one may be intolerable for another. Life may be preferable to death for some, but death may be more merciful than some kinds of life to others. Some ascribe SOL as a value or moral standard of religion, though it should be noted that most religions have higher values as well. Life as the highest good would be seen as idolatry for some traditions.

Relativism. This is the doctrine that morals or ethics are related to the culture in which they are found. Thus there are no universally valid moral standards. Proponents of this view do not usually realize that they are promoting a universal standard that they believe is relative. Kohlberg and others have pointed out several dozen moral precepts that are found in all or most human societies and, in this sense, are universal. These may be expressed differently, however, and relativists note that different societies and subcultures have different values as well.

Rights. Rights involve a claim, usually upon others. They may be legal or ethical or both. A legal right gives a privilege, such as driving a car, that may be conditioned by a corresponding requirement to obey the laws. In a larger sense, one might have a right to be left alone, and others have an obligation to respect that privacy, again within the limits of the law. The right to be left alone might be considered a negative right. Civil rights are often a matter of law. The guarantee of civil rights has been a major concern in recent decades. Moral or ethical rights may be written into law, but they may also be apart from or higher than the law. People who practice civil disobedience in the face of what they consider a bad law often appeal to a higher law, perhaps of nature or of God. In the "Declaration of Independence," Thomas Jefferson said, "We hold these truths to be self-evident, that all men are created equal, that they are endowed by their creator with certain unalienable rights, that among these are life, liberty, and the pursuit of happiness . . ." The last three may be interpreted as implying that people have a right to health care, for without it, they might not live, they might not have liberty, and they might not be able to pursue happiness. This is a positive right, implying that someone, such as health care providers, has a duty to provide the health care. Others dispute the right to health care, however, especially since part of health depends on one's choice of lifestyle. The unalienable aspect suggests that these rights are a natural part of life that no one can take away. Perhaps one should say, "that no one should take away." Reality may differ from the ideal. Right to life or sanctity of life is part of the abortion debate. The rights of the fetus are heavily debated. Some do not think the fetus has rights, whereas others think the rights are relative to the rights of women. The anti-abortion position generally favors the rights of the fetus.

Rule Deontology. The system of ethics described under *Deontology.*

Rule Utilitarianism. Rule utilitarianism claims that some ethical rules (deontology) have been found to have greater utility than no rules at all. The commitment, however, is not to the rules for their own sake but for their contribution to the utilitarian ethic.

Sanctity of Life. Life is the highest good. Sheer existence is valued without regard to the quality of life, physically, socioeconomically, or in any other way. A modified SOL ethic would consider extreme deficiencies in the QOL and/or place the SOL within a hierarchy with God or one's country or one's family or some other commitment having a higher value. SOL is a main feature of the abortion debate, as noted under *Quality of life* and *Rights.*

Self-Determination. See *Autonomy.*

Situational Ethics. This is an act utilitarianism in which right and wrong are determined by or in relation to the situation. The concept is especially associated with Joseph Fletcher, though he is but one of its proponents. He also has a rule—the loving thing to do—that could justify calling his position rule utilitarianism or even a monistic (one-principle) deontology.

Supererogation. The Latin *rogare* means "to ask." Super "asking" is above or beyond the call of duty. In Roman Catholicism, saints are those who have performed works above and beyond their own salvation. These become merits in the treasury of saints available to others. Nursing has been considered in this category. Some distinguish between the work actually contracted as a duty and the caring or compassion traditional to nursing as the supererogation—that which is beyond payment or contract. As noted under *Beneficence,* some see a duty to do no harm and consider doing good as supererogation.

Teleology. The Greek word *telos* means "the end." A teleological ethics is represented by the aphorism, "The end justifies the means." The focus is on the consequences, and the term "consequentialism" is sometimes used interchangeably with teleology. Utilitarianism is an example of such a system, and sometimes it is also used interchangeably. As noted in the text, utilitarianism may be a universalist form of the teleological ethic. Egoism, ethical elitism, and ethical parochialism are suggested as less than universalist forms.

Universality. At first glance, this term takes in the universe. In practice, it refers to the human race and, on rare occasions, other forms of life and other aspects of existence. Kant's deontology is a universalist ethic. Some see utilitarianism as universalistic also, at least in contrast to other forms of teleological ethics.

Utilitarianism. This is the ethical system often paired and contrasted to deontology in philosophical ethics. As noted under *Teleology,* utilitarianism is concerned with the end or the consequences or the purpose in ethics. As noted under *Universality,* it may be seen as the universalist form of teleological ethics. Utilitarianism is sometimes summed up by the aphorisms, "The end justifies the means," and "The greatest good for the greatest number." The good may be expressed as that which has the greatest utility or that which brings the greatest happiness or the greatest pleasure. The latter is not necessarily hedonistic. The pleasure may be self-centered or altruistic, physical pleasure, reading a book, doing something for others. The system can be traced back to Jeremy Bentham (1748–1832) and John Stuart Mill (1806–1873).

Values. Simon and Clark define values as a set of personal beliefs and attitudes about the truth, beauty or worth of any thought, object, or behavior. Chapter Four lists seven criteria for values in value clarification theory.

Annotated Bibliography

American Nurses' Association. Clinical and Scientific Sessions 1979. Kansas City, MO: American Nurses' Association, 1979.

This volume includes community health, gerontological, maternal and child health, medical–surgical, psychiatric and mental health nursing. It opens with Anne J. Davis' "Theoretically Realistic," and Rita J. Payton's, "Pluralistic Ethical Decision Making."

American Nurses' Association. Code for Nurses with Interpretive Statements. Kansas City, MO: American Nurses' Association, 1976.

This revision of the 1950 code for nurses shifts from loyalty to the physician to accountability to the patient. The Interpretive Statements expand the detail each of the 11 points in the *Code*. A new set of interpretive statements is in process.

American Nurses' Association. Ethics References for Nurses. Kansas City, MO: American Nurses' Association, 1982.

This is a comprehensive bibliography on concepts of ethics, the nursing role, nursing education, and such issues as informed consent, death and dying, reproduction and genetics, behavior control, and the allocation of resources. Separate sections are on government publications and audiovisuals.

American Nurses' Association. Guidelines for Implementing the Code for Nurses. Kansas City, MO: American Nurses' Association, 1980.

One concern of this overview is the profession's obligation to the public that all service rendered by its members is of high quality. The reality of life is that there will always be those who stop being really professional, who stop learning, and whose ethical practice is unacceptable. One way of dealing with these problems is through law. Another is the discipline of the organization. Education is another. This includes initial and continuing education. While state and national groups can encourage both positively and punitively, the ultimate responsibility is with the individual.

American Nurses' Association. Perspectives on the Code for Nurses. Kansas City, MO: American Nurses' Association, 1978.

The six papers were presented at the convention in June 1976. They present perspectives of history, education, practice, administration, research, and philosophy. These essays are excellent background for understanding the development and use of the Code.

Annas, G.J. The Rights of Hospital Patients: The Basic ACLU Guide to a Hospital Patient's Rights. New York: Avon, 1975.

This is a handbook of the American Civil Liberties Union. Rights overlap the two areas of morals or ethics and law. Some of these rights are written into law. Others are part of informed consent, autonomy, transplants, and so on. The special chapters on women and children are very helpful. Annas does not pay much attention to nurses, but he notes on page 15 that patients are cared for by nurses 99 percent of the time.

Arras, J., and Hunt, R. (Eds.) Ethical Issues in Modern Medicine, 2nd ed. Palo Alto, CA: Mayfield, 1983.

Arras has redone this second edition of a work first published in 1977. It is so extensively redone, it is a new book. The vast changes are a reminder of the fast moving nature of bioethics, some of it newer than this morning's newspaper. Arras has selected essays on professionals, abortion, euthanasia, experimentation, genetics, public policy, and justice. Along the way he recommends additional reading. A special listing offers journals and audiovisuals in the field.

Bandman, E.L., and Bandman, B. (Eds.) Bioethics and Human Rights. Boston: Little, Brown, 1978.

The views of these insightful pieces range from personal opinion to well-documented studies. The essays discuss the nature of rights, genetics, abortion, and the rights of children, parents, nurses, patients, and prisoners. National and international rights are included. This is probably the best volume available on the topic of rights.

Barry, V. Moral Aspects of Health Care. Belmont, CA: Wadsworth, 1982.

Barry discusses health care professionals (HCP), including nurses and physicians. His is one of few balanced approaches in terms of HCPs. The theory section includes the present climate, the distinctions between values and priorities and law, as well as the traditional philosophical ethics. He considers the HCP in the context of the system and in relation to patients and special issues, such as abortion, euthanasia, experimentation, and the allocation of resources.

Beauchamp, T.L., and Childress, J.E. Principles of Biomedical Ethics, 2nd ed. New York: Oxford University Press, 1983.

The authors suggest that case studies tend to be disconnected so it is difficult to see the relationship of one to another. In contrast, they offer their volume on the principles that both create and illuminate the dilemmas. While referring mainly to physicians and researchers, they claim, "Most of the issues that we raise may be redescribed in virtually identical terms for nurses. The same moral principles and rules govern nurses as well as physicians." After an introduction to theory, they consider autonomy, beneficence/nonmaleficence, and justice. Professional relationships, ideals, virtues, and integrity round out their presentation. The second edition updates the bibliography, expands the case studies from 14 to 35, and includes extensive revision of the text.

Beauchamp, T.L., and Walters, L. (Eds.) Contemporary Issues in Bioethics, 2nd ed. Belmont, CA: Wadsworth, 1982.

This is one of the finest selections of articles among the many edited texts on the market. A new essay in this second edition on ethical theory by Beauchamp is a minicourse in the subject. A new chapter on personhood considers this much-debated subject. A new chapter on disclosure includes articles on truth, informed consent, and confidentiality as part of patient–professional relationships. Other sections include life and death, allocation and policies, and research. The traditional concerns of abortion, euthanasia, and so on are well represented. Nurses are not but the ANA Code is included as well as the Royal College (England) of Nursing's concern with ethics and research.

Benjamin, M., and Curtis, J. Ethics in Nursing. New York: Oxford University, 1981.

This is an excellent introduction to the subject, with 30 case studies for practice. After the opening chapters on theory, the focus is on relationships with patients, physicians, other nurses, institutions, and public policy.

Benoliel, J.Q., and Berthold, J.S. Human Rights Guidelines for Nurses in Clinical and Other Research. Kansas City, MO: American Nurses' Association, 1975.

Nursing responsibilities are changing in research as in health care in general. Ethical guidelines are offered here for the nurse along with mechanisms for the protection of rights. The interface of law and ethics is also discussed.

Brody, H. Ethical Decisions in Medicine. Boston: Little, Brown, 1976.

The author considers the usual bioethical issues but in the context of moral reasoning and alternative ethical methods. Among his appendices is one on "Criteria for Determining Quality of Life." Joseph Fletcher calls this the first modern textbook in medical ethics written by a physician for medical students. The concern is for making decisions rather than following rules or physician etiquette.

Callahan, D., and Bok, S. (Eds.) Ethics Teaching in Higher Education. New York: Plenum Press, 1980.

The opening chapter surveys a century of teaching ethics in the American undergraduate curriculum. Other essays discuss goals, pluralism and indoctrination, moral psychology, evaluation, teaching ethics in professional schools, paternalism, and whistle blowing. While the discussion is in general terms rather than specific to nursing, it is relevant for the concerns of ethics in nursing.

Carlton, W. "In Our Professional Opinion . . .": The Primacy of Clinical Judgment over Moral Choice. Notre Dame: University of Notre Dame Press, 1978.

The author worked on the staff of two hospitals. As an insider, she became aware that ethical choices are often made under the guise of clinical judgments. The persons making the choice are not always aware of the distinction. The moral of the story is that clinical judgments are not value free.

Cassell, E.J. The Healer's Art: A New Approach to the Doctor–Patient Relationship. Philadelphia: Lippincott, 1976.

The art is to treat patients rather than diseases. Cassell tries to see things from a patient's perspective. One of his concerns is overcoming the fear of death.

Childress, J.F. Priorities in Biomedical Ethics. Philadelphia: Westminster, 1981.

Childress discusses paternalism, death, research, the allocation of scarce resources, and technology. These subjects have priority—they require attention before others. Others might choose other priorities, and Childress himself has (see Beauchamp and Childress), but these are certainly important subjects. He justifies mild paternalism in the sense of caring for patients who may not be able to care for themselves.

Childress, J.F. Who Should Decide? Paternalism in Health Care. New York: Oxford University Press, 1982.

Childress notes the ongoing tension between the autonomy of the patient and the paternalism of the professional. The latter has a duty to benefit others even as one has a duty to respect others. This means informed consent, but it does not mean indifference to health care needs. Intervention is justified not only when patients request help but at times when they do not, as in suicides or incompetency. He does not deal with the "Who decides?" among health care providers, institutions, or society.

Connery, J. Abortion: The Development of the Roman Catholic Perspective. Chicago: Loyola University Press, 1977.

The author surveys the history of the Church's position to mid-20th century. He sees a clear and consistent teaching against abortion from conception even as he documents those Catholics who thought otherwise.

Curtin, L., and Flaherty, M.J. Nursing Ethics: Theories and Pragmatics. Bowie, MD: Brady, 1982.

The first half of the book considers human rights and the relationship of nurses to patients, families, society, the institution, and other health care professionals. The second half is a series of case studies with analysis and commentary.

Davis, A.J., and Aroskar, M.A. Ethical Dilemmas and Nursing Practice, 2nd ed. Norwalk, CT: Appleton-Century-Crofts, 1983.

The first half of the book provides an overview of ethics. The second half considers issues like abortion, mental retardation, public policy. Examples of dilemmas are presented for discussion in a closing chapter.

Davis, A.J., and Krueger, J.C. Patients, Nurses, Ethics. New York: American Journal of Nursing, 1980.

A series of essays focus on research. One section covers government regulations and institutional review boards (IRB). Four articles are on informed consent, including role conflict. Specific populations considered are women prisoners, the dying, fetuses, children. Five appendeces provide copies of the ANA *Code,* the ANA *Human Rights Guidelines in Research,* procedures for a human subjects committee, sample consent forms, and an experimental subject's bill of rights.

Donnelly, G.F., Mengel, A., and Sutterly, D.C. The Nursing System: Issues, Ethics, and Politics. New York: Wiley, 1980.

The authors claim there is more than one way to do things. They expose "the paradoxes and confusions in the nursing system and in the nursing role as it focuses on issues universally identifiable to nurses." For them, the conflict is a source of growth. Debate and discussion stimulate creativity. They use the *koan* ("What is the sound of one hand clapping?") to add to that stimulation of thought. They also draw on myths, such as that of Sisyphus, who spent eternity rolling a boulder up a hill only to have it roll back down so he had to start over. Nursing is like that, they suggest. They ask such questions as, "What is the balance between altruism and the nurse's own security?" They ask disturbing things—for example, whether nursing is a profession and how professionals relate to each other as illustrated by the pecking order in nursing.

Duncan, A.S., Dunstan, G.R., and Welbourn, R.B. (Eds.) Dictionary of Medical Ethics, rev. New York: Crossroad, 1981.

This is a collection of essays on a wide ranging number of topics such as African medicine, hospital chaplains, nursing, the World Health Organization, as well as the more usual topics of abortion, confidentiality, contraception, informed consent, suicide.

Ehrenreich, B., and English, D. Witches, Midwives, and Nurses—A History of Women Healers, 2nd ed. Old Westbury, NY: Feminist Press, 1973.

This is controversial consciousness-raising worth considering for the professionalization of women in health care. Women have been systematically excluded from the physician role. Witches were burned, midwives banned, and nurses allowed only when they made it clear they would serve physicians and not challenge authority or profits.

Emmet, D. The Moral Prism. London: Macmillan, 1979.

Light coming through a prism separates into different colors. So moral thought separates into different views. Here are sane thoughts about those differences in terms of political morality, science, the esthetic, religion, existentialism, the good. This is a valuable context for bioethics. One response to pluralism is to dismiss it. Here is the effort to understand.

Ethical dilemmas in nursing—A special AJN supplement. American Journal of Nursing, 1977, 77(5):845-876.

This is a very useful collection of essays about nurses and ethics. Authors include Levine, Romanell, Johnson, Cawley, Lestz, Yeaworth, the Bandmans, Churchill. The focus is on dilemmas, which are illustrated by actual incidents.

Feldman, D.M. Marital Relations, Birth Control and Abortion in Jewish Law. New York: Schocken Books, 1978 (original 1968).

Reform and Conservative Judaism are more liberal than Orthodox Judaism. The focus here is on the latter's traditional views. There is considerable variety in these.

Fenner, K.M. Ethics and Law in Nursing: Professional Perspectives. New York: Van Nostrand, 1980.

Fenner examines the interface between these overlapping concerns in health care. She includes the historical perspective and extends her survey to include values clarification. Specific issues are considered under the rubric of "social issues," which takes in racism and sexism as well as the usual abortion, behavior control, death and dying. Exercises and suggestions for further reading make the volume even more helpful.

Fletcher, J.F. Humanhood: Essays in Biomedical Ethics. Buffalo, NY: Prometheus Books, 1979.

This a collection of Fletcher's articles published between 1968 and 1978. They cover happiness, goodness, distributive justice, fetal research, abortion, infanticide, euthanasia, suicide, experiments on humans. The lead article sets forth 20 criteria for humanness, beginning with intelligence. The nature of personhood is, of course, a vital concern in such areas as abortion and euthanasia.

Fletcher, J.F. Morals and Medicine. Princeton: Princeton University Press, 1954.

Fletcher reviews rights, truth-telling, contraception, and euthanasia. Historically, this volume is significant as an early Protestant view that acknowledges Roman Catholic efforts in bioethics. Fletcher here considers himself a personalist in contrast to either utilitarianism or deontology. In other writings, he presents himself as an act utilitarian.

Fletcher, J.F. Situation Ethics. Philadelphia: Westminster, 1966.

The theme of this often quoted text is that the situation determines what is right or wrong. At the same time, Fletcher offers a standard, "What is the loving thing to do?" This is usually taken as a deontological ethical principle. The controversial storm over the book turned on the denial that traditional rules, such as that against adultery, were necessarily wrong. Other categories, such as contraception, abortion, euthanasia, are also opened for discussion.

Foltz, A.-M. An Ounce of Prevention: Child Health Politics Under Medicaid. Cambridge: MIT Press, 1982.

This is a case study of the early and periodic screening, diagnosis, and treatment program of Medicaid (EPSDT). The study is divided into two subcases: Texas and Connecticut. The program is deemed a failure in the latter state because it never started. It is considered a success in Texas because children were screened and then referred to private physicians. If they could not afford the latter, the children went untreated. Throughout her case studies, the author shows how politics, money, and power interact. In Texas, the medical society was able to control the referral process and thus allowed the program to go that far. Eventually the program was cut. It started out as a health measure but ended up as a welfare measure. When the federal government withheld $12 million out of $18 billion to enforce care for the poor, the states objected. This is a valuable review of the pitfalls of public policy.

Francoeur, R.T. Biomedical Ethics: A Guide to Decision Making. New York: John Wiley & Sons, 1983.

After an overview of ethical systems, there are 11 chapters on techniques for making ethical decisions. The second half of the book consists of exercises to practice the techniques. The techniques include triage, cost-benefit, decision tree, decision matrix, consensus.

Fromer, M.J. Ethical Issues in Sexuality and Reproduction. St. Louis: C. V. Mosby, 1983.

Fromer opens with a review of ethical theory. She continues with homosexuality, contraception, population ethics, abortion, genetics, reproductive technology, fetal research, and infants as human beings. Ethics is a matter of rationality, whereas beliefs are illogical. Not all would agree, but her attempt to provide a rational approach to sexuality is helpful. Sex research and therapy are new in today's world. Both raise issues about competency, confidentiality, and the cost-benefit ratio as well as the adequacy of scientific methods. She notes that homosexuality is not unnatural. While adultery is traditionally immoral, it is widely practiced and receives less and less condemnation. She suggests the condemnation of homosexuality stems from a fear she calls "homophobia." She notes that while the world suffers a population explosion, 20,000 people a year are having children by means of artificial insemination. She notes the problem of the quality of life issue in ethics is that there is no solution.

Gilligan, C. In a Different Voice: Psychological Theory and Women's Development. Cambridge: Harvard University Press, 1982.

Gilligan notes the exclusion of women from theory building psychological research. She cites Freud, Piaget, and Kohlberg as examples. She goes on to suggest that women have a different moral development from males. The primary ethic of women is an ethic of care rather than an ethic of justice. The morality of rights emphasizes separation, whereas the morality of responsibility emphasizes relationship. While males must separate from their mothers, women are free to remain in relationship. The core data she cites from her own work shows women developing through several of Kohlberg's stages after they separate from their fathers or male partners. This is a groundbreaking work of special importance for nursing that has sometimes been seen as having an ethic of caring.

Gustafson, J.M. Protestant and Roman Catholic Ethics. Chicago: University of Chicago Press, 1978.

The author looks at historic divergences of the two traditions, practical moral reasoning, the philosophical and theological bases of the two, and ends with a look into the future. While there are wide divergences in both traditions, there is perhaps more that unites the two than separates them.

Hardin, G. Mandatory Motherhood: The True Meaning of "Right to Life." Boston: Beacon Press, 1974.

Biologist Hardin thinks women should have a choice on abortion. This is a strong prochoice statement that sets forth the issues.

Haring, B. Ethics of Manipulation: Issues in Medicine, Behavior Control and Genetics. New York: Seabury Press, 1975.

Father Bernard presents the traditional Catholic teachings in relation to Protestant traditions. Manipulation is any use of modern technology that endangers human dignity and freedom.

Harrison, B.W. Our Right to Choose: Toward a New Ethic of Abortion. Boston: Beacon Press, 1983.

Theologian Harrison surveys the history, theology, and politics of abortion. The result of her carefully documented study is in the title of the book. One of the problems she highlights is that ethicists, especially male and celibate males at that, push their abstract moral claims without regard to the real individual people involved. It is a bit like being interested in a disease or an ethical issue like autonomy but never considering the person who has the illness or who is supposed to exercise the autonomy.

Harron, F., Burnside, J., and Beauchamp, T. Health and Human Values: A Guide to Making Your Own Decisions. New Haven: Yale University Press, 1983.

The emphasis here is on the reasoning process in decision making. The authors' concern is not to provide the answers to bioethical issues but to aid the reader in deciding for herself or himself. The topics are the usual—abortion, euthanasia, informed consent, genetics, the right to health or health care.

The Hastings Center Report.

This journal is published by the Institute of Society, Ethics, and the Life Sciences, Hastings-on-Hudson, NY 10706. It is the best journal in the field for staying abreast of current events in ethics. There are reports, analyses, and think pieces. The coverage of nursing is very limited. For nursing ethics, one must hunt down the articles in the various nursing journals.

Holmes, H., et al. Birth Control and Controlling Birth. Holmes, H. The Custommade Child. Both volumes are subtitled, "Women-Centered Perspectives." Clifton, NJ: Humana Press, 1981.

These two books come from a symposium on the subject. The ethical dimensions of public policy and politics are noted. These often work to the detriment of women, both as health care receivers and providers. Holmes notes that while the public ethics of the health care system is for such things as truth-telling, justice, and beneficence, the real ethics are greed, power, status, and self-protection. In health care, here is feminist consciousness raising at its best.

Illich, I. Medical Nemesis. New York: Pantheon Books, 1976.

Illich focuses on iatrogenic illness—that which is caused by medical care. His solution is to get rid of the entire system. Stay home, save money, and be healthier. An ancient prayer asks for salvation from the physicians. In "One Flew Over the Cuckoo's Nest" the patients needed salvation from "Big Nurse." Illich can make one angry or make one think. The former may perpetuate the problems, whereas the latter might help with the solution.

Jonsen, A.R., and Garland, M.J. (Eds.) Ethics of Newborn Intensive Care. Berkeley: University of California Press, 1976.

Symposium (1974) participants were agreed that it may be right at times to withhold or even withdraw life support. The text considers policy and both clinical and social concerns.

Jonsen, A.R., Siegler, M., and Winslade, W.J. Clinical Ethics: A Practical Approach to Ethical Decisions in Clinical Medicine. New York: Macmillan, 1982.

An ethicist, a physician, and a lawyer combine their wisdom to produce a pocket guide to ethics. In the tradition of the medical consultation, they offer guidance to the practitioner. The four sections of the text consider medical intervention, including decisions to terminate intervention, the preferences of patients, the quality of life, and external factors, such as research and the allocation of resources.

Kelly, L.Y. Dimensions of Professional Nursing. New York: Macmillan, 1980.

Chapters 17 to 22 are on legal rights and responsibilities. Overall, this is one of the most comprehensive volumes in the field.

Kieffer, G.H. Bioethics: A Textbook of Issues. Reading, MA: Addison-Wesley, 1979.

The usual concerns of genetics, reproduction, euthanasia, experimentation, and behavior control are here. The author is also concerned with future generations, the natural world, the population explosion, science, and society. He holds a theory of evolutionary ethics. Not all will agree with this perspective, but the text is one of the best single-author volumes on the market.

Kohlberg, L. Essays on Moral Development. Volume One: The Philosophy of Moral Development. San Francisco: Harper & Row, 1981.

This is the first systematic presentation of Kohlberg's philosophy. He provides some new material by way of introduction and comment, but for the most part, this is a collection of previously published essays. The theory has been superseded by his later work at a number of points, which is distracting, but the overall value of the text remains high. He may be that rarity in human affairs in presenting his ground, where he is coming from, before presenting the data of his psychological work scheduled for Volume Two. Here he talks about his concern with justice and beyond, with preliminary remarks on the implications for education, scheduled for full treatment in Volume Three. All of it is of value for nursing, current and future.

Kosnik, A., et al. Human Sexuality: New Directions in American Catholic Thought. New York: Paulist, 1977.

This volume was commissioned by the Catholic Theological Society of America. The committee reviews the science, church history, and the Bible for perspectives on sexuality. A pastoral guidelines section covers marital, nonmarital, and homosexual relations. Free sex is not approved, but there is a new openness to sexuality that goes far beyond traditional views.

Kubler-Ross, E. (Ed.) Death, The Final Stage of Growth. Englewood Cliffs, NJ: Prentice-Hall, 1975.

This collection of articles reviews the positive aspects of death, how to deal with death, testimonies, religious views including Jewish, Hindu, and Buddhist. The author suggests that nurses may be unhelpful through overcommitment to institutional roles. Creative listening is a major way to be helpful.

Kubler-Ross, E. On Death and Dying. New York: Macmillan, 1969.

Anyone who works with the dying or their families will find this volume helpful. It is Kubler-Ross' basic work in which she spells out the five stages of death. Some observers disagree with her perspective, and alternate views need to be kept in mind.

Levine, C., and Veatch, R.M. (Eds.) Cases in Bioethics from the Hastings Center Report. Hastings-on-Hudson: Hastings Center, 1982.

The cases are grouped in seven categories: reproduction, patient–physician relationships, mental health, death and dying, research, scarce resources, policy. Each case is presented along with two or more commentaries. This is a valuable resource for the study of bioethics.

Little, D., and Twiss, S.B. Comparative Religious Ethics. San Francisco: Harper & Row, 1978.

A general discussion of religion, morality, and law is applied to the Navajo, the Gospel of St. Matthew, and Theravada (Southern) Buddhism. A good bibliography expands the usefulness of the text. Nurses may not meet too many Navajo or Theravada Buddhists, but in our pluralistic society, this is an obvious possibility. More importantly, this is a good beginning for considering other cultures in health care ethics.

Mercer, R.T. Perspectives on Adolescent Health Care. Philadelphia: J.B. Lippincott, 1979.

Someone said that adolescence is not a disease! It is a normal part of human life. Special concerns remain for this stage of human development. Health care providers and other workers with teens will find this text helpful, especially in the areas of the health care system, sexuality, pregnancy, and general health.

Midgley, M. Heart and Mind: The Varieties of Moral Experience. New York: St. Martin's Press, 1981.

Midgley is concerned with the whole person. We must break the conceptual barriers that have divided the heart and the mind, values and facts, culture and individual, human nature and human freedom. She compares freedom and heredity, feelings and reasoning, objectivity and subjectivity. While academic specialization fragments the picture, she is trying to put it together. The basic content of this text is of value for nursing with its concern for the whole person, for health as well as illness.

Mohr, J.C. Abortion in America: The Origins and Evolution of National Policy, 1800–1900. New York: Oxford University Press, 1978.

Readers may be surprised to find that abortion became an issue as a political football kicked around, not by religious groups, but by the AMA. Mohr claims the organization used it as a rallying cry to gain members and political power and to put the irregulars out of business. Prior to 1875, abortion before quickening was so common it was advertised in religious journals. With a few setbacks, organized medicine managed to get all the states to pass laws against it by 1875. The appeal was racist and anti-Catholic. It is of course a controversial interpretation, but Mohr's documentation is strong. It is a reminder that issues as seen today may not be the way the issues started out, as documented elsewhere for contraception—a largely Protestant legal maneuver before the Supreme Court ruled it a matter of privacy.

Moore, T.D. (Ed.) Ethical Dilemmas in Current Obstetric and Newborn Care. Columbus, Ohio: Ross Laboratories, 1973.

This is a report of the 65th Ross Conference on Pediatric Research. Dagmar Cechanek represented the nursing perspective, and Joseph Fletcher and Robert M. Veatch represented ethics. Presentations and discussion considered legal and administrative procedures, the ethics of treatment vis a vis consequences, pregnancy, abortion, postnatal care, and who decides.

Munsey, B. (Ed.) Moral Development, Moral Education, and Kohlberg: Basic Issues in Philosophy, Psychology, Religion, and Education. Birmingham, AL: Religious Education Press, 1980.

Authors agree and disagree with Kohlberg. Along the way, various aspects of development are considered. The text ends with a response from Kohlberg himself that updates his research to that point. This is an excellent text to see and to understand the issues in moral development.

Munson, R. Intervention and Reflection: Basic Issues in Medical Ethics, 2nd ed. Belmont, CA: Wadsworth, 1983.

An introduction on theory precedes four parts on termination, rights, controls, resources. The first considers abortion, infanticide, birth defects, and euthanasia. The second includes paternalism, experimentation, and informed consent. Controls include behavior control, genetics, and reproduction. Resources considers allocation and the right to health care. Munson presents a case or cases, an introduction to each section, selected essays on the subject, and decision scenarios in which the reader participates in a bioethical decision. It is an excellent combination of approaches and method. The 2nd edition has additional cases and scenarios, revised sections, new presentations, such as that on reproductive control, and an updated bibliography.

Murchison, I., Nichols, T.S., and Hanson, R. Legal Accountability in the Nursing Process, 2nd ed. St. Louis: C.V. Mosby, 1982.

Too often, people live in fear of the law. In health care, it is the fear of malpractice lawsuits. The actual number of such suits is relatively small. The authors suggest that the law can be a positive force for health care. It can support independent nursing action. The law can also define nursing conduct, a reminder that nurses need to be involved in shaping that law and standards of nursing practice. The content covers nurse–patient relationships, autonomy–accountability, employer–employee responsibilities, the meaning and mythology of consent, standards of care, legal duties, do good, and do no harm. The 2nd edition adds a chapter on the nurse as a court witness besides updating with recent cases.

Muyskens, J.L. Moral Problems in Nursing: A Philosophical Investigation. Totowa, NJ: Rowman and Littlefield, 1982.

Nursing has assumed more and more responsibility in the new technology of health care. Muyskens sees a real urgency in the need for moral discussion in nursing. He opens with professional codes, the Hebrew–Christian moral tradition, the logic of decision making, and moral principles. He goes on to discuss the role of the nurse vis a vis physicians, clients, the profession, employers, and society. Specific nursing situations include abortion, defective neonates, the dying, the aged, the chronically ill.

Oden, T.C. When Shall Treatment be Terminated? New York: Harper & Row, 1976.

After the Karen Ann Quinlan case, a group of lawyers and ethicists gathered to assess the situation. Their guidance is to favor the patient. When in doubt, continue treatment, but this is not an absolute dictum.

Pence, G.E. Ethical Options in Medicine. Oradell, NJ: Medical Economics, 1980.

The author does not think that studying ethics will make a person more moral. He hopes it will help people think more clearly about the moral aspects of health care. His major concern is Aristotelian virtue. "Phronesis" or "good judgment" is the key or master virtue. Intellectual virtue comes through study, but practical virtue comes through practice. To this Aristotelian view, he adds Aristotle's concern for friendship and the concepts of honesty and love. All of society need these. Physicians also need the virtues of humility, compassion, and respect for good science. Good physicians are temperate, competent, courageous, just, and have phronesis.

Piaget, J. The Moral Judgment of the Child. New York: Free Press, 1965.

This version of a 1932 classic will be helpful to nurses working with children. Piaget is notoriously difficult to read but well worth the effort. Other child development specialists do not always agree with Piaget, but his influence remains and is apparently growing.

President's Commission for the Study of Ethical Problems in Medicine and Biomedical and Behavioral Research.

The Commission produced a number of volumes over several years. Among them are Screening and Counseling for Genetic Conditions: A Report on the Ethical, Social, and Legal Implications; Whistleblowing in Biomedical Research: Policies and Procedures for Responding to Reports of Misconduct; Making Health Care Decisions: The Ethical and Legal Implications of Informed Consent in the Patient–Practitioner Relationship, 3 vols; Securing Access to Health Care: The Ethical Implications of Differences in the Availability of Health Services, 3 vols; Deciding to Forego Life-sustaining Treatment: Ethical, Medical, and Legal Issues in Treatment Decisions. The volumes are all published by the US Government Printing Office, Washington, D.C.

The titles basically reflect the contents of these extremely valuable reflections. Some observers consider them the present consensus of American society. This may be the closest we have come to such a consensus, though plurality remains the closer description for this society. It is regrettable that so few nurses were involved by the Commission, although at one point the Commission did convene a panel of nurses to discuss the issues.

Purtillo, R.B., and Cassell, C.K. Ethical Dimensions in the Health Professions. Philadelphia: W.B. Saunders, 1981.

The authors do not cover all 268 health care professions, but they give a good introduction to bioethics. In addition to the usual theories on ethics, they ask "What is a professional?" Part of their answer is that a professional not only knows what and how but why. They see professions as autonomous. Nursing is a profession struggling for more autonomy. They offer a fourfold procedure for ethical decision making: gather relevant information, identify the dilemma, decide what to do, and complete the action. One of their case studies is a nursing situation that includes putting the job on the line. Nurses who are unwilling to do this have already made their ethical decision. For the authors, the welfare of the patient is paramount. They see professional health care as an ethic of care.

Ramsey, P. Ethics at the Edges of Life: Medical and Legal Intersections. New Haven: Yale University Press, 1978.

Protestant ethicist Ramsey is sometimes seen as more conservative than Roman Catholics, whose work he acknowledges and draws upon. He opposes quality of life (QOL) decisions and any form of euthanasia, passive or active. At the same time, he does not think we should prolong dying for those who are actually terminally ill.

Ramsey, P. The Patient as Person: Explorations in Medical Ethics. New Haven: Yale University Press, 1970.

The theme is a growing one—health care should treat the person and not the disease. That may be an interesting liver in Room 562, but, more importantly, there is a person in Room 562. Our first concern should be with the person.

Rawls, J. A Theory of Justice. Cambridge, MA: Harvard University Press, 1971.

Rawls considers five principles of justice: general, universal (see Kant), public, orderable (conflicting claims), and final (beyond law or custom). He does not give practical directions, but his discussion of the theory continues to have a major influence.

Reich, W.T. (Ed.) Encyclopedia of Bioethics. New York: Free Press, 1978, four vols.

The 285 authors provide 314 essays on definitions, issues, religious views, and so on. Its size (2000 pages) and price ($200) make it a library item rather than the usual personal possession, but it is the most comprehensive publication in bioethics. In general, the coverage is well balanced among liberal and conservative and other alternate views.

Shannon, T.A. (Ed.) Bioethics. New York: Paulist Press, 1976.

Shannon presents the Roman Catholic tradition, but his selections are from across the board. The essays are drawn from all traditions, though there is a slightly liberal tilt to the collection.

Shelly, J.A. Dilemma: A Nurse's Guide for Making Ethical Decisions. Downer's Grove, IL: InterVarsity Press, 1980.

Shelly presents a Christian nurse's perspective on the issues. While this perspective is more conservative than some, she presents a balanced view of the issues. The first half of the book is concerned with theory, and the second half presents a series of case studies. Her fourfold decision making process includes clarifying the personal context, defining the problem, proposing alternatives, and evaluating the alternatives.

Steele, S.M., and Harmon, V.M. Values Clarification for Nursing, 2nd ed. Norwalk, CT: Appleton-Century-Crofts, 1983.

While the first edition focused on issues, this new version focuses on persons—the nurse, the patient, society. The major context, as the title implies, is values clarification. The goal is self-understanding in a time of rapid change. The effort is to present a rational approach to the decision making process. Some say the approach is not as objective as its proponents sometimes claim. However, for the distinctions between values—personal and professional, professional and patient, health care systems and the larger society—this is an invaluable work for nursing.

Steinfels, P., and Veatch, R.M. (Eds.) Death Inside Out. New York: Harper & Row, 1974.

These articles focus on the revolutionary changes in attitudes toward death that have taken place in Western culture in recent decades. Death is not seen as more natural though there are still those—patients and health care providers—who want to hold it off as long as possible. Sometimes this helps people live while dying, and at other times, it prolongs the dying.

Tate, B.L. (Ed.) The Nurse's Dilemma: Ethical Considerations in Nursing Practice. Geneva: International Council of Nurses, 1977.

Case studies are drawn from around the world. A helpful set of questions is presented for all situations. The text is organized around the *ICN Code for Nurses: Ethical Concepts Applied to Nursing, 1973*. The volume should be in every nurse's library.

Thompson, J.B., and Thompson, H.O. Ethics in Nursing. New York: Macmillan, 1981.

After an introduction to ethical theory, the authors follow the life cycle. When nurses specialize, they tend to do so in particular areas. Here are chapters on the ethics of family planning and genetics, contraception, abortion, neonatology, childhood, the adult years, and the elderly. A guest chapter by Lucie Young Kelly presents the legal perspective. Case studies allow the student or practitioner the option to consider the ethical dimensions of nursing, or one can use personal experiences. Extensive footnotes and an annotated bibliography offer further depth beyond the basic presentation.

Uustal, D.B. Values in Ethics: Considerations in Nursing Practice: A Workbook for Nurses. South Deerfield, MA: D.B. Uustal, 1978.

The exercises are designed to help one identify and clarify one's own values. They include the various situations that can arise in nursing practice. The book would be best used in relation to a volume on theory and the history of values or in a context where these are known and presented along with the exercises.

Veatch, R.M. Case Studies in Medical Ethics. Cambridge, MA: Harvard University Press, 1977.

The 112 cases are drawn from those presented in *The Hastings Center Report* as part of their ongoing series. Veatch presents a capsule summary of theory and the usual topics of genetics, contraception, abortion, transplants, behavior modification, experimentation, informed consent, death and dying. This is a good text for the case study method of studying ethics. The ICN volume is more appropriate for nurses.

Walton, D.N. Ethics of Withdrawal of Life-Support Systems: Case Studies on Decision Making in Intensive Care. Westport, CT: Greenwood Press, 1983.

This is one of the most intensive analyses available in this area of bioethics. The author writes for the nonspecialist by giving a review of ethical theory and recent, highly publicized cases. He follows with cases on brain death and vegetative states, patient, family, and physician decision making. The closing chapters consider the process of decision making and the ethical principles involved.

Wilson, J., and Cowell, B. Dialogues on Moral Education. Birmingham, AL: Religious Education Press, 1983.

This is a cleverly done dialogue between Socrates and Cephalus, who represents the moral majority. The latter's son represents the relativist position. In the process, the dialogue covers natural and divine law, relativity, tastes, wants, wisdom, reasoning, moral aptitude, and the reason for morality in the first place.

Woods, N.F. (Ed.) Human Sexuality in Health and Illness, 2nd ed. St. Louis: C.V. Mosby, 1979.

This is an important book for nurses working with adolescents, pregnancy, and abortion. The tendency is to avoid sexuality until problems arise. A healthier approach is to care for the whole person.

Index

A

Abortion
  attitudes toward, 17, 116, 192, 201
  case studies, 196, 201
Absolute duty, 14, 217. *See also* Duties
  and obligations
Abuse, case studies, 200, 202
Accountability
  definition, 217
  professional, 13, 96, 207
  role of nurse, 13, 194, 206, 207
Act deontology, 37, 217
Act utilitarianism
  definition, 30, 218
  ethical system of, 30–31
Advocacy/patient advocate, 52
Allocation of scarce resources
  case studies, 110, 198, 199, 202–203,
    207–208
  concept of social worth in, 10
  definition, 218
  ethical issues in, 115, 120
  nurse's role in, 107

American Medical Association (AMA)
  Principles of Medical Ethics, 131,
    210–211. *See also* Codes of ethics
American Nurses' Association (ANA)
  Code for Nurses, 12. *See also*
    Codes of ethics
  duties and obligations, 14–16,
    160–161
  historical background, 11–12
  professional values in, 32, 60, 63, 76,
    83, 131–132, 145–146, 174, 222
  use in decision making, 60, 132–133,
    134, 166
Applied ethics, 5, 7, 218. *See also*
  Normative ethics
Autonomy/self-determination. *See also*
  Rights
  case studies, 103–104, 192, 204, 205
  concept of, 91, 132, 138, 145–146
  definition, 218
  patient, 76, 103–104, 106, 125, 126, 134,
    194
  use in decision making, 177–178

B

Beliefs
definition, 78, 218
ethics and, 124, 129, 135
values and, 77-78, 135-136
Beneficence
definition, 126, 218-219
ethical concept of, 125, 126
use in decision making, 177-178
Bioethics, 8, 219. *See also* Ethics
Biomedical technology
decisions on use, 146-147
definition, 219
ethical issues raised by, 9-10, 38, 75,
115, 198

C

Categorical imperative (Kant), 33-34,
219
Clinical judgment, 6, 75, 91
Codes of ethics, 11-17
AMA Principles of Medical Ethics, 11
ANA Code for Nurses, 12
definition, 219-220
development of, 9, 11
Hippocratic Oath, 11
ICN, 11
professional values in, 11
Cognitive disequilibrium, 220
Confidentiality
definition, 220
patient information and, 118
nurse's role in, 118
Consensus ethics
definition, 18, 31, 220
President's Commission and, 76
Consequentialism, 220. *See also*
Deontology
Contract theory, 36-37, 221
Cost-benefit ratio. *See also* Risk/benefit
definition, 221
use in decision making, 10, 176-178
Cultural transmission, 58, 221

D

Decision making, ethical
capacity for, 109, 158-159, 197
communication and, 118
ethical dilemmas in, 94-97, 172
models of, 97-99, 105, 177-178, 213-215
moral justification and, 172
nurses and, 60, 97, 157-158, 160-161,
162, 178-179
patients and, 156-157
process of, 1, 27, 89, 92-93, 97-99, 108,
171
team, 60, 96, 159
trends in, 153-154, 156, 161
values and, 1, 84
Defining the Issues Test (DIT)
description of, 61-64, 222
use of, 138
Deontology
definition, 31, 222
ethical system of, 27, 31-37
use in decision making, 174-175, 181
Descriptive ethics, 5, 222
Distributive justice, 222-223. *See also*
Allocation of scarce resources
Duties and obligations
concept of, 14-15
professional, 110, 127, 141

E

Egoism, ethical, 27, 28, 223
Ethical, 93. *See also* Ethics
Ethical decision making. *See* Decision
making, ethical
Ethical dilemma
definition, 94
criteria of, 94-97
Ethical elitism, 28, 223
Ethical issues, 32, 121-122
Ethical parochialism, 28, 223
Ethical pluralism
decision making and, 176
definition, 55, 223

Ethical principle. *See also* Deontology
  definition, 229
  examples of, 32-33, 80
Ethical theory, 27, 223
Ethical universalism
  definition, 28, 224
  Kant and, 219
Ethic of caring
  definition, 145
  nursing as, 83, 228-229
Ethics. *See also* Bioethics
  definition, 4-5, 7, 224
  history of, 8-9, 123
Euthanasia, 224

F
Fraternal charity, 225

G
Golden Rule
  definition, 42
  ethics and, 42-43, 126, 181

H
Hierarchy of values
  decision making and, 95, 182
  ethics and, 148-149
Hippocratic Oath, 11, 63, 126

I
International Council of Nurses (ICN)
    Code of Ethics, 209-210
Informed choice (client), 96, 110, 119,
    134, 138, 153, 156-157, 194, 203,
    204, 205, 206
Informed consent
  age of, 199-200
  case studies, 196-197, 199-200, 201, 204
  definition, 225
  history of, 126-127

legal concept of, 200-201
relationship to ethical decision
    making, 76, 116
Intuitionism
  definition, 225
  ethical system of, 27, 34-36
Is-ought, 10, 38-39. *See also* Naturalistic
    fallacy

J
Judeo-Christian traditions
  ethics and, 42-126
  natural law and, 37-40
  rule ethic and, 5, 33
Judgments About Nursing Decisions
    (JAND), 63
Justice and fairness. *See also* Rawlsian
    theory of justice
  definition, 225
  Kohlberg and, 5, 56, 66
  Rawls and, 36-37

L
Law of double effect, 226

M
Maternalism, 3, 76, 179. *See also*
    Paternalism
Medical ethics, 7, 226. *See also* Ethics
Metaethics, 5-6, 226
Moral agent
  definition, 226
  nurse as, 63-64
  person as, 6, 7
Moral development. *See also* Stages of
    moral development
  concept of, 35, 56-60, 78
  women and, 64-67
Moral justification, 27, 172
Moral Maturity Quotient (MMQ), 61
Moral philosophy, 54

Moral reasoning
    definition, 90
    ethical decision making and, 89–92,
        104–105, 185–186
Moral relativism, 58, 227
Morals (morality). *See also* Moral agent
    definition, 4–5, 6, 19–20, 227
    source of, 42, 49
Moral theology
    definition, 40, 227
    ethics and, 40–43

N

Naturalistic fallacy, 38–39, 227–228
Natural Law
    definition, 227
    ethical system of, 37
    use in decision making, 175–176, 181
Nonmaleficence
    case studies, 125, 175
    definition, 126, 228
Normative ethics, 5. *See also* Applied
        ethics
No treatment decisions, 106, 197–198,
        199, 200, 204, 205
Nursing Dilemma Test (NDT), 63–64
Nursing ethics. *See also* Ethic of caring
    characteristics of, 5, 9, 68, 82–83
    concept of, 7, 68
    definition, 228–229
    NDT, 63–64

O

Ordinary/extraordinary means, 14,
        224–225
Obligation, 229. *See also* Duties and
        obligations

P

Paternalism. *See also* Maternalism
    concept of, 229
    ethical decision making and, 76, 96

Patient's Bill of Rights, 15
Patient's rights (client), 96, 108, 125, 126,
        192, 193, 196, 197, 198, 200, 202,
        203. *See also* Rights and
        responsibilities
Piaget's theory of Cognitive
        development, 49–51
Piaget's theory of equilibrium, 50, 81
Pluralistic decision making model, 176,
        215
Prima facie, 5, 229
Primum non nocere, 32. *See also*
        Nonmaleficence
Professional
    definition, 13, 93
    duties and obligations, 14–15
    rights and privileges, 15–17
    roles and responsibilities, 13–14

Q

Quality of life
    case studies, 192, 199, 205
    definition, 10, 194, 229–230

R

Rawlsian theory of justice, 36–37
Respect for persons, 124, 125, 136,
        139
Rights and responsibilities. *See also*
        Patient's rights
    definition, 230
    employer's, 207
    health care, to, 15
    human, 16
    professional's, 13–14, 15–17, 110, 125,
        202, 203
    societal, 116–117
Risk/benefit (ratio), 176–178. *See also*
        Cost–benefit ratio
    case studies, 107, 198
Rule deontology, 37, 222, 230
Rule utilitarianism, 30, 31, 230